Other books coauthored by Mike Samuels (with Hal Z. Bennett):
The Well Body Book
Spirit Guides: Access to Inner Worlds
Be Well

By Mike and Nancy Samuels:
Seeing with the Mind's Eye: The History, Techniques and Uses of Visualization
The Well Baby Book

Mike Samuels, M.D., and Nancy Samuels

The well child book

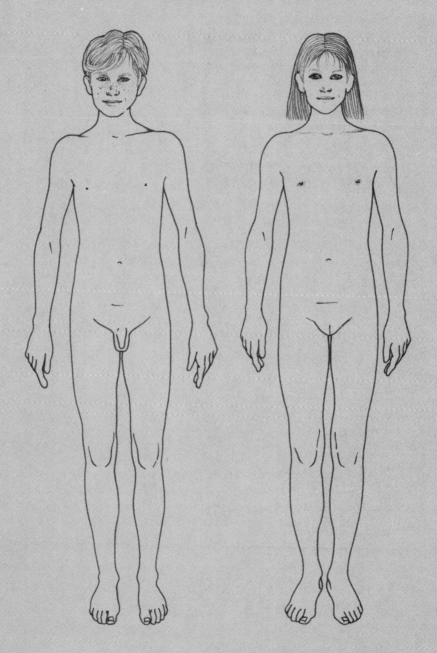

Illustrated by Wendy Frost

Summit Books   New York

Section I epigraph from Swami Prabhavananda and Frederick
Manchester, translators, *The Uphanishads,* New York: New Ameri-
can Library, 1961. Section II epigraph from "Can You Picture
That," *The Muppet Movie,* by Paul Williams and Kenny Ascher, ©
1979 Welbeck Music Corp., used by permission, all rights
reserved. Section III epigraph from "My Favorite Things," *The
Sound of Music,* © 1959 Rodgers and Hammerstein II, Williamson
Music, Inc., owner of publication and allied rights.

Photograph of Wendy Frost and family, page 400, courtesy of Seiji
Kakizaki. All other photographs are from the collection of Mike
Samuels and Nancy Samuels.

Published by SUMMIT BOOKS

A Simon & Schuster Division
of Gulf & Western Corporation

Simon & Schuster Building
1230 Avenue of the Americas
New York, New York 10020

SUMMIT BOOKS and colophon
are trademarks of Simon & Schuster

Design and layout by Clint Anglin and Stanley S. Drate

Manufactured in the United States of America

10 9 8 7 6 5 4 3 2 1

First edition
Library of Congress Cataloging in Publication Data

Samuels, Mike.
   The well child book.

   Bibliography: p.
   Includes index.
   1. Children—Care and hygiene.   2. Parent and
child.   I. Samuels, Nancy.   II. Title.
RJ61.S2795   613'.0432   81-21345
ISBN 0-671-40063-0 cloth   AACR2
ISBN 0-671-43893-x pbk.

To our children, Rudy and Lewis, for whom this book is written, and to our parents, who give us help and support.

Acknowledgments

We would like to thank all the people who made special contributions to this book—Jim Silberman, our publisher, for his continued support of the projects we choose to undertake, and Paul Bresnick, our editor, for his confidence and organization in helping to put the book together.

We especially want to thank our illustrator, Wendy Frost, for her friendship and her ability to give visual form to our ideas. She has a special gift for drawing children of all ages who are healthy and appealing and for doing medical drawings that don't make kids say "Ooh, gross!"

And finally we wish to thank all the people who gave their time to our boys while we worked on the myriad details of the book. Laurie, Linda, Florence and Iggy, Hope, Wen, and Greg, Elizabeth, Carol, Donna, Karen, and Terry O'Connor.

Contents

Creating health and illness / How stress makes illness more likely / Stress-related illnesses / Life events and illness / Feelings of discontent and illness / How parents' attitudes affect their children's health / Effects of social support / Family styles and health / Relaxation creates health / Relaxation relieves stress / Relaxation techniques / Visualization / Visualization techniques / Ways of dealing with children's behavior to relieve family stress / Classroom styles and stress / Community styles and stress / Bioprograms and the world

Food makes the body / The parent as the "gatekeeper" / Other influences on children's food habits / Nutrition and childhood illness / How childhood nutrition affects adult illness / Other nutritional trends—special diets / Toward an optimum diet

The chemical environment / Chemicals and cancer / How chemicals cause cancer / A personal cancer plan for families / Smoking and cancer / Alcohol and cancer / Sunlight, radiation, and cancer / Diet and cancer / Drinking water and cancer / Industrial chemicals and cancer / Consumer products and cancer

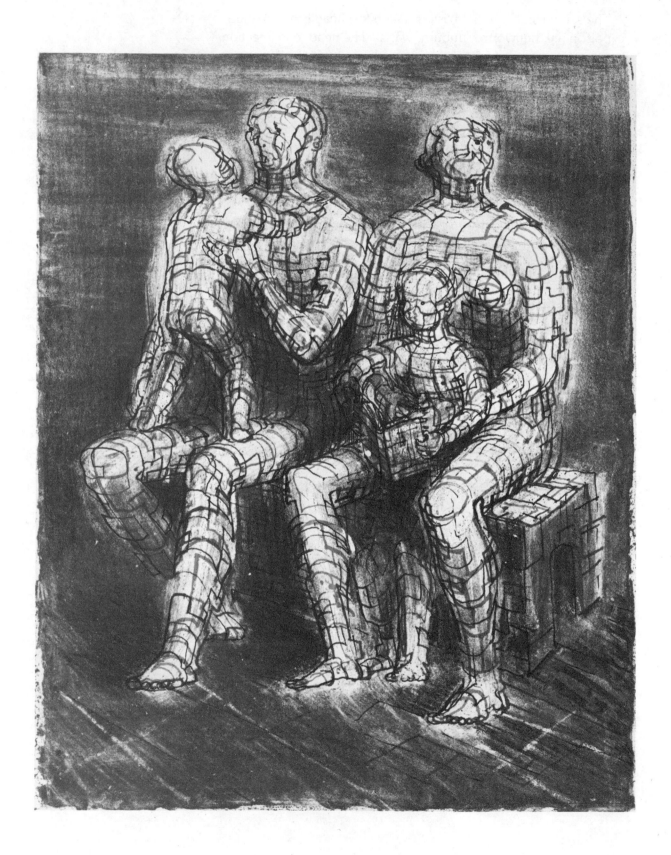

Introduction

We hope *The Well Child Book* will be more than a book. We hope it will be a *family activity*—something to be experienced as well as read. To achieve this goal we have divided the book into three sections.

The first section is designed to be read by parents. Its purpose is to show how profoundly health is affected by stress, nutrition, chemicals, rest and exercise and, more specifically, to acquaint parents with how family life affects children's illnesses. Since new scientific evidence points to the fact that over half of childhood illnesses and accidents can be eliminated merely by managing stress better, Section I provides activities and relaxation/visualization exercises that can help parents make their homes less stressful. And because illness is affected by diet, rest, and exercise, this section also contains information on optimizing diet, avoiding chemicals, and getting balanced rest and exercise. The purpose is to show parents how radically they affect their children's health and how they can make that effect a positive one.

The second section of *The Well Child Book* is intended for children. That is, it is designed for parents to read and discuss with their children, though in many cases older children will be able to read it alone. We suggest that parents of very young children skip complicated words and some of the steps in long explanations. Parents may even want to read the text themselves and simply discuss the illustrations. Section II teaches children how their bodies work, emphasizing how the body normally functions and heals itself. Also, this section explains to children what causes illness and how they can help to prevent it through relaxation, visualization, good nutrition, rest, and exercise—what children can actually do to stay healthy. To communicate the information we have used a variety of visual and exploratory techniques as well as words. There are drawings, charts, things to do, experiments to try, photographs, and works of art.

We feel that Section II is the core of our book. It is revolutionary in that it attempts to actively involve children in creating healthy bodies. Our belief is that by teaching children about health at an early age we can guide them toward lifelong patterns that will promote health and prevent many medical problems they might otherwise have. The information in this section should immediately help to lessen childhood accidents and minor illnesses. Children don't want to be sick any more than adults do.

Family life can be patterned to create healthy children.

Moore, Henry. Family Group. 1950. Lithograph on plastic, printed in color. $11\frac{1}{4} \times 8\frac{5}{8}$". Collection, The Museum of Modern Art, New York. Gift of the artist through School Prints, Ltd., London.

When made aware of specific things that will lower the chances of illness, they are happy to do them. In fact, they often are eager to share their newfound understanding. For example, our seven-year-old learned that when he had a stomachache before going to sleep (one of the most common physical complaints of children his age), it was probably due to worrying about something he had to do the next day. He knows now that if he can figure out what's worrying him and express it, his stomachache goes away. What this means is that he no longer fears stomachaches because he has learned what causes them and how to control them. In a different medical context, such stomachaches might have been treated with antacids or possibly diagnostic X-rays. By looking at the stomachaches as a message about his relationship to the world, the family was not only able to cure the stomachaches, but also was able to use the illness as a positive force for change. Getting to the root cause prevented possible serious illness (such as an ulcer), taught him something important about dealing with stress, and also gave him feelings of strength and competence. We believe it is of great importance to teach children such basic skills in learning how to read messages from their bodies.

In the final section of the book we deal with treating illness. Section III is designed for parents and children to use together. Here we discuss the common illnesses of the years between 5 and 12. The discussions are specifically oriented to what the children and their parents can do to prevent and treat illness. We explain, in a way that children can understand, what the illnesses are about. Our aim is to convey understanding and relieve worry. Scientific studies have shown that when parents understand children's illnesses, the children sense this, and all their symptoms are less severe and disappear faster. A major goal of this section is to reduce first-time and repeat doctor visits. Studies have shown that a *large* number of doctor visits (45 to 55 percent) are due to worry about the *possibility* of illness. We hope that by explaining and reassuring we can save both the parents and the children the expense and trouble of these unnecessary visits.

The three sections of the book, taken together, create a unified family approach to childhood health. We wrote this book because we have two young children who are susceptible to all the usual physical complaints and minor illnesses of childhood, and who look to us for support and explanation. Because of our long-term involvement with and dedication to self-help and holistic medicine, we became involved with teaching our children about health both when they were sick and when they were well. To get an even broader idea of children's understanding and questions, we taught some of the material in our older boy's school, in classrooms from kindergarten to sixth grade. We were delighted to find that most children were very interested in the health of their bodies, enjoyed the lessons, and had an endless supply of questions.

Children mean many things for all of us. They are truly our future, but they are also our link with the past. They provide us with some of our highest moments of joy, as well as with some of our most profound moments of doubt and frustration. They continually ground us to the realities of day-to-day life, but at the same time they allow us to soar by giving us some of our most special moments. In these moments we join our children in the here-and-now and experience beauty in the simplest things. This gives us a glimpse of how arbitrary our view of reality is.

It has been said that children are our teachers, and they really can be in terms of illness. The illnesses of our children are often inseparable from our own experiences. When our children are ill, we are ill, and we must strive to understand what is happening. Their illness is often a reflection of our own unfulfillment and lack of knowledge about ourselves. Conversely, by making our children healthy, we heal ourselves and grow.

We feel this view of childhood illness is a very positive one. The fact that these ideas are now being demonstrated scientifically in extensive research is exhilarating. We would rather view health in this way than to view illness as events out of our control that force us to deal with an impersonal medical establishment.

This book is about changing people's views of childhood illness. It is about realizing that we are all continuously involved in the health of our families, and that by our very actions we can profoundly affect this health. Our book is both an adventure and an experiment: an adventure because it provides things to actually do that will enable us to change; an experiment because such a book has never been done before. The text, pictures, activities, games, and exercises will help us and our children to look at our bodies differently for the rest of our lives.

How this book is arranged

Section I—For parents

Who gets sick and why

Family styles—how stress, nutrition, and exercise can affect children's health

Section II—For children

How the body works, grows, and heals

What causes illness

How to prevent illness through relaxation, visualization, good nutrition, and exercise

Section III—For parents and children

Learning about treating and preventing common illnesses and accidents

Who the doctor is and what he or she does

What common drugs do

Preventive medicine —for parents

"To darkness are they doomed who worship only the body, and to greater darkness they who worship only the spirit. They who worship both the body and the spirit, by the body overcome death, and by the spirit achieve immortality."

In the Sanskrit this verse is exceedingly obscure. Commentators explain it variously, and not very clearly.

> —Swami Prabhavananda and Frederick Manchester, translators, Isha Upanishad, The Uphanishads

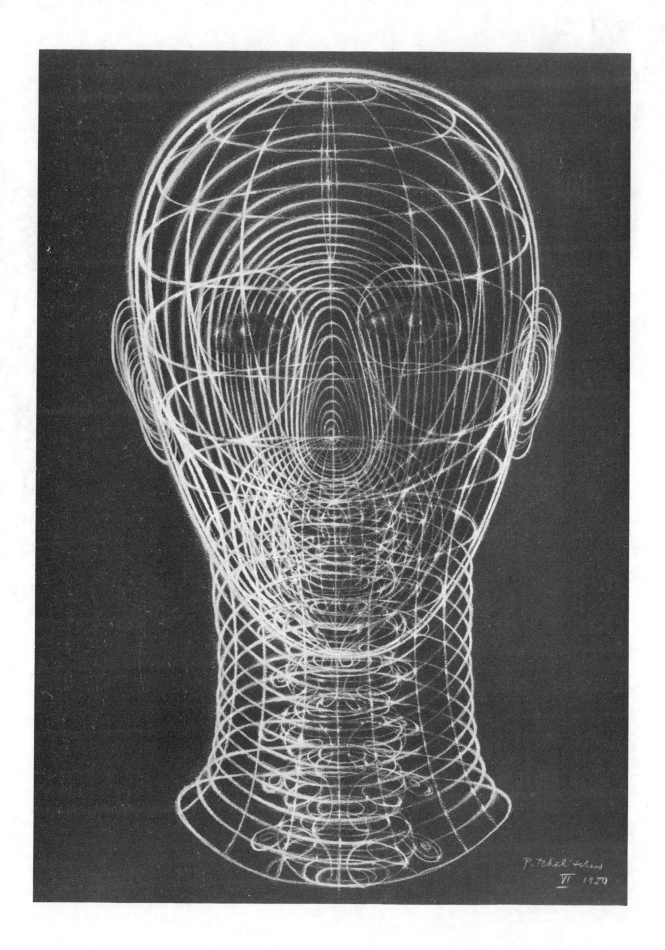

P. Tchelitchew
VI 1950

Preface

This book is about childhood health, but in a larger sense it deals with people's relationship to their bodies and their world. By the time children are twelve, they have established patterns of experience and interaction that will form the basis of how their bodies will serve them over a lifetime.

Childhood is a time of prodigious learning, much of it unconscious. In a metaphorical sense, children are engaged in crystallizing a physical body from a mental image. This mental image grows out of their interaction with all of their daily experiences. Researchers are discovering that particular kinds of experience are more likely to produce health. And by health we mean both mental and physical well-being. We can no longer look upon a person's mind and body and spirit as being separate in terms of health. Our culture has tended to make us believe they are separate, just as it has tended to reinforce the idea that the sole cause of disease lies in organisms that are outside of the body and beyond our control. In truth we have amazing control over our bodies if we will accept this idea and learn about it. What's happening now in research is that scientists are beginning to find out how mental images affect body physiology. When the spirit feels at home, the body is healthy.

Many cherished scientific notions are being reexamined. The most forward-thinking scientists no longer even believe that the body ends with the skin, or that it functions as if it were separate from the world outside. Physicists tell us that all molecules, including those of our bodies, are "indefinite," that they are constantly in motion. The picture that emerges of the human body, as of all other matter, is one of a vibrating field that has no exact boundaries. Our bodies are constantly exchanging their component substances with the outside world. We breathe in air, take in chemicals through our skin, ingest foods, and excrete byproducts through a miraculous process that has been developed over a period of 15 million years.

We are all affected by external organisms and agents with which we come into contact. Our bodies are host to a multitude of substances, some healthful, some not. The way our body reacts to these substances is not predetermined simply by what they are. For example, everyone who comes in contact with meningitis does not contract the disease. In fact, almost everyone at some time or another is host to meningitis bacteria. Yet fewer than one person in 100,000 ever becomes ill with meningitis. What this means is that we must take into account factors other than external agents when we think about the cause of illness.

We create our physical bodies from the mental images we have of ourselves.

Tchelitchew, Pavel. Head VI. 1950. Colored pencil on black paper. Sheet: 19⅞ × 13¾". Collection, The Museum of Modern Art, New York. Gift of Edgar Kaufmann, Jr.

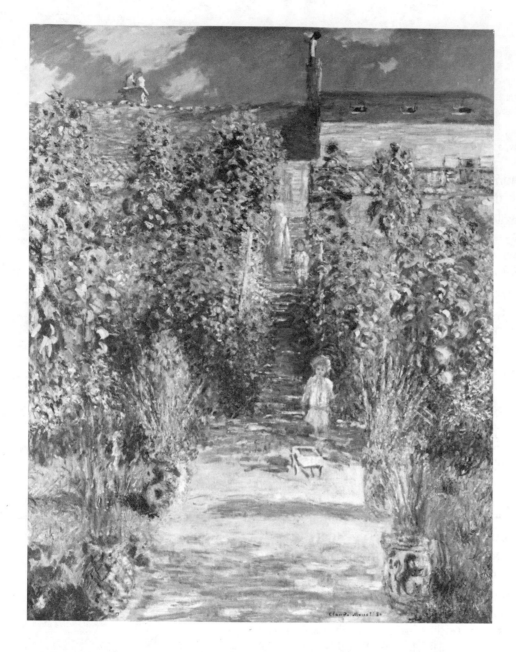

The human body is a vibrating energy field that overlaps with the fields around it.

Monet, Claude. The Artist's Garden at Vétheuil. *1880. Oil on canvas. 59⅝ × 47⅝". Ailsa Mellon Bruce Collection, 1970, National Gallery of Art, Washington.*

As doctors have long known, the physical state of the host affects resistance to disease. The healthier people are, the less likely they are to be adversely affected by external substances. Part of our human inheritance is a subtle and effective immune system. Movies taken through electron microscopes show the amazing energy and complexity of our white blood cells, the *lymphocytes*. These cells can be seen to move about, amoeba-like, in a purposeful fashion, surrounding and engulfing dangerous substances of all kinds, including cancer cells.

Scientists are also realizing that our bodies are affected by our life habits and day-to-day events. Life habits include the kinds of food we eat, the chemicals we ingest, and the kinds of rest and exercise we get. Scientists are also finding that the body's resistance to illness is strongly influenced by life events. Family discord, loss of a friend or relative through relocation or death, and other stressful events tend to undermine the body's natural defenses. Children who are under stress are two-to-three times more likely to become ill or have accidents.

Current research even indicates that attitudes about life affect health. If people *perceive* an event as stressful, the efficiency of all their homeostatic (self-regulating) mechanisms is lessened. If people *perceive* the same event as challenging or exciting, they are not adversely affected by it. People who view their whole lives as unfulfilling or beyond their control are much more likely to become ill. Clearly, inner imagery has direct effects on the body. If people see themselves as sick, they can become ill or even die. A most striking example of this is "taboo death." This phenomenon occurs when a tribal witch doctor or figure of reputed power puts a "curse" on an individual. Very often that person does die. Scientists have found that death occurs because the people, believing they have no power to reverse the curse, unconsciously send impulses down the vagus nerve, actually stopping the heart from beating. On autopsy, no sign of organic illness is found. The mechanism of death is the person's mental image that he or she is going to die. Conversely, positive images of living and achieving goals optimize the heartbeat and the immune response and help to create good health.

Understanding the mind/body/outer world interconnections enables us to make choices and effect changes that can profoundly alter our health. At the molecular level, we need to realize that we are affected by all the substances we come into contact with: food, air, water, and industrial products. For example, certain chemicals like nitrosamines can actually penetrate cells, slide into the DNA helix in the nucleus, and share its electrons. This chemical bond confuses the cell's normal pattern of replication and causes it to become cancerous. Usually, what happens next is that the body's lymphocytes recognize the confused cell, move into the cell, and actually attempt to heal it. If the cell cannot be repaired, the lymphocytes eliminate it. This process goes on a million times a day in every body, dealing with a wide variety of foreign substances. In the course of the body's functioning, this is simply normal, everyday housecleaning and mopping up. The question then becomes how can we best help our body go about its normal housekeeping operations? First, we need to avoid those substances most likely to cause disease. Next, we need to maintain our bodies at their optimum by eating the most nourishing foods, breathing the purest air, and getting the kind of exercise that increases strength and balance.

These factors will certainly make it easier for our immune systems to operate and help lighten their load. But all of this will not prevent us from becoming ill if we are unhappy, dissatisfied, or under stress. For our bodies to function optimally, we must have a balanced life. Scientists now know that stress or even the perception of stress actually suppresses the ability of our lymphocytes to clear our bodies of foreign substances, repair

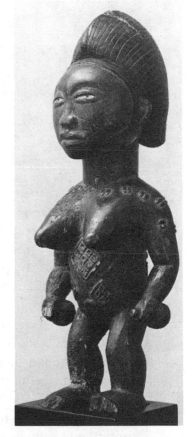

Taboo death is an example of a person dying because of a strong mental image.

African. Standing female. 19th–20th cent. Wood. Height: 38.5 cm. The Metropolitan Museum of Art, New York. The Michael Rockefeller Memorial Collection of Primitive Art, Gift of Nelson A. Rockefeller, 1964.

Levels of the world around us

External

Energy	Light and sound
Molecules	Atoms, electrical and magnetic energy, molecules
Chemical compounds	Air, chemicals, and food
Small life forms	Microorganisms: viruses and bacteria

Internal

The body	Rest and exercise of the body
The mind	The mind's perception of stress
Imagery	The mind's perception of the world
Spirit	The oneness

diseased or damaged cells, and kill dangerous invaders or cells. Thus every time people work to eliminate chronic stress, learn to ease a daily time of family tension, and/or learn to handle inevitable stress successfully, they are actually "immunizing" themselves against disease. In this context, conscious relaxation and positive imagery become extremely important medical tools, both in preventing and healing disease. If our bodies are relaxed and we are holding a positive image in our minds, then our blood flow, hormonal secretions, breathing, heartbeat, and lymphocyte activity all function optimally for healing.

We all have information inside us about how to live in accord or harmony with the universe. Scientists now think that this information is in the DNA of every cell in our bodies. It is the job of one part of the body—the limbic system and hypothalamus of the lower brain—to send this information to our conscious mind. The information often comes in the form of dreams, images, or subtle body feelings.

Beyond these inborn programs for harmony, we enter a state which we experience as bliss. This experience is without images and is most similar to deep sleep or meditation states where the mind is blank. In this state, time and space disappear and the most profound healing takes place. Yet it remains out of reach of scientific medicine. People glimpse the state in their highest moments, through religion, art, and music. The state of bliss, which represents the most powerful point on the healing continuum, is as useful and available to us as any of the other healing tools. In these time-less moments it is likely that our bodies bring together *all* of the healing

Keep well

Avoid dangerous chemicals.

Eat the best foods, breathe the best air.

Exercise.

Deal with stress—relaxation and imagery soothe the spirit.

tools—all stress disappears, all the body's cells and molecules balance, and the body, instead of using energy, is energized. These moments are truly beyond understanding; they are simply to be experienced and felt. At these moments we free our 15 million-year-old healing mechanism to function at its best.

This inborn mechanism is more powerful than any medical treatment—in fact, medical treatments rely on the body's healing, self-sustaining mechanisms to be effective. Antibiotics, the greatest advance of twentieth-century medicine, do not "cure" diseases in and of themselves. Antibiotics lower the number of pathogenic (disease-causing) bacteria so that the body's lymphocytes can work effectively. In an operation, the surgeon skillfully sews layers of tissue, but he doesn't "heal" the incision. Similarly, the orthopedist aligns broken bones and secures them with a cast, but he doesn't "knit" the bones together. Finally, immunizations by themselves do not prevent us from getting specific diseases; they prepare the body's lymphocytes to recognize specific viruses or bacteria and turn out large amounts of special antibodies that can lock onto the foreign organisms and render them harmless. Similarly, when we learn to understand and work with the relationship of body/mind/external environment, we are maximizing our immune system's ability to work effectively. Such a "mental immunization" is as real as any vaccine and is likely to play as important a role in future medicine.

Chapter 1

Stress

Creating health and illness

For the last fifty years Western medicine has viewed disease as solely caused by factors beyond a person's control: germs, an inherited predisposition, birth defects. Dr. Lewis Thomas has said, "Most illnesses are blind accidents that we have no idea how to prevent. . . . We are beset by plain diseases, and we do not control them; they are loose on their own, afflicting us unpredictably and haphazardly." [1] This model is beginning to be abandoned in the face of mounting evidence that people do more to affect their own health than they have ever dreamed. In fact, it may be that people actually create and can heal their own illnesses.

Illness seems to have its basis in people's perceptions of themselves and the outside world. This new view of disease grew out of several innovative lines of research that came to light in the 1950s. One was the physiology studies of Walter B. Cannon, Hans Selye, and others. They proved without a doubt what heretofore had been disbelieved—that perceptions in the mind affect the body. The second line of research was the work primarily of Lawrence E. Hinkle, which dealt with the fact that people do not become ill equally or randomly; people become ill when they *perceive* their life situations as negative and unchangeable.

Out of these beginnings have come whole new fields of medicine based on an extensive body of research. Fields like behavioral medicine, sociobiology, psychophysiology, psychoneuroendocrinology, and holistic medicine have grown out of these roots. All of this information together has led to the first basic understanding of how a person's perception of the world causes illness.

How stress makes illness more likely

The physiological mechanisms between brain and body that lead to illness are complex, but they can be explained fairly simply. Thoughts in the mind excite nerve cells in the brain, which in turn send impulses out through the autonomic part of the nervous system. Autonomic nerves go to the skin, the digestive system, the heart and blood vessels, the lungs, virtually to the whole body. Perhaps most importantly they go to the adrenal glands and cause the secretion of hormones that regulate heartbeat, breathing, and muscle tension. Thoughts in the mind also cause the pituitary or "master" gland to send out hormones that affect the adrenal, sex, and thyroid glands.

The body's most immediate response to any perception is through the *autonomic nervous system,* which is divided into two parts. The excitement of one part, called the *sympathetic nervous system,* basically results in tension and action. These reactions have been called "the fight-or-flight response," and are described as trembling, chills, pounding heart, stomach in knots, and so on. Such feelings arise in situations of sudden fear, for example, when people hear a car behind them or feel their ladder

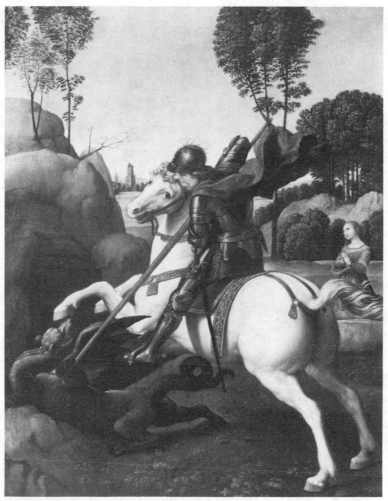

The body responds to situations of sudden danger with the fight-or-flight response.

Raphael. Saint George and the Dragon. *1504–6. Oil on wood. 11⅛ × 8⅜". Andrew W. Mellon Collection, National Gallery of Art, Washington.*

The fight-or-flight response

Heart rate speeds up.

Blood vessels of the heart open up.

Blood pressure rises.

Stored glycogen is broken down to blood sugar.

Bronchioles leading to the lungs widen.

Pupils of the eyes widen.

Extra blood is sent to the skeletal muscles.

Blood is directed away from the skin and digestive system.

Cell metabolism goes up by one-half.

tipping. Stimulation of the other part, the *parasympathetic nervous system,* leads to a general lessening of body tension. This reaction has been called the "relaxation response," and the body-feelings associated with it are described as calm and tranquil, quietly radiant, warm with happiness, and so forth. These feelings arise when people are engaged in quiet, pleasurable activities like lying in the sun, listening to peaceful music, or going for a leisurely stroll.

As soon as the sympathetic nervous system is aroused, the body's adrenals and pituitary and thyroid glands release powerful hormones. The most familiar of these hormones, adrenalin (epinephrine) and nor-adrenalin (nor-epinephrine), produce a sudden burst of energy and galvanize a person to action. These hormones are produced by the inner core of the adrenal gland, the medulla. The cortex or outside of the adrenal produces another set of hormones, which affects the body's equilibrium in a more subtle way. Cortisone is the best known of this second group. These hormones play a critical role in keeping the body in balance. They help to maintain the right levels of sugar, potassium, sodium, and chlorine. In infection or allergy they also control the amount of inflammation—swelling, redness, heat, and pain.

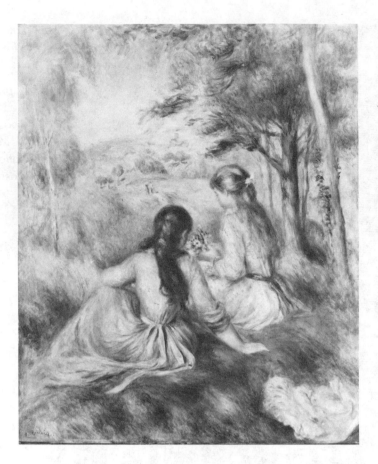

These same hormones that help us to react in urgent situations and that help maintain the body's chemical balance can, under certain circumstances, contribute to illness. When people experience unusually prolonged stress, they produce abnormally high levels of adrenalin, nor-adrenalin, cortisone, thyroid, and other hormones. These high levels cause body changes that contribute to all kinds of illness. First, just the presence of large amounts of these hormones in the blood raises blood pressure. This in turn causes microscopic tears in artery walls, and cholesterol plaques anchor to the tears. Buildup of plaque narrows the walls of the arteries, which impedes blood flow and leads to both stroke and heart attack. In addition, adrenalin and nor-adrenalin control the release of lipids (fats) into the bloodstream. When these hormones are circulating in high levels, more fats are released into the bloodstream and become attached to the arteries. This sequence is a graphic picture of how the perception of stress can alter the body's natural balances and lead to illness.

Not only do high levels of stress wear down the body by direct damage to the tissues, they also suppress the body's immune system. This makes people more susceptible to all kinds of infection, and even cancer. Ordinarily the lymphocytes, a type of white blood cell, work to keep the body healthy. They produce antibodies in response to various antigens—

The relaxation response

Heart rate slows
down.

Blood pressure
drops.

Cell metabolism
slows.

Breathing slows.

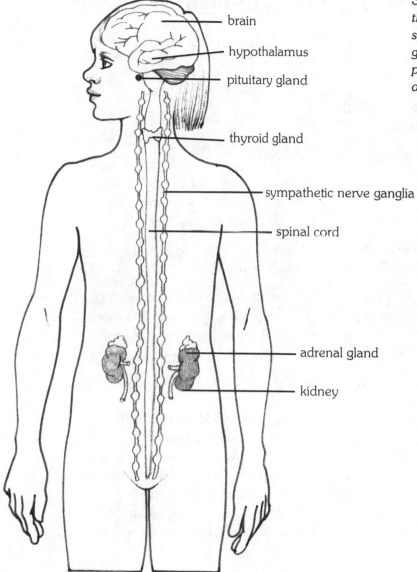

brain

hypothalamus

pituitary gland

thyroid gland

sympathetic nerve ganglia

spinal cord

adrenal gland

kidney

Stressful thoughts stimulate the sympathetic nervous system and the adrenal glands. If such stimulation is prolonged, it can cause disease.

viruses, bacteria, cancer cells, and foreign substances. The antibodies either render the antigens harmless or they act directly to kill them. Other lymphocytes then break down and remove the debris.

It has long been known that people under stress have less resistance to disease, but it was only recently that there was information on why this was so. First, high levels of adrenal hormones, as part of their role in controlling swelling and inflammation, naturally suppress the whole immune system. They lower the lymphocytes' ability to recognize foreign substances and produce antibodies. Second, studies show that the sympathetic part of the autonomic nervous system, which is excited by stress, is directly linked to the immune system. When animals' sympathetic nervous

Hormonal effects of the fight-or-flight response

Gland	Hormone produced	Effect of hormone
Pituitary	ACTH (Adrenocortico-tropic)	Stimulates adrenal cortex
Pituitary	Thyrotropic	Stimulates thyroid gland
Thyroid	Thyroxine	Steps up metabolism in all cells; raises output of heart; excites nervous system
Adrenal medulla	Epinephrine	Reinforces the effects of all the other hormones
Adrenal cortex	Cortisol (hydrocortisone)	Increases glucose in the blood; increases use of protein; increases use of fat; keeps lysosomes in the cells from breaking and dissolving cells; reduces antibody formation

systems are damaged, their ability to produce antibodies is radically lowered. The sympathetic nervous system actually has nerves that lead to the spleen and the thymus, two organs that are involved in the production and growth of lymphocytes. Third, scientists are now postulating that the hypothalamus, a part of the brain, is directly involved in the immune response because there is great activity there when antibodies are being produced. Damage to the hypothalamus also lowers antibody production.

Stress-related illnesses

There is a large and growing body of studies relating stress to the onset and course of illness. Not all people who are under stress get ill, but there is no doubt that stress is an underlying factor that sets off many illnesses, and the likelihood of a stressed person getting ill is much greater.

One of the early, impressive studies that alerted the medical community to the effects of stress was done by Dr. Lawrence E. Hinkle on several thousand people who worked for the telephone company. The group was chosen because for years the company had maintained excellent records on employee health. Hinkle was surprised to find that illness was not spread randomly among the employees or over the years. Twenty-five percent of the people had 50 percent of all the illness; another 25 percent of the people had less than 10 percent of all the illness. This was true

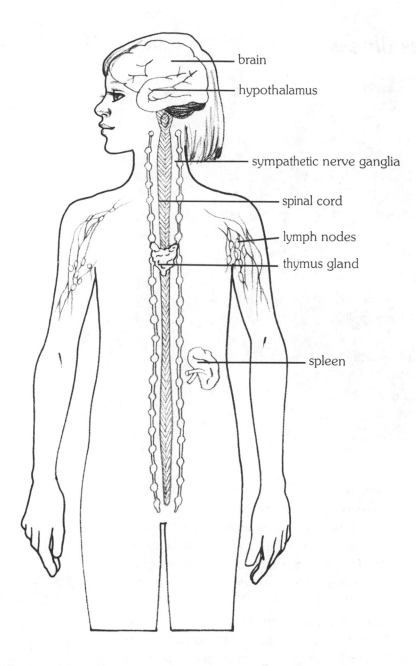

- brain
- hypothalamus
- sympathetic nerve ganglia
- spinal cord
- lymph nodes
- thymus gland
- spleen

Stressful thoughts stimulate the sympathetic nervous system and depress the production of antibodies by the thymus, spleen, and lymph nodes.

regardless of how severe the illness was or where it was in the body. Hinkle also found that people's illnesses occurred in "cluster years," that is, one-third of their illness occurred in one-eighth of the time studied. Often, individuals would suffer from several seemingly unrelated illnesses, all within a relatively short time.

When questioned, the only factor that was different between healthy individuals and those frequently ill was that the sick people described themselves as having family and job problems. These people felt limited in the choices they could make, and felt that their needs and drives were unsatisfied. Hinkle found that "illness occurs when people perceive their life situations as unsatisfying, threatening, overdemanding and productive of conflict—and no adaptation could be made." [2] Hinkle defined "perceiv-

How stress causes illness

When people perceive they are under stress, their bodies react with tension:

1. their brain sends out impulses to the nervous system that
2. directly stimulate the heart, muscles, and stomach, to tense and
3. the adrenal glands secrete hormones that increase the general level of tension, thereby
4. causing direct tissue damage, like tears in artery walls.

When people perceive they are under stress, their immune systems become less effective:

1. their brains send impulses out to the nervous system that
2. lower the thymus's and spleen's ability to produce lymphocytes and
3. the adrenal glands secrete hormones that lower the lymphocytes' ability to produce antibodies, thereby
4. lowering the body's ability to detect and eliminate bacteria, viruses, and cancer cells.

ing'' as the way a person received and evaluated information in their world. He believed that people's perceptions created ''the state of the host'' that fostered the disease. Based on his research, Hinkle concluded that the ''reaction of man to his life situation has an influence upon all forms of illness, it plays a role of significance in at least one-third of all episodes of disease regardless of their nature or location, their cause or severity.''[3]

Another study done by pediatrician Dr. Roger Meyer directly relates stress to illness in children. Meyer studied a group of basically healthy children and kept track of the incidence of strep throat over a period of time. First he did throat cultures on all the children and discovered that 30 percent of all the well children had strep bacteria present in the throat, but showed no symptoms of illness. From this he concluded that ''peaceful coexistence [between the child and strep bacteria] is the rule, disease is the exception.''[4] Like Hinkle, Meyer tried to isolate the factor that caused the individual to become ill. What he found was that one-fourth of the children's strep throats followed a family crisis. An ill child was four times as likely to have just experienced a stressful episode as was one of the well children. Meyer concluded that stress increases the probability of a child's getting a strep throat.

Dr. Klaus J. Roghmann more recently did a study on the effects of stress on *any* illness in children. The probability of illness on the day of a stress

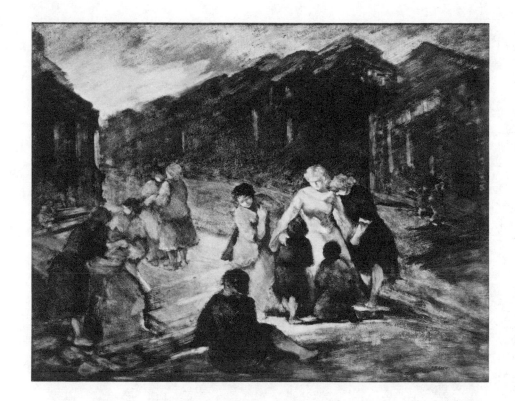

episode is approximately double for both mothers and children. The day *after* a stressful episode, the probability of a mother or child becoming ill was even higher—three times more likely than normal. Roghmann also found that families under stress were more likely to visit a doctor whether or not they were actually ill. Roghmann defined stress as "any event perceived by the family as upsetting." Most often the stressful episode involved either family fights or job tensions that required some coping behavior or adaptation. Roghmann concluded that "the greatest future challenge lies in controlled trials or methods to reduce internal stress. This would reduce acute illness and doctor visits. [The way to do this would be to] reduce external stress and/or 'immunize' people against inevitable life crises by strengthening their ability to handle stress without becoming physically or mentally ill." [5]

Life events and illness

One of the greatest contributions to stress research was the work done by Seattle psychiatrists Thomas H. Holmes and Richard H. Rahe. Basically, Holmes realized that stressful life events seemed to make it more likely that people would become ill, and that the illness would not be limited to one type of disease or organ system. Like Hinkle, he found that both infectious diseases and accidents did not occur evenly throughout the population, but occurred in a relatively small number of people during short periods of time. Also like Hinkle, Holmes found that these periods of

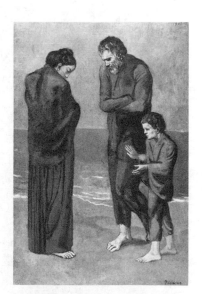

Stress scale for children

Different life events produce varying amounts of stress for children—the more points, the greater the stress. The chart is arranged in order of how frequently the events occur.

Life events	Preschool Age	Elementary Age	Junior high Age
Beginning nursery school, first grade, or high school	42	46	45
Change to a different school	33	46	52
Birth or adoption of a brother or sister	50	50	50
Brother or sister leaving home	39	36	33
Hospitalization of brother or sister	37	41	44
Death of brother or sister	59	68	71
Change of father's occupation requiring increased absence from home	36	45	42
Loss of job by a parent	23	38	48
Marital separation of parents	74	78	77
Divorce of parents	78	84	84
Hospitalization of parent (serious illness)	51	55	54
Death of a parent	89	91	94
Death of a grandparent	30	38	35
Marriage of parent to stepparent	62	65	63
Jail sentence of parent for 30 days or less	34	44	50
Jail sentence of parent for 1 year or more	67	67	76
Addition of third adult to family (e.g., grandparent)	39	41	34
Change in parents' financial status	21	29	40
Mother beginning to work	47	44	36
Decrease in number of arguments between parents	21	25	29
Increase in number of arguments between parents	44	51	48
Decrease in number of arguments with parents	22	27	29
Increase in number of arguments with parents	39	47	46
Discovery of being an adopted child	33	52	70
Acquiring a visible deformity	52	69	83
Having a visible congenital deformity	39	60	70
Hospitalization of yourself (child)	59	62	59
Change in acceptance by peers	38	51	68
Outstanding personal achievement	23	39	45
Death of a close friend (child's friend)	38	53	65
Failure of a grade in school		57	62
Suspension from school		46	54
Pregnancy in unwed teen-age sister		36	60
Becoming involved with drugs or alcohol		61	70
Becoming a full-fledged member of a church/synagogue		25	28
Not making an extracurricular activity you wanted to be involved in (i.e., athletic team, band)			49
Breaking up with a boyfriend or girlfriend			47
Beginning to date			55
Fathering an unwed pregnancy			76
Unwed pregnancy			95

Used by permission from *Journal of Pediatrics* 83: 119 (1973).

illness were related to the people's moods and their ability to adapt to change.

Borrowing a technique from psychophysics, Holmes and Rahe set up a *relativity scale of life events,* ranking situations in terms of the amount of stress they engendered and the amount of coping they required. They asked hundreds of people to assign a relative number value to all kinds of life events, assessing which were the most stressful and required the greatest readjustment. The scale ranged from 1 to 100. Getting married was used as a reference point and was arbitrarily assigned a value of 50. Other life events that were used included divorce, separation, pregnancy, loss of a job, moving, death of a friend or relative, Christmas, and traffic tickets. What Holmes and Rahe found was that people's responses were not random. There was remarkable agreement among people of different professions and backgrounds.

Studies showed that life events totaling 150 points within a one-year period meant that a person had a fifty-fifty chance of developing an illness or health change in the next year, whereas a score of 300 points increased the likelihood of illness to 90 percent. Holmes and Rahe found that people with high life-changes had statistically five times as great a chance of developing health problems as those with little life-change had.[6] Now that factors such as attitude and family support have been taken into account as well, the original Holmes-Rahe scale has become an even more accurate tool in the statistical prediction of illness.

Since Holmes's pioneering work, R. Dean Coddington and J. Stephen Heisel have devised special scales for children of different ages. Like the Holmes-Rahe scale, these new scales are accurate prognosticators of illness, but they deal with a different set of life events. Instead of losing a job or getting married, the scale deals with events such as birth of a sibling (50 points) and starting or changing school.[7] The researchers studied a broad range of illnesses from minor to serious, including children in hospitals as well as in outpatient clinics. They found that children who were sick were three times as likely to have experienced more frequent or serious life events in the year prior to the onset of their illnesses.[8] In another study that evaluated children for high stress and then followed them at weekly intervals, it was found that the children with high stress figures were three times as likely to have accidents, both severe and minor, as the children with low stress figures.[9]

It is ironic that Hippocrates, the Greek father of modern medicine, said more than 2,000 years ago, "It is changes that are chiefly responsible for diseases, especially the greatest changes, the violent alterations."

Feelings of discontent and illness

Life events require people to make adaptive decisions, and attitudes toward these events contribute to whether the body stays well. Just as feelings of discontent and lack of control make a person more likely to get ill, so a belief that one gets ill all the time actually increases the likelihood of illness.

The effects of attitude on resistance were dramatically shown in a study by Dr. George G. Jackson on the common cold. Jackson introduced cold virus into the throats of a number of healthy, young volunteers. To everyone's surprise, he found that only one-third of the volunteers caught a cold. Moreover, chilling, fatigue, and lack of sleep did not affect the number of colds or who got sick. These results were further evidence that people do not simply "catch a cold," and that the presence of disease organisms is not the sole cause of illness. The only difference Jackson could find between those volunteers who got sick and those who did not, was that the sick ones had a different mental attitude toward themselves and toward disease. The people who did not get colds did not believe they would get sick (all expressed the feeling that they almost never got sick), and had few worries on their minds at the time of the study. Contrastingly, the people who got sick said that they frequently got colds *and* had problems they were worrying about with no satisfactory resolution in sight.

Jackson's next study was a creative and unusual one that was destined to change the way people thought about illness. He took the people who claimed to have frequent colds (five or more a year) and sprayed their throats with distilled water, which he said contained cold virus. Of the volunteers, 26 percent came down with clinically diagnosable colds, complete with running nose, headache, fever, cough, and so on.[10] This study has been replicated using other illnesses. In an equally striking study, distilled water was sprayed in the throats of asthmatics who were told that "you are breathing something that usually gives you asthma." Nineteen of the forty patients in the study immediately experienced difficulty breathing and began wheezing.[11] In a similar study, people who were highly allergic to poison ivy were stroked with a leaf said to be poison ivy (but which, in fact, was not). Real poison ivy developed in some of these subjects.[12]

In this chapter we have discussed a group of experiments designed to determine what kind of person gets ill. The studies show that basically the people who become ill are those with a certain mental attitude toward themselves and their ability to handle life crises. Researchers found that people who perceive themselves as dissatisfied, alienated, and out of control are most likely to get ill. Conversely, those who describe themselves as successful, happy, and optimistic are least likely to get ill.

Scientists are learning *who* gets ill from epidemiological studies of thousands of people and *how* people become ill from studying the physiology of the nervous, endocrine, and immune systems and their interconnections. To parents, this knowledge is a gift—it gives them the ability to do things that will increase their children's likelihood of staying well. Since we know that stress and self-perception are linked to a major portion of the illnesses of childhood, we as parents can now work out ways to lessen stress for ourselves and our children, and to greatly improve the ability to cope with it.

Ages when children commonly get certain illnesses or symptoms

4 years	Lots of colds
	Stomachaches when upset
	Needs to urinate often when upset
	Frequent accidents when upset
5 years	Occasional stomachaches or vomiting because of disliked foods
	Feet hurt when tired
	May get sick after starting school
	Stomachaches connected with school demands
	Face and head hurt when washing and combing
6 years	Frequent sore throats
	Stomachaches at school time
	Broken arms
	Face and head hurt when washing and combing
7 years	Headaches when tired or excited
	Legs and knees ache when tired
	Rubs eyes a lot
	Gets very tired, stretches and yawns
8 years	Improved health
	Increased allergies
	Headaches, stomachaches, and increased urination when the child has to do something not liked
	Frequent accidents
	Broken legs
9 years	Improved health
	Many symptoms when the child has to do something not liked
	Feels dizzy
10 years	Worries about health occasionally

Adapted from the Gesell Institute's *Child Behavior* by Frances Ilg and Louise Bates Ames (New York: Harper & Brothers, 1955).

Characteristics of people who get ill, and people who don't

Likely to get ill	Unlikely to get ill
Crisis-ridden	Hopeful
Under stress	Has a purpose in life, a reason
Dissatisfied	for being
Discontented	Optimistic
Unhappy	Trusting
Resentful	Has high self-esteem
Unsatisfied	Has high congruity with peers
Threatened	Successful
Out of control	Excited
Under demands	Interested
Loaded with responsibility	Happy
Worried	Satisfied
Depressed	Stimulated
Frustrated	Involved
Helpless	Has high social standing
Lonely	Has stable social structure
Grief-stricken	Has sense of cohesion, agree-
Confused	ment
Abandoned	Receives social support
Lacks positive feedback	Receives positive feedback

Parents' attitudes and their children's health

Throughout the early childhood years, the family is the most basic social unit with which the child comes into contact. Not only does the family provide most of the child's social interactions and experiences, it determines to a large extent how the child will view those interactions, then and later.

From the beginning, parents teach children how to regard their bodies, to take pleasure in some sensations, to be concerned or even frightened by others. Parents unconsciously pass on their feelings about their bodies and about health and illness. If parents feel they have little control over their bodies or think that they are always ill, then that is the attitude they will give to their children, even when the children are infants. As children grow up, go to school, and branch out into the world, they experience other ways of regarding their bodies, but their parents' views remain their dominant grounding. The basic program that parents give to the child, consciously and unconsciously, starts with two messages: (1) You are always well, *or* you are always sick; and (2) you have control over your

Do you perceive yourself and your family as healthy?

Are you sick always, often, little, never?

Is your wife or husband sick always, often, little, never?

Is your first child sick always, often, little, never?

Do you have total, a lot, some, little, or no control of your health?

body, both mentally and physically, or you do not—you are a passive victim who can only fear illness. These statements present the extremes, when in truth most parents fall somewhere in between.

In a similar way, parents teach their children a life view built upon the way they perceive reality. Parents label experiences for their children by their own reactions to situations. Like their attitudes toward their bodies, parents express their life attitudes both consciously and unconsciously, in verbal language and body language. The parent who presents a happy, interested life to the child gives that child reason to be healthy rather than ill. If a parent perceives events around him as being annoying, frustrating, or basically negative, the child will learn to perceive the world in a similar way. Such stressful thoughts tend to lower resistance and increase the likelihood of all illness. This kind of tuning actually begins in utero, when the mother's stress hormones cross the placenta and affect the baby.

In addition to teaching the child how to perceive stress, the parents create stress or calm by the way they set up the household. Although there are times when all parents feel that stress originates with the child, basically the control of the situation lies with the parent. By becoming alert to stressful situations that are about to occur and stepping in with appropriate action, parents can relieve many moments of tension.

Take control of your health

Stress has an effect on whether you are well.

You can begin to deal with stress.

Illness occurs for limited periods of time and the periods will end.

Decide to make this a "healthy time."

Decide that you are now a healthy person who rarely will get ill; the ill time is over.

Decide to play an active part in keeping yourself healthy.

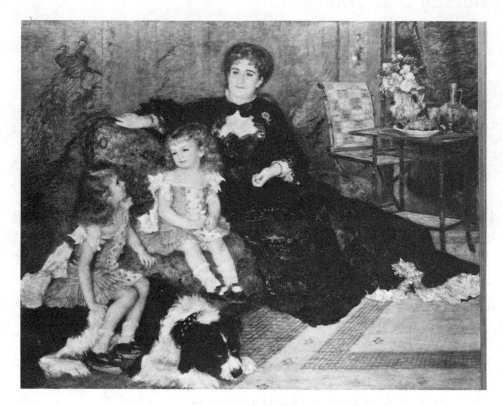

A parent who has a relaxed, happy home life is helping to make her children healthy.

Renoir, Pierre-Auguste. Madame Charpentier and Her Children. *1878. Oil on canvas. $60\frac{1}{2} \times 74\frac{7}{8}$". The Metropolitan Museum of Art, New York. Wolfe Fund, 1907.*

The pioneering psychiatrist Carl Jung believed that children are more powerfully influenced by their parents' unconscious feelings than by their words and actions. Moreover, Jung said that "What usually has the strongest effect on the child is the life which the parents . . . might have lived . . . which they have always shirked."[13] Jung thought this was due to "the extraordinary infectiousness of emotional reactions." He believed in the "identity of the psychic state of the child with the unconscious of the parents." The younger the children, the less separate and unique are their personalities and the more they depend on and reflect their parents' personalities. Young children are remarkably open and sensitive, and they readily pick up the conflict and tension of unresolved areas of their parents' lives.

Reading this, it may be easy for a parent to feel guilty and over-whelmed. *Please do not!* Blaming yourself does not help the children; if anything, it adds to whatever stress and negativity they feel. Parents are who they are in part because of the way they were raised. We do not single-handedly create our view of ourselves and our bodies. So blame is neither justified nor useful. What will make the situation better is positive change. But how can parents overcome their unconscious attitudes in a short time?

Actually, it's not even necessary. The most important thing is for parents to accept themselves as they are. Their new awareness of the situation will immediately start to bring about change. Frances G. Wickes, a child psychiatrist who worked with Carl Jung, treated children with night terrors,

Become aware of areas of tension

Relax and let images come into your mind.

Examine your family life, job, where you live, your view of yourself, your past.

Simply let the images float by, but try to become aware of areas of tension or frustration.

phobias, and extreme fears of parental separation. Wickes observed that the children's symptoms often disappeared when the parents simply faced up to their areas of tension or problems. "The child then intuits the strength, courage, and honesty that come from a real attempt at understanding." [14]

Another example of how only little change in the parents might exert a tremendous positive influence on their children's health and well-being comes from a study done at Yale–New Haven Medical Center by Dr. James K. Skipper. Skipper's study showed that simply reassuring parents by giving them a small amount of factual knowledge dramatically improved the recovery of children after tonsillectomy. In the study, children who were being admitted for routine tonsillectomies were divided into two groups. A control group was treated in the normal way (with a minimum of information). Nurses gave the mothers in the experimental group 20 minutes of explanation of what the operation was and what would happen to their child—several minutes on admission, several directly before the operation, and several before going home. Aside from the nurses who gave the explanation, no one else knew the difference between the two groups.

The results Skipper found were truly remarkable. After the operation the children from the experimental group had lower temperatures (less fever), lower pulse rates, lower blood pressures, were able to urinate sooner, had less nausea and vomiting, drank more fluids, and, on the whole, had a much faster recovery while they were in the hospital. When they went home, the experimental group continued to have faster recoveries. The children ate more easily, had less fear of doctors, slept better, cried less, were less infantile, and had fewer follow-up visits to doctors for continued medical problems. Members of the experimental group were diagnosed as healed quite a bit before members of the control group. To explain the results Skipper postulated that "the mother is a prime factor in determining whether changes in the child's emotions and behavior will be detrimental or beneficial to his treatment and recovery. If the mother were able to manage her own stress and be calm, confident, and relaxed, this might be communicated to the child and ease his distress." [15]

If Skipper had invented a drug that helped heal children after surgery as well as this, it would have been hailed as a major discovery. Yet all Skipper did was give the *parents* (not even the children) a few minutes of explanation, without asking them to do anything. Indeed, none of the parents *did* anything that the experimenters could see would cause the results.

Skipper thought that the prepared mother might naturally be making more rational decisions and adapting better to the stress of the situation by engaging in "imaginative mental rehearsal" during which the work or worry can occur. Another name for imaginative mental rehearsal is visualization. Since the time of the study, visualization has come to be an important medical tool (see pages 57–61 and 256–271).

Effects of social support

Whatever the prepared mothers did is classified under the heading of "support." Support is a relatively new term in the health care field. It consists of anyone or anything that makes a person feel better, function better, or be more optimistic. Support leads people to feel loved and cared for, raises their self-esteem, and makes them feel they are part of a group. It can come from intimate relationships with family or friends, jobs or hobbies that give people positive feedback, or a system of beliefs that gives meaning to life. One of the most important health discoveries of recent years is that social supports actually protect one from illness during periods of stress. In terms of health, support is the functional opposite of stress. The more support people have, the greater their protection. High amounts of support protect people almost *completely* against stress-related illness. If stress is a poison, then support is the antidote.

The first study on support was done by Katherine Nuckolls in 1972. Nuckolls studied several hundred pregnant women in terms of stress (using the Holmes-Rahe scale) and social support. To measure support, she asked the women questions about their perception of themselves, about their marriage and living conditions, and their extended family and community. The questionnaire dealt with intimacy, happiness, religion, economic support, and friendship patterns. Nuckolls found that women with high life-change scales (Holmes-Rahe) had one-third fewer complica-

A community that supports its members has lower illness rates than a community without support.

Park, Linton. Flax Scutching Bee. *1885. Oil on bed ticking. 31¼ × 50¼". National Gallery of Art, Washington. Gift of Edgar William and Bernice Chrysler Garbisch, 1953.*

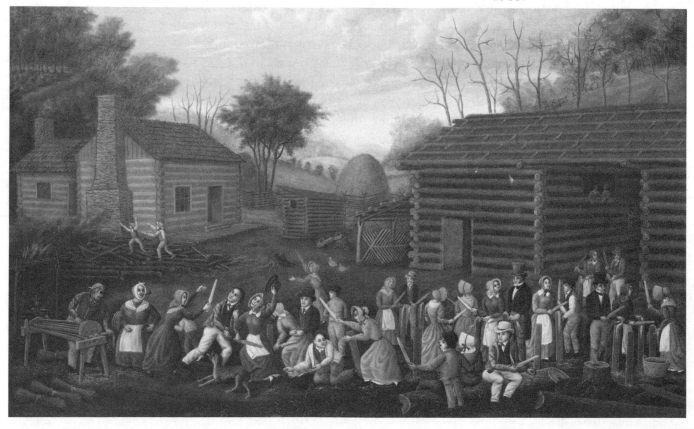

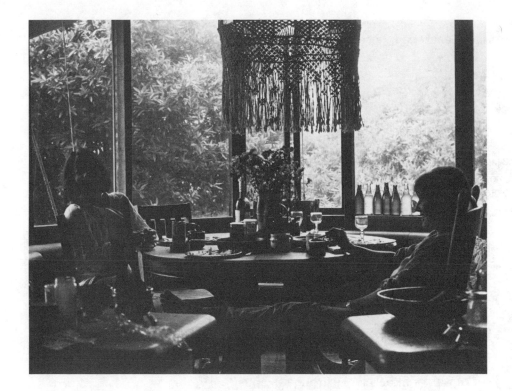

People who have daily contact with close friends have lower incidences of illness, depression, and family problems than people who don't have such social support.

tions in pregnancy and delivery if they also had high support. "Susceptibility to illness and illness outcomes is in some part a function of the balance between the individual's personal and social resources and the social milieu to which he is forced to adapt." [16]

Another study was done by Dr. G. W. Brown on a group of English housewives. [17] Brown set up a scale to evaluate the extent to which the housewives had people with whom they could discuss their problems. The A group had daily intimate contact, the B group once a week, the C group less than once weekly, and the D group not at all. Brown found that depression, serious illness, and major family problems were most frequent in B, C, and D women, and almost never occurred in the A-group women.

Yet another study, by Dr. Sidney Cobb, dealt with how a group of men with arthritis responded when their plant was closed and they lost their jobs. [18] Cobb found that men with low social support had ten times as many arthritis flare-ups as men with high social support.

During the Vietnam War a remarkable study was made by Dr. Peter G. Bourne concerning how a group of medical corpsmen responded to the incredible stress of dangerous combat rescues. [19] Normally, because of stress, people in danger have very high levels of the adrenal hormone cortisone. But the group Bourne studied had lower levels of cortisone than the average person who was not in combat. The only explanation Bourne could find for these results was that these corpsmen were members of a tremendously cohesive group and felt that their work was very important.

Do you have enough support?

Do you confide in someone each day, once a week, less than once a week, never?

Do you feel secure in your environment each day, once a week, less than once a week, never?

Do you feel that you have some control over your environment each day, once a week, less than once a week, never?

Do you feel that people approve of you each day, once a week, less than once a week, never?

Do you have an intimate relationship with someone each day, once a week, less than once a week, never?

Does your support come from family, friends, community?

Do you feel you have enough money? Usually? Sometimes? Never?

Do you have a strong set of personal beliefs? A strong religious affiliation?

The famous child psychiatrist, René Spitz, studied the illness patterns of children in a foundling home and a state nursery. Both of the institutions had excellent hygiene in terms of general cleanliness and formula preparation. The children in the home were cared for by nurses, those in the nursery were cared for by their mothers. What Spitz found was that the infants raised by nurses were retarded in their growth, were much more susceptible to disease, and had a higher mortality from all diseases.[20]

It has even been found that support affects patterns of serious illness. A group of studies was made in Roseto, Pennsylvania, an Italian-American community that was extremely cohesive and had strong family ties with a village in southern Italy. The average person in Roseto had a very fatty diet and was obese. Despite these predisposing factors, the death rate from heart attacks in Roseto was less than half that in surrounding communities. Relatives who moved *out* of Roseto had higher rates corresponding to outside communities.[21]

In the context of teaching parents things they can do to increase the health of their children, these studies are almost earthshaking. They show that people do not have to do anything complicated, technical, or unenjoyable to improve their health. Parents only need to have a basic knowledge of diseases in order to reduce fear and increase their coping ability, and they need to understand how stress and support function in terms of preventing or increasing the likelihood of illness of all kinds.

Family styles and health

So far we have discussed in fairly general terms how a child's health is affected by its social environment. But what specifically are the factors that make up the child's social world? First and foremost there is the family, later the school, and finally the community. The new field of medical sociology has undertaken to make some sense out of the huge number of complex factors that make up the social environment and to see how these factors relate individually to the child's health.

One of the basic theories of medical sociology is that environments, like people, have unique "personalities." Thus, two families living side by side, using the same schools and community resources, can have totally different family personalities. School-age children are particularly aware of how different each friend's family life is. Many adults notice that other families are radically different from theirs in feelings, goals, and illness patterns. The more a family becomes aware of its own personality and patterns, the more it can evaluate which patterns are positive and make conscious decisions to strengthen them.

Medical sociologists now analyze specific environments, for example, the family, in terms of a fascinating group of dimensions. They look at three broad categories—*relationships, personal development,* and *system maintenance and change. Relationship* dimensions have to do with "the extent to which people are involved in the environment, the extent to which they support and help one another, and the extent to which there is spontaneity and free and open expression among them." [22] This includes such characteristics as a sense of belongingness, togetherness, feelings of friendship or love for other members, sense of commitment, concern and help for others, ability to freely discuss personal problems, laughter, warmth, and physical expression. The opposite end of this spectrum deals with the amount of conflict, sense of separateness, individuality, lack of mutual support or commitment to or communication with the group, and amount of rejection, hostility, or indifference. The *personal development* dimension describes "the basic directions along which personal growth and self-enhancement tend to occur in the particular environment." The characteristics include goals and purposes such as independence, self-sufficiency, achievement, ambition, competitiveness, interest in intellectual and cultural activities (lessons, discussions, courses, performances, reading matter), recreational interests, and religious and ethical values. *System maintenance and change* dimensions "evaluate orderliness, the clarity of expectations, the degree of control, and the responsiveness to change." Characteristics include how organized the social unit is, the degree of defined duties and chores, planning and scheduling of activities, budgeting, neatness and cleanliness, strictness, and definition of rules.

Many of the characteristics described above have been studied in relation to children's mental and physical health, as well as to their behavior. A study by Thomas Prendergast [23] examined health and illness patterns of high school students in the context of relationships with their parents. Prendergast found that in a highly controlled family, with a tense father,

Every family has its own personality or style. Some styles promote health, some contribute to illness.

John Singleton Copley. The Copley Family. 1776–77. Oil on canvas. 72½ × 90⅜". National Gallery of Art, Washington. Andrew W. Mellon Fund.

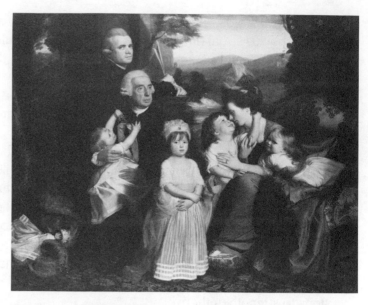

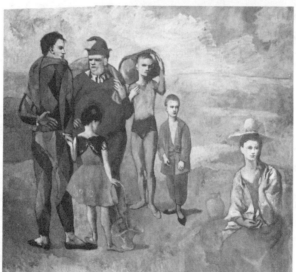

Picasso, Pablo. Family of Saltimbanques. Late 1904– late 1905. Oil on canvas. 83¾ × 90 ⅜". Chester Dale Collection, 1962, National Gallery of Art, Washington.

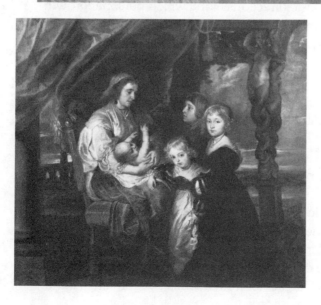

Rubens, Peter Paul. Deborah Kip, Wife of Sir Balthasar Gerbier, and Her Children. 1629–30. Oil on canvas. 65¼ × 70". National Gallery of Art, Washington. Andrew W. Mellon Fund, 1971.

Evaluating your family style

Relationship dimensions

Do family members feel as if they "belong"?

Is the family a unit?

Does the family do things together?

Do family members help each other?

Do family members discuss problems with other family members?

Does your family have laughter and warmth?

Is there much conflict?

Is there much hostility?

Personal development dimensions

Do members work independently?

Is intellectual work pursued—sciences, music, art?

Does school work receive emphasis?

Are grades important?

Does the family go to church/synagogue or celebrate religious holidays?

Personal change dimensions

Are there rules at home?

Are there duties and chores?

How much of the day is planned?

How neat is your house?

How strict is home discipline?

Is your family competent?

Is there pride at home?

Do things work?

Do people communicate with each other?

illness and doctor visits were greatest. Families highest in tension and rejection had the greatest number of accidents.

Another study, by Virginia Bordman, dealt with how family competence related to all kinds of illness in 7- to 11-year-old children.[24] Family competence was based on participation, communication, pride, and so on. Bordman found that children from close, confident families were much less likely to be ill with accidents or infections. Interestingly enough, the parents of these families also tended to be healthier and lost less time from work.

Perhaps the most remarkable finding of Bordman's study was that families with several children under five were much less likely to rate their family as competent and much more likely to have older children who were ill. This association between preschool children and greater illness has been reported in a number of other studies. Pediatricians have been aware of this correlation for some time. They have tended to attribute it to the fact that preschoolers have not yet built up their immunity through repeated exposure to the many different viruses and bacteria. But now there is some question as to whether the stress of life with preschoolers doesn't contribute significantly to family illness patterns.

Still another way to study a family is to look at the personal style of one of its members and to see how that style affects the amount of stress the whole family experiences. Studies have been done on how the father's attitude toward responsibility and work pressure affect heart disease. People under heavy responsibility have higher levels of adrenal hormones and higher heart disease rates. Dr. Ray H. Rosenman and Dr. Meyer Friedman found that aggressive, ambitious, time-oriented people, whom they labeled as Type A, had six times the incidence of heart disease as people who did not share these characteristics.[25] Even children with these behavior patterns show body changes that are linked to heart disease. Type A children had 6 percent higher cholesterol levels than other children. It is clear that Type A behavior tends to put stress on the whole family and probably helps create what anthropologists call a "tough" culture, that is, a culture whose very nature is hard on its members. Characteristically such a culture fosters competitiveness, tension, and dissatisfaction among its members. In a tough culture it's very hard to ever achieve goals and very few people ever reach high positions. Western industrial society is considered by anthropologists to be a very tough culture, as evidenced by such factors as drug and alcohol abuse, suicides, and aggression. For example, if a corporation puts sole emphasis on being the president, or a classroom on being the best student, then everyone else is made to think less of himself and/or is under tremendous pressure to get to and stay on top. The more challenging an environment is, the more likely people are to assume Type A characteristics and become ill. A study on Benedictine monks illustrates this point very well. Monks who were heads of schools and seminaries had two to three times as many

Are you or members of your family heart-disease personalities (Type A)?

A Type A person

Struggles against time

Is vocally explosive and accentuates words

Always moves and eats quickly

Is impatient

Has a lot of trouble waiting in lines or in traffic

Tries to do several things at once

Always tries to steer conversations to his or her own topics

Feels guilty when relaxing

Doesn't see beauty around himself or herself

Schedules more than can be done

Challenges other Type A's

Clenches fists

Feels speed and efficiency are essential for success

Evaluates everything in numbers

A Type B person

Is free of all Type-A habits

Doesn't suffer from time urgency

Isn't impatient

Isn't hostile

Doesn't need to brag

Can play for fun and relaxation

Can relax without guilt

Can work without agitation

Adapted from *Type A Behavior and Your Heart,* by Meyer Friedman, M.D., and Ray H. Rosenman, M.D. (Greenwich, Conn.: Fawcett Crest, 1974).

How tough is the cultural milieu in which you live?

Is your society large or small?

Are positions throughout a hierarchy accepted as equal or just praised at the top?

Can you get the highly valued objects of your culture easily?

Can most people get highly valued objects of your culture easily?

Can most people easily achieve goals that are respected?

Is there pressure at your job to get to the top?

heart attacks as their brothers who ate the same diet but never left the monastery.[26]

A huge cross-cultural study done by Dr. James Henry and Dr. J. C. Cassell[27] showed that the average blood pressure is much lower in people with a stable, traditional culture or people who are well-adapted to their particular subgroup. What seems to cause blood pressures to rise is the stress of cultural disintegration, and the need to change and adapt without adequate resources or social support.

Relaxation creates health

Just as stress creates a physiology of illness, so relaxation creates a physiology of health. Dr. Herbert Benson found that by simply telling people to sit comfortably, relax, and concentrate on a single thing, their blood pressure, heart rate, oxygen consumption, metabolism, and level of cortico-hormones would be lowered.[28] Benson termed this physiology the *relaxation response* and postulated that it was the opposite of the *fight-or-flight response*. This healthful change in physiology is due to a lowered sympathetic nervous system and adrenal gland activity.

Other researchers have shown that mental relaxation and yoga methods lowered blood pressure by 20 points in people with high blood pressure, dropped their serum cholesterol by almost a fifth, and cut their drug usage in half.

In addition to treating high blood pressure, relaxation is also being used to treat anxiety. The psychiatrist Helen De Rosis says, "[anxious] people describe their insides quivering. They can't stay still, or they feel like they've got a motor running."[29] Anxiety can manifest itself physically in various ways and there doesn't necessarily have to be anything organically wrong. "You can have gastro-intestinal pain, cardiac distress, or pulmonary distress. You can have aches and pains, headaches, backaches or leg aches," says Dr. De Rosis. The physiology of anxiety is the same as the physiology of stress—the fight-or-flight syndrome described earlier. The sympathetic part of the autonomic nervous system is aroused and this arousal results in muscle tension, increased heart and breathing rate, and high levels of adrenal hormones. As De Rosis says, "You actually have the muscles all ready to go—and yet you're probably sitting in a chair or working at a desk. There's an incompatibility. You're ready to go, but holding yourself back."

In his pioneering work on muscle physiology, Edmund Jacobson discovered that the physical sensations of relaxation actually are contrary to and inhibit the physical sensations of anxiety. Relaxation eliminates the uncomfortable confusion of being primed for action but not knowing what to do and replaces anxiety with a calm, peaceful feeling of being in harmony. Researchers in behavior therapy have found that when people are relaxed they have much less of a reaction when faced with anxious or stressful stimuli. Furthermore, when a stressful stimulus is repeated, people become less and less anxious each time; when people are not relaxed, they become just as anxious each time the stimulus is repeated.

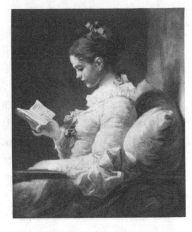

Relaxation replaces anxiety with a calm, peaceful feeling.

Fragonard, Jean-Honoré. A Young Girl Reading. 18th cent. Oil on canvas. 32 × 25½". National Gallery of Art, Washington. Gift of Mrs. Mellon Bruce in memory of her father, Andrew Mellon, 1961.

Relaxation relieves stress

Relaxation is a basic tool for relieving stress and preventing all manner of stress-related illnesses. For example, many families have a period before dinner during which there's always stress and fighting. If the parents are generally tense and anxious, a full-blown family fight can result from a spilled glass of milk. This kind of situation increases tension in every family member. The mother might respond by developing a tension headache, the father's blood pressure might rise and remain elevated, the child who spilled the milk might fall off his bike the next day, and another child might have a nervous stomachache that night and develop a G.I. flu the next day. This imaginary scenario illustrates in a slightly exaggerated way how illness can be related to an event that everyone perceives as stressful.

If the family is generally relaxed, they are unlikely to perceive a spilled glass of milk as a stressful event; in fact, the situation might actually be regarded with a certain amount of humor. Even if the family happens to be tense or tired, a problematic situation may be avoided if family members are able to see what is happening and make a conscious decision to relax. What might result is that the milk will be cleaned up, the incident will be resolved, and the family might go on to a discussion of the day's events. When a situation is successfully resolved, tensions will ease and the kind of physical symptoms described in the first scenario will not develop. In fact, the family's feeling of calmness will serve to relieve residual levels of tension in the muscles around the mother's forehead, lower the father's blood pressure from his normal work level, and relax the sibling's nervous stomach and allow antibodies to be produced against the G.I. flu going around. Finally, the child who spilled the milk would be relieved at not having provoked a family incident and would not be so distracted the following day as to get into a bike accident.

Relaxation is becoming one of the major tools of psychology and medicine. It is being used in treatment of hypertension (high blood pressure), heart arhythmias, headaches, asthma, anxiety and stress-related illnesses like ulcers, preparation for surgery and follow-up, natural childbirth, insomnia, muscle and joint pain, systematic desensitization of fears and phobias, and in all types of psychotherapy.

Relaxation is deceptively simple. Nevertheless researchers have discovered that relaxation leads to profound physiological changes that result in a state that is quite different from people's everyday one. Relaxation is characterized by turning inward and concentrating on one's own body and mind rather than on external events. Inherent to the relaxed state is a certain feeling of detachment; that is, a lack of concern for how one is doing—as Dr. Wolfgang Luthe says, "a casual, relaxed attitude involving minimal or no goal-directed voluntaristic efforts in the sense of energetic striving, and apprehensive, tension-producing control of functions leading to the desired result." [30]

This inward-directed lack of striving has a very special effect on the body's nervous system. At the very least, it produces the relaxation response. What this means physiologically is that the body switches from a hypothalamic sympathetic adrenal arousal to a hypothalamic parasympathetic adrenal turn-off. In a sense relaxation takes place when the body turns off the system that alerts to external change or danger and turns on a system that puts the body on a self-regulating, minimum-maintenance, self-healing mode. During relaxation, heart rate, respiratory rate, oxygen consumption, and carbon dioxide production drop. [31]

Some medical thinkers claim a great deal more for relaxation. For example, Itzhak Bentov, a biomedical researcher, postulated that during relaxation an altered state of consciousness occurs in which one's mind enters a reality where space and time are different. In this reality, Bentov believes that our minds act independently of our bodies and can travel anywhere and learn anything.

The physiology of relaxation

Muscles are relaxed and muscle blood flow drops.

Breathing slows.

Oxygen consumption drops.

Elimination of carbon dioxide drops.

Heartbeat slows.

Blood pressure drops.

Cardiac output drops.

Skin resistance increases.

Brain waves change to alpha and theta.

Blood lactate drops.

Adrenal hormone levels drop.

Blood flow to bowels increases.

Relaxation techniques

Anyone can learn to relax by following a set of written instructions. Recent research shows that the maximum effects of relaxation can be achieved with only four to eight hours of instruction and twenty minutes of practice a day. There are as many methods for learning to relax as there are instructors. No one method has proved to be superior, and, in fact, they are all rather similar. The common aspects that have been found to be most helpful are (1) a set of clear instructions and a belief in them, (2) a comfortable position so muscles can relax, (3) a passive attitude of *allowing* relaxation to take place, (4) a quiet place, and (5) deep, regular breathing. Many also find it useful to tape record the instructions or have someone read them out loud.

Before trying to relax it is quite helpful to try an exercise designed to increase awareness of small amounts of muscle tension. Very often our muscles are slightly contracted and we are not even aware of it. The more nervous and tense we tend to be, the more likely we are to be unaware of constant, low-level tension that we have come to accept as normal.

To feel muscle tension, lie in a comfortable position with your hands resting at your sides. Raise one hand slightly by bending it at the wrist and you will feel muscles in the top of your forearm contract and tense. If you let your hand go limp, these muscles will relax and your hand will drop. With practice you will become aware of the subtle difference in feeling between a contracted muscle and a relaxed one. If you're not sure of the tension, rest the fingers of your other hand lightly on top of your forearm and feel the muscle contract when you raise your hand.

What are your tense areas?

Everyone has certain areas or muscles that get tense when they are nervous or under pressure. Here are the most common areas to check out for tension:

Eyes

Jaw

Neck and shoulders

Lower back and pelvis

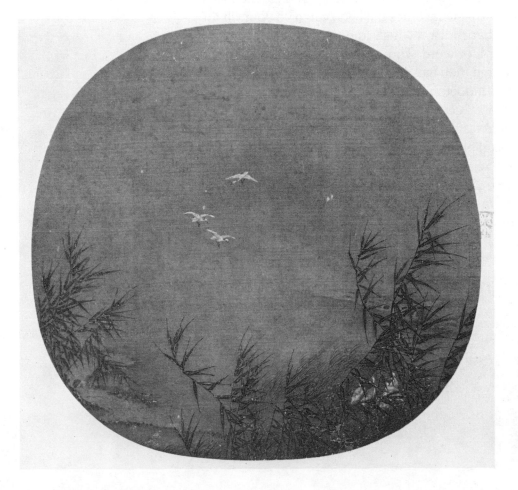

Most people are frequently distracted by thoughts that suddenly cross their mind, just as birds fly across the sky.

Chinese. Landscape with Egrets. *Sung Dynasty (960–1279). Ink, light color on silk. 9¹⁵/₁₆ × 10⁵/₁₆". The Metropolitan Museum of Art, New York. Fletcher Fund.*

Just as it is useful to know what muscle tension feels like in order to relax, it is also important to learn what a passive attitude is. An ancient yogic exercise called "counting breaths" teaches concentration and can help everyone understand how the mind works. When you count breaths you quickly realize that thoughts constantly enter your mind one after another and that you have little control over the occurrence or nature of those thoughts. We all have had similar experiences when we tried to solve a problem, only to find our minds constantly wandering to other concerns.

To count breaths, sit in a comfortable position and concentrate on your breathing. Simply count "one" on inhale and "two" on exhale. When extraneous thoughts come to mind, and you lose track of counting, simply return to the count. Most people find that their counting is frequently interrupted, often with thoughts of how poorly they're doing or errands they have to do.

The most popular current technique for teaching relaxation is *autosuggestion*, which generally can be taught in a short time. Usually the teacher recites the directions slowly while those learning do the exercise. After they know it, they can give themselves the instructions mentally. In doing the exercise below, for example, you can have someone read you the exercise slowly, or you can tape record the exercise and play it back or simply read the exercise over several times until you can give yourself the instructions mentally. The basic idea is what's important, so the exercise needn't be memorized word for word. Those who are unfamiliar with this kind of exercise may find that they feel a little awkward at first and wonder if anything is happening. But doctors can measure actual muscle relaxation and other physical changes even if you yourself don't notice anything. Each time you do the exercises, you will become more aware of the subtle feelings of deepening relaxation.

Here is an example of a relaxation exercise that uses autosuggestion: Find a tranquil place where you won't be disturbed. Lie down with your legs uncrossed and your arms at your sides. Close your eyes; inhale slowly and deeply. Pause a moment. Then exhale slowly and completely. Allow your abdomen to rise and fall as you breathe. Do this several times. You

When to do a brief relaxation exercise

During stressful times in the household (before dinner, before bed)

After stressful times (after the kids go to school, after a family fight)

During planned rest times (coffee break, lunch hour)

More often during high-stress periods

More often when you feel as if you might be getting sick

now feel calm, comfortable, and more relaxed. As you relax, your breathing will become slow and even. Mentally say to yourself, "My feet are relaxing. They are becoming more and more relaxed. My feet feel heavy." Rest for a moment. Repeat the same suggestions for your ankles. Rest again. In the same way, relax your lower legs, then your thighs, pausing to feel the sensations of relaxation in your muscles. Relax your pelvis. Rest. Relax your abdomen. Rest. Relax the muscles of your back. Rest. Relax your chest. Rest. Relax your fingers. Relax your hands. Rest. Relax your forearms, your upper arms, your shoulders. Rest. Relax your neck. Rest. Relax your jaw, allowing it to drop. Relax your tongue. Relax your cheeks. Relax your eyes. Rest. Relax your forehead and the top of your head. Now just rest and allow your whole body to relax.

You are in a calm, relaxed state of being. You can *deepen* this state by counting backward. Breathe in; as you exhale slowly, say to yourself, "Ten. I am feeling very relaxed. . . ." Inhale again, and as you exhale, repeat mentally, "Nine. I am feeling more relaxed. . . ." Breathe. "Eight. I am feeling even more relaxed. . . ." Seven. "Deeper and more relaxed. . . ." Six. "Even more. . . ." Five (pause). Four (pause). Three (pause). Two (pause). One (pause). Zero (pause).

You are now at a deeper and more relaxed level of awareness, a level at which your body feels healthy, your mind feels peaceful and open. (It is a level at which you can experience images in your mind more clearly and vividly than ever before.) You can stay in this relaxed state as long as you like. To return to your ordinary consciousness, mentally say, "I am now going to move. When I count to three, I will raise my left hand and stretch my fingers. I will then feel relaxed, happy, and strong, ready to continue my everyday activities."

Each time you relax, by any method, you will find it easier and relax more deeply. The sensation of relaxation may be experienced as tingling, radiating, or pulsing. You may feel warmth or coolness, heaviness or a floating sensation. When you have practiced a method of relaxation several times, you may be able to relax deeply just by breathing in and out and allowing yourself to let go.

Visualization

Relaxing and concentrating on mental images is now an important technique in medicine. This process is called *visualization*. Through visualization people can get in touch with inner feelings, envision goals for the future, and make changes in their lives to harmonize with their feelings and accomplish their goals. Actually people visualize all the time without even realizing it. They picture things in their mind's eye, see events from the past, envision plans for the day, picture the solutions to problems they are working on in art, science, and everyday life. Although most people visualize constantly, they don't make conscious use of this skill.

A brief relaxation exercise

Whenever you feel tense, take several slow, deep breaths, let your whole body be still, and sink into the feelings of relaxation.

When people visualize peaceful scenes, they heighten feelings of relaxation.

Hokusai, Katsushika. Waterfall of Amida. *18th–19th cent. Print. 14½ × 10″. The Metropolitan Museum of Art, New York.*

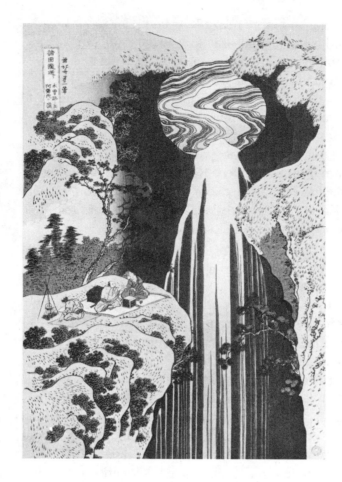

Daubigny, Charles-François. The Farm. *19th cent. Oil on canvas. 20¼ × 32″. Chester Dale Collection, 1962, National Gallery of Art, Washington.*

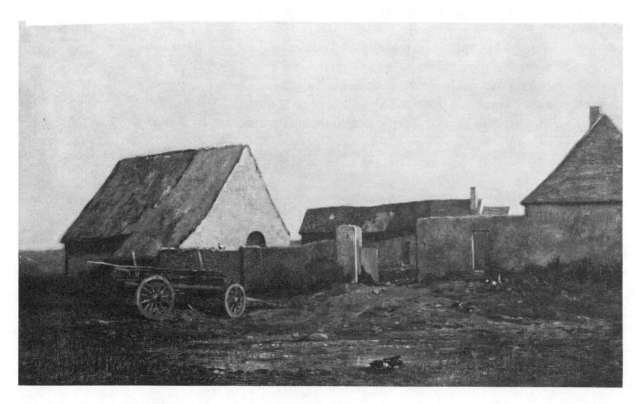

Potentially, visualization is one of the most useful tools we have to improve our lives. With practice, visualization becomes even more powerful. Age-old visualization techniques in religion and medicine are being discovered anew and adapted to many fields. Meditation helps people relax and clear their minds; visualization allows them to use this clear mental space to learn more about themselves and improve their lives.

The visualization state is actually an extension of the relaxation state. In a sense, they are inseparable because when people are letting themselves relax, they are probably picturing letting go with some kind of relaxed image. When people imagine lying in a meadow, their bodies relax. When people relax and picture an image in their mind, they can feel the image with all their senses.

Scientists have found that the same nerve and muscle pathways that are involved in a *real* action are also involved when a person *pictures* that activity in their mind. The more vividly people can picture a situation in their imagination, the more their body reacts as if it's actually happening.

Researchers have now recorded changes in almost every physiological system in response to visualization. When people picture a delicious meal, they actually begin to produce saliva. When they picture running for a train, their heartbeat and respiration rise dramatically and small electrical impulses are detectable in their running muscles. When they picture themselves in a peaceful scene such as lying on the beach, when they feel the warm sand and sun, hear the waves, and smell the salt, all the physiologic results of relaxation are heightened considerably. Heart rate, breathing rate, oxygen consumption and muscle tension drop as much as 25 percent.[32]

Doctors studying *autogenic therapy*, a German medical technique involving visualization, have demonstrated other physiological changes in response to imagery. An interesting finding in autogenic research is that any area of the body that people pictured as warm went up in temperature and blood flow. When people "in passive concentration" repeated to themselves, "My right arm is heavy" and "My right hand is warm," a large group of changes took place. An interesting one was the change in Galvanic Skin Response (GSR), the factor measured in lie detector tests. GSR is known to be an accurate reflection of sympathetic nervous system activity. GSR rises when a person is worried, aroused, alert, emotional, or under any stress. GSR drops dramatically when people picture a peaceful scene. Anyone who can learn to visualize a peaceful scene has a powerful tool for reducing stress and preventing illness.

Visualization techniques

We think visualization techniques fall into two basic categories—receptive and programmed. *Receptive visualization* involves clearing the mind and then letting images arise spontaneously. It provides access to inner feelings

Some physiological changes measured during autogenic training

Heart rate drops.

Blood pressure drops in hypertensives.

EKG changes in heart patients.

Skin temperature increases.

Breathing rate decreases in asthmatics.

Stomach contractions improve.

Intestinal filling and movement improve.

Insulin requirement decreases in diabetics.

Labor is shorter in childbirth.

and ideas. It is one of the fundamental tools used in all forms of psychiatry, and it can be used to get in touch with feelings about parenting. *Programmed visualization* involves choosing and holding images, rather than just letting them arise. Concentrating on particular images has specific effects on people's mental and physical states and on their lives. Thus programmed visualization is useful in achieving goals and making changes.

We will give instructions for both programmed and receptive visualization. The instructions are simple and easy to follow and your ability to perform them will improve with repetition. Before doing the exercises, you should be familiar with the relaxation exercise just described. In fact, we suggest that you do the entire relaxation exercise as a preface to both visualization exercises. As you become accomplished at relaxation, you will find that the abdominal breathing will be enough.

Here is a receptive visualization for getting in touch with feelings: find a quiet space where you will be undisturbed, a place where you feel at ease. Make yourself comfortable. Let your eyes close. Breathe in and out deeply, allowing your abdomen to rise and fall. As your breathing becomes slow and even, you will feel relaxed. Imagine the relaxation in your whole body deepening by stages. You are now in a state in which your mind is clear and tranquil. You can visualize vividly and easily. Your mind is open and receptive. Imagine your mind is like a screen and you can see images relating to your feelings about being a parent. You can look at these images as long as you wish. Some images will make you feel good, some images will make you feel uncomfortable. Simply note the images; do not dwell on the emotions. Each time you visualize in this way,

How to use receptive visualization to get in touch with inner feelings

Visualize how you'd like to spend your time at work, at home.

Visualize how you'd like family relationships to be—how you'd like your children and mate to treat you, how you'd like to treat them.

Visualize what would be the most pleasurable family vacation or weekend you can imagine.

Visualize things you could do to improve problem areas in your personal life, your family life.

Visualize what situations make you or your family members sick, healthy.

the images will be clearer and flow more easily. To return to your ordinary state, count slowly from one to three, and gently move some part of your body. Allow yourself to return slowly, and open your eyes when you feel ready to do so. You will now feel rested, calm, and ready to evaluate and interpret the images that have come into your mind.

Here is a programmed visualization exercise: find a place that will be undisturbed, a place where you feel at ease. Make yourself comfortable. Let your eyes close. Breathe in and out deeply, allowing your abdomen to rise and fall. As your breathing becomes slow and even, you will feel relaxed. Imagine the relaxation in your whole body deepening by stages. You are now in a state in which your mind is clear and tranquil. You can visualize vividly and easily. Imagine your mind is like a screen and you can see any image you choose. The image may be something you have seen, something you have imagined, something you would like to happen. Scan the image with your mind's eye and notice small details. The more closely you look at the image, the clearer and more vivid the details will become. When you visualize a scene, imagine you are really there. *Look* at your surroundings, *listen* to the noises, *smell* the air, *feel* the breeze. Be there. Enjoy all the sensations of the positive visualization you are holding. Experience your visualization as long as you wish. To return to your ordinary state count slowly from one to three, and gently move some part of your body. Allow yourself to return slowly, and open your eyes when you feel ready to do so. You will now feel rested and calm. You will be able to return to the positive image you held more and more readily each time you visualize it.

People invariably end such an exercise with a sense of well-being and energy. Many find that the visualizations that they "program" in advance eventually do come about.

Visualize yourself in loving scenes with your family.

Visualize yourself and family members enjoying and doing well at things that are important to you, to them.

Visualize yourself and family members as strong and healthy.

Ways of dealing with children's behavior to relieve family stress

One of the most important stress-producers for parents is their child's behavior at times. Parents become upset and anxious if they feel that their child is behaving in an "unsociable" way. A child may be excessively wild, noisy, stubborn, or withdrawn. If this happens only in isolated instances, most parents have no trouble dealing with it and do not consider it a problem. If such behavior happens frequently, parents may come to label the behavior as problematic and wonder if they are handling the situation in the best or most effective way. At this point parents would normally look to friends and relatives for guidance. With our highly mobile society and the dissolution of the extended family, this becomes harder and harder to do. Often, parents themselves have had little previous experience with young children (either younger siblings, nieces or nephews, or friends' children), so they have very little firsthand knowledge of how to deal with such problems. The result is that parents tend to do what *their* parents did. For adults who have mixed feelings about their own parents, this leads to increased stress and anxiety.

Unfortunately, most doctors have not been trained to deal with behavioral problems. But forward-thinking pediatricians are now coming to recognize that such problems are a larger concern for most parents than colds, and can cause stress and thereby result in physical illness. Tension is not necessarily limited to a particular parent or child, but can affect all members of the family. The new family-practice model maintains that all members of the family are tied together and react both individually and collectively to stressful family situations. A specific crisis will cause a physical or mental illness in one member that in turn will be "communicated" to the other members, each of whom will react individually in either a healthful or nonhealthful way, depending upon the personalities of particular members and their relationships with one another.

To stop such a cycle of stress, discomfort, and illness, physicians are advising families to change behavior patterns that lead to these situations. There are three basic tools that doctors use. First, they recommend that parents read popular books like the Gesell Institute's *Child Behavior* in order to become better acquainted with normal child behavior at different ages. Then parents can be more reasonable and more confident in their responses to their children. For example, in *Child Behavior*, Dr. Frances Ilg and Louise Ames describe a seven-year-old as "morose, mopey, and moody." At seven a child is "more likely to complain than rejoice" and "tends to feel that 'Nobody loves me.'" Ilg and Ames end by saying that the seven-year-old's "good days will steadily increase in number as he gets older." The book is based on observation of a very large number of children and can be extremely reassuring to parents during their child's moody stage. If parents know that sevens tend to mope and complain, they are able to help the child at this stage rather than to become angry, frustrated, and guilty.

The second thing that progressive doctors recommend is that parents make specific changes in their own actions in order to bring about positive changes in their child's behavior. Dr. R. W. Chamberlain says that the "common denominator of all these approaches appears to be helping the individual identify his frequently occurring behaviors that set the general tone of the relationship in question, and helping him become aware of the typical situations that call these behaviors forth."[33] Once parents have identified and spotlighted specific problem situations they can often figure out how to change or even avoid the situation until they or the child can cope with it better.

Chamberlain says that parents and children sometimes develop vicious

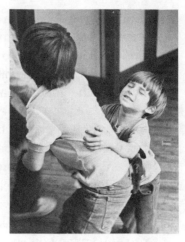

Sibling rivalry and fighting are a cause of stress and illness in many families.

Typical ages, stages, and growth rhythms

The Gesell Institute suggests that common rhythms occur in growing up; periods of equilibrium alternate with disequilibrium.

3 years	Loves to conform, share, is cooperative and easygoing
	Is secure, likes people, loves language
	Is positive, at equilibrium, good company
3½ years	Insecure, in disequilibrium, uncoordinated
	May fall, tremble, stutter, get cross-eyed, bite nails, cry, whine, become jealous
4 years	"Out of bounds," hits, breaks things, is profane, angry, defiant, boastful
	Imaginative, brashly confident
5 years	"Delightful equilibrium," reliable, stable, well-adjusted, secure
	Likes to stay at home with mother
6 years	Tumultuous, emotional, negative, cannot accept criticism, has vigor and energy; is ready for anything, is worst with mother, is rigid, wants own way
7 years	Withdrawn, complains, retreats, morose, mopey, moody, frowns
	Likes to be alone, likes to watch others, likes television
	Likes to touch and explore, demands much of self
	Feels persecuted and that people are "unfair"
8 years	"Meets the world," can accept failure, expansive and speedy, busy and active, sensitive, wants relationships
9 years	Independent, likes friends more than family, perfects skills, takes failure hard
	Worries, complains, has many physical complaints when work has to be done
	May rebel
10 years	Obeys, is pleased with parents and world, friendly, flexible, at equilibrium

Adapted from the Gesell Institute's *Child Behavior* by Frances Ilg and Louise Bates Ames (New York: Harper & Brothers, 1955).

circles of behavior that can be identified and interrupted. He identifies two basic kinds of vicious circles. In one, the parent gives out increasing punishment to try to eliminate unwanted behaviors and the child increasingly resists. In the other, the parent is overprotective or overpermissive with the child and comes to allow the child to make increasing demands in regard to structuring a problematic situation. An example of the punishment-resisting circle would be a child refusing to eat the right kinds of foods and then either being spanked, ignored, or made to sit at the table for long periods. The problem can be alleviated by having the mother recognize the circle, lessen her food demands, *consistently* deal with aggressive behavior by putting the child in his room, and spend more time with the child in pleasurable situations.

There are many other examples of parent-altered behavior in stressful situations in the popular parenting literature. Not only can these books help parents with so-called behavior problems, they will also contribute to improving the family's overall health. *Parent Effectiveness Training* by Thomas Gordon[34] suggests that parents communicate their *feelings* to children rather than order the children around or let the children do whatever they want. Gordon's method consists of *active listening,* and *"I" statements* to the child. In active listening the parent listens attentively to the child's problem and responds in a way that will help the child get insight into the problem. The parent might say, "It sounds as if you feel that . . ." "I" statements communicate the parent's own feelings, rather than assign blame. A mother might say, "I'm unhappy when the house is messy," rather than "You always leave everything in a mess!" Gordon also suggests making changes in routines so that it will be easier for children to behave well—giving them something to do while waiting for an appointment, scheduling meals when they are usually hungry. All parents naturally do these things sometimes, but many do not do them in an organized way. Too often when parents themselves feel depressed or under stress, they respond to a situation too quickly with too little concern for the child's feelings. If parents can add some new responses to their repertoire, they can use them in stressful times and eliminate potential fights before they arise.

Child development researchers have identified a number of times and places that cause strife in many families. Parents most frequently complain about mornings before school, the time before dinner, bedtime, shopping, car travel, and eating out. The more parents can do to anticipate these occasions and take steps to deal with them, the less stress they will have in their lives. For example, if a child always has problems getting off to school without whining or crying, the parents may try waking the child earlier so there is time to talk and play as well as get ready for school.

The third way that doctors are attempting to help parents reduce the stress of child rearing is by using behavior therapy. The basic premise of behavior therapy is that behavior is *learned;* that is, when people do something that is followed by something they enjoy, they'll do it again,

Identify your own problem times

Do you regularly feel tension, have crying times, or yell in your house . . .

When getting up

At breakfast

Before school

After school

Before dinner

During dinner

Before bed

Shopping

At friends' houses

Before babysitting

While traveling

Eating out?

and, conversely, if they don't enjoy what happens after an act, they won't repeat it. Historically, this premise is based on Pavlov's work with animals, in which he found that dogs who were fed when a bell was rung eventually would start to salivate at the sound of the bell even if there was no food. The animals learned to associate a set of events with a particular stimulus, and always reacted in the same way to that stimulus.

All parents naturally use reward and punishment to affect their children's behavior. Technically, rewards are called *positive reinforcers.* They include such things as food, warmth, attention, praise, money, and treats like candy or toys. Psychologists call punishments *negative reinforcers.* Criticism, ignoring, making fun of, and spanking are all negative reinforcers. Doctors are now trying to teach parents to be behavior therapists for their own children. The goal is to make the positive and negative reinforcers used by parents function to benefit the parents and the children.

Maxine Schoggen[35] did a remarkable study of 9,000 parent-child interactions in which the parents wanted the children to behave in a certain way. A very high number of times the parents' reactions to the children's behavior were neutral rather than positive or negative; they rarely rewarded *or* punished the child for complying or noncomplying with their wishes. If parents want their children to obey them, they need to make their wishes better known and to respond more clearly to the children's behavior with either a positive or negative response.

Doctors have suggested that in problematic times parents must look to their own behavior to see how they are inadvertently stimulating and/or reinforcing their child's undesirable behavior. First the parents are told to identify the *specific* problem behavior to which they objected. Then the parents are instructed to totally ignore the behavior (if it is not too dangerous or disruptive) and to respond approvingly to other behavior. Initial experiments by Robert G. Wahler[36] showed sudden dramatic improvement in the child's behavior when mothers followed these instructions in an experimental setting. But if ignoring the child's behavior doesn't work, another technique, called "time out," can be applied: the parents send the children to their room for five minutes with the instruction not to come out until they can refrain from the objectionable behavior.

A third behaviorist technique involves having parents keep a careful record of both good and problematic behavior. Good behavior earns points or stars, while bad behavior is just noted or given a minus. A chart is kept in a highly visible place so that the children, as well as the parents, are aware of how things are going. Children may simply accumulate points or stars, or they may work toward a larger goal such as a visit to the zoo after earning a certain number of stars. Similarly, too many objectionable-behavior-points might result in loss of privileges—loss of allowance or suspension of television for a time. What is important is that the children clearly understand the rules in advance and know what behavior is objectionable and what is not, as well as what the rewards and punishments will be.

Classroom styles and stress

Young children's families make up by far the largest part of their world. But as they grow older they begin to spend more time away from their own family. They begin attending school for longer and longer times and they spend more and more time in the company of their peers. This time outside the home comes to have profound effects on their image of themselves and ultimately on their health. Just as demands and interactions between people can produce learning or stress in the home, so can they produce these effects in the classroom. The same sociological dimensions that are used to describe family personalities can also be used to describe classrooms. Classrooms that have high involvement, that foster personal relationships between students and between student and teacher, and that have great teacher support of the students, tend to foster high student satisfaction and a low absence rate due to illness. Classrooms that are competitive and intellectually challenging may teach a child more, but foster more stress and a higher illness-absence rate if there is not a strong underlying sense of support.

Children tend to be more comfortable in classrooms that reflect their family style—that is, children from homes that place a high value on productivity and achievement are most likely to be comfortable in competitive, intellectually challenging classrooms, and children from families that have high personal involvement in relationships tend to do better in classrooms that foster strong support, friendship, and personal interactions. Not only children, but also parents can become aware of the tone of a particular classroom simply by spending some time in it. If parents feel their children are out of tune with the class they're in, they have several options. They can make their observation known to the teacher and also explain the situation to the children and give them as much support and encouragement as possible at home. Support can include helping the child with homework, taking a keen interest in the classroom, and making the children's outside activities as rewarding as possible. If a child shows signs of tremendous stress—either excessive anxiety about school or repeated illness that seems to correlate with times of high stress in the classroom—parents should consult with the school and consider moving the child to another class more in harmony with his or her personality. Teacher-student matching seems to be more important now than previously since there is such variation in teaching styles (as well as in family styles). Many schools offer parents some choice in classroom assignments. In such instances the ideal solution is to have parents consider their child's needs before he or she is assigned to a class. Particularly when a child's health is involved, most schools will make every effort to accommodate concerned parents who make their feelings known early.

Another cause of stress in the classroom is a child's maturational readiness for schoolwork in relation to peers. Whenever children move into a radically different situation—changing from nursery school to kindergarten, or from lower to middle school, or suddenly having longer hours or a much heavier load—they are likely to reflect these disruptions in their

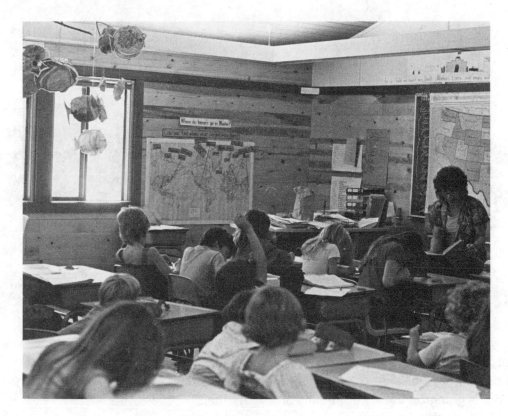

Children tend to have the least stress and be the most comfortable in classrooms that reflect their family style. Such low-stress situations result in fewer absences for illness during the school year.

bodies and their attitudes. It is somewhat akin to an adult switching jobs or being promoted to a more responsible position. Some children may greet the changes joyfully, others may find them difficult. Children who are under stress may be more tired, crankier, cry more easily, and be less interested than usual in their after-school activities. When the stress becomes acute, children may complain of nervous stomachaches, plead to be excused from going to school, and have lower resistance to all kinds of infectious diseases. Sometimes the cause of children's anxiety does not relate to the classroom itself, but only to a specific aspect of school: teasing on the bus, a bully in the playground, problems with lunch or toileting, or fear of testing. In such instances parents can help children by encouraging them to talk about the problem. Once that is defined, parents can work with children to figure out an effective solution. Solving such problems will often do more to prevent stomachaches and colds than a visit to the doctor.

Community styles and stress

The next level of interaction for children is with their community. Such community interaction is directed and moderated by the parents for many years. The more involved and comfortable parents feel in a community, the more community resources they will take advantage of, and the more

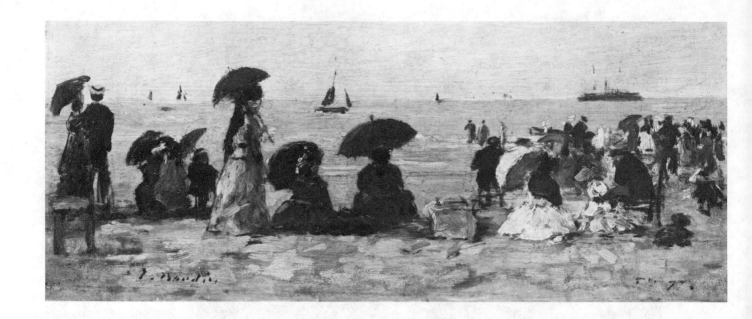

their children will directly and indirectly feel themselves a part of the community. The more people have a sense of belonging, the more they feel in harmony with what is going on in the community and with others' goals, the more defined and accepted their roles are in the community, the less stress they'll experience, and the healthier they will be.

A number of community variables are unavoidably stressful. Overcrowding, air pollution, noise, high crime, lack of personal safety, lack of beauty and human facilities, and impersonal spaces all increase stress. Many of these are characteristic of inner-city ghetto areas. And it is not surprising that these very areas have much higher rates of all illnesses and accidents. In fact, medical sociologists now speculate that these rates may be the result of stress rather than simply a result of poverty. While many families are not in a position to live wherever they choose, they can make efforts to create a harmonious existence in their community by establishing personal relationships with similar people; by creating a clear, orderly home; and by seeking out whatever positive resources the community does offer especially for children—parks, libraries, zoos, museums, and friendly local shops.

The more people feel in harmony with their community, the less stress they'll feel.

Boudin, Eugène. The Beach. 1877. Oil on wood. 4¼ × 10". Ailsa Mellon Bruce Collection, 1970, National Gallery of Art, Washington.

Bioprograms and the world

Beyond the community, every child has a sense of place or purpose in the world. In large part, the way children view the world reflects the way their parents see the world. Just as children's minds are affected by their family life and community, some scientists feel they are also affected by the past and the future. The past affects children and their families by contributing the coded message of human experience. Through evolutionary history, social patterns have been created that contribute to human learning, growth, happiness, and health; and to harmony with the environment. For example, when a baby is born and looks into its mother's eyes, a "bond" forms between the two that strongly fosters the mother's taking care of the baby and the baby's learning how to nurse. Later the baby forms an attachment to its mother that promotes maximum care and early learning. The traditional roles of mother caring for the child and father providing for the family are underlaid by a social structure which, through patterns of people, architecture, and family styles, supports the parents' roles.

Some scientists believe that the historical usefulness of these behavioral patterns has been retained by nature in the form of bioprograms in the brain's hypothalamus and limbic system. It has been found in animal studies that the more that bonding, attachment, parenting styles, and cultural density and structure are disturbed, the more stress the animals experience and the sicker they become.

People are aware of such bioprograms through intuitive feelings that are believed to originate in the right side of the brain, the right lobe of the cerebrum (see page 193). Some researchers are now theorizing that the cerebrum acts like a receiver, picking up thoughts from other areas of the brain and possibly even from outside the brain. They postulate that thoughts are like holograms—three-dimensional pictures created by light-wave interference patterns. Neural events that start nerves firing in the brain require so little energy that they can be triggered by wave force fields that are outside the body.[37] These fields are radiated by every person and even by the earth, sun, and stars.

Where cultures are disrupted, illness rates are high.

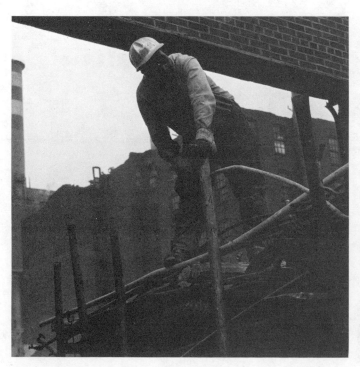

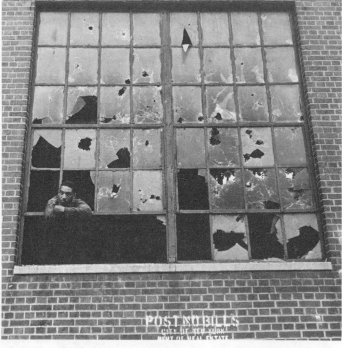

Physicists studying quantum mechanics have long known that at very high or low velocities time becomes distorted and, in a sense, almost stops. This is the basis of Einstein's relativity theory and nuclear physics in general. Many people have had the experience of "time slowing down" or seemingly stopping during thought. Parapsychologists have found that clairvoyance, telepathy, and psychokinesis experiments do not obey the laws of time and that psychics can sometimes read the past and the future. One popular theory for such altered states of consciousness is that they occur at the specific point during the body's vibrations when the body's energy wave changes direction.[38] At this point it is postulated that, in accordance with the laws of physics, the mind goes into a timeless space in which information (another form of energy) from past, present, or future can be received by the brain. Thus information about the future of man's evolution can be glimpsed in the right brain as intuitions or feelings.

Presently the culture and family are undergoing great change in Western society. People find themselves out of harmony with the three-million-year-old bioprograms from the hypothalamus. Almost everyone feels the stress of this disharmony. At the same time people feel impelled toward the future—the nature of which seems uncertain. Perhaps the only way to resolve the stress thus engendered is to look inward to catch an intuitive glimpse of the future. This does not necessarily mean "reading" the future so much as discovering harmonious patterns for the present.

Chapter 2

Nutrition

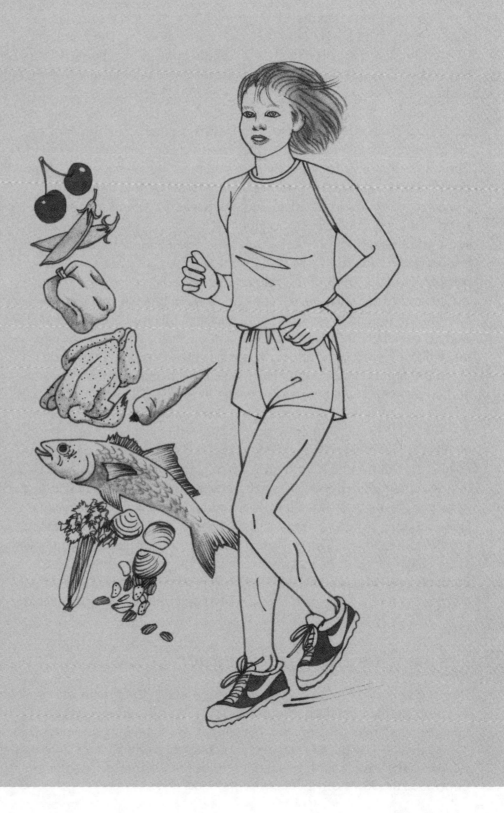

Food makes the body

People's bodies are composed of atoms, which in turn make up molecules. The area between the electrons and the nucleus of the atom is space that is pulsing with various energy fields—magnetic, electrical, gravitational. These units of energy and mass are organized into more and more complicated structures: first, simple molecules like water; next sugars; then complex proteins, fats, and carbohydrates. These building blocks are joined together in more exquisite forms of organization to make hormones, tissues, and organs. The organs are joined together to form our bodies.

The second law of thermodynamics states that all organized systems tend toward disorder over time. Our bodies maintain their remarkable order by continually taking in energy from outside themselves in the form of organized molecules from air, water, plants, and animals. The breakdown of these organized molecules releases their stored energy and provides molecules to maintain and create new structures in the body. Each and every molecule throughout the body is replaced continually—some within a matter of hours, some within days, some within years. Our bodies retain their form with the aid of a template, or program, held (probably) in the DNA of the cells and in our minds.

Our bodies are somewhat like a grid or mesh into which molecules are fitted for an indefinite period of time and then released and replaced. The body is excellent at this, and the fitting and releasing of the molecules takes place largely without our conscious control. In fact, if the body is given the approximate number of molecules it needs, it is highly flexible and creative and can generally maintain itself well. The part that we consciously play in all this is the selection of food and other substances that we invite or allow to enter our bodies. A thousand or even a hundred years ago our choices were limited, easy, and almost automatic. Essentially each culture had a food-growing or gathering pattern that had been handed down over generations. There were no man-made chemicals, and what people ate was based largely on intuition and what was available. Diets certainly weren't based on a scientific analysis of which substances produced health or disease. Today, however, there's almost an unlimited availability of foodstuffs that contain highly variable amounts of basic nutrients and other chemicals. There is rapid change in food substances themselves and a significant breakdown of old cultural patterns of eating.

The parent as the "gatekeeper"

Like the parents of a thousand years ago, present-day parents still provide the food for their children. But present-day parents must choose and analyze what their children eat. While no one will deny that nutrition affects health, few people can agree on what the correct diet is. Views now range from eating at least a minimum of basic nutrients to consuming enormous amounts of vitamins and proteins.

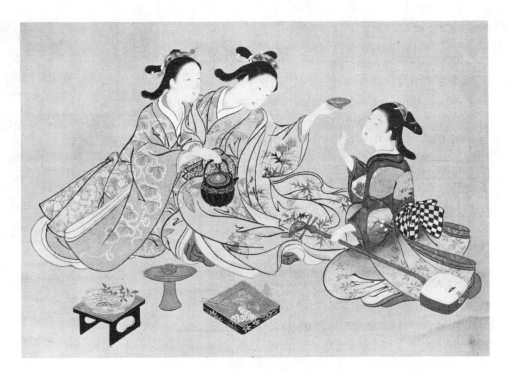

In the past, every culture had its own pattern of eating that was handed down from generation to generation.

Sukenobu. Three Girls Having Tea. *18th cent. Watercolor on silk. 21½ × 25". The Metropolitan Museum of Art, New York. Exchange, 1952, funds from various donors.*

Nutrition is the most controversial area of preventive medicine. Everyone would agree that children need basic daily amounts of proteins, carbohydrates, fats, vitamins, and minerals. Beyond that, there is almost no agreement and very few studies have been done with correct scientific methods. Even worse, there is tremendous emotionalism and fanaticism connected with each diet, and a most remarkable tendency for adherents of a particular diet to claim it can cure everything—all ills, depression, and misbehaviors.

One of the main theories of this book is that illness is caused by the combination of *many* factors in a person's life, and rarely by just *one* factor. This is especially true of a factor as general as nutrition. A person's food habits are irrevocably tied to his or her mental attitude, geographical location, upbringing, exercise, finances, and so on. Nutritional studies are just beginning to deal with these underlying factors, and they are finding that such factors can be just as important as what foods people actually eat.

Children's food patterns are basically established in their homes, at an early age. Although more and more men are sharing the household chores equally with their wives, it remains generally true that in most families the mother is the one who chooses the food. In nutritional terms, she is the *gatekeeper*. She decides what food will be in the house, shops, and prepares the food. There may be input from the father and the children (influenced by TV ads and the array of goodies at the local store), but the kitchen is generally the mother's province. And studies have shown that what the homemaker buys is dependent on her cultural background, educational level, attitude, and social class.[1] What children learn is a "good" diet is transmitted directly from their parents. And what children learn about food in early childhood generally determines their food habits throughout their lives. Much of children's attitudes toward food are already established by five years, but it is definitely possible to set up a new environment geared to health after a child has reached five.

Miriam A. Lowenberg, a respected nutritional researcher, gives these suggestions to parents: (1) The "gatekeeper" is in charge because she provides the food. It's difficult for children to eat too much of one thing if the mother doesn't buy it or if she buys it in strictly limited amounts. (2) Parents need to analyze their own food habits and decide which of them they want to pass on to their children. (3) If parents change their own undesirable eating patterns, their children will also. Changes should be introduced gradually, and in a stepwise fashion. If changes are too quick or too sweeping, parents are likely to encounter resistance and resentment from their child.[2]

Several studies have shown the importance of the mother's attitude toward the child's *actual* daily intake of vitamins and nutrients.[3] The more a mother knows about food values, the more likely she is to have a positive attitude toward meal planning and balancing. The more knowledgeable the mother is about nutrition, the greater the child's intake of calcium, iron, riboflavin, and ascorbic acid. The more permissive parents are about food, the less nutrients the children actually consume. When mothers regulate the children's food intake more, the children definitely consume more proteins, vitamins, and minerals.

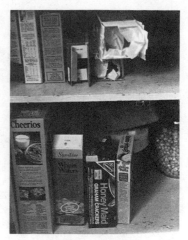

It's difficult for children to eat large quantities of nutritionally empty foods if such foods are not kept in the home.

Other influences on children's food habits

What conditions a child's food preferences besides the parents' habits and regulations? At present there are many influences in the outside world that predispose us toward a diet high in sugar, fats, and refined foods. School-age children are found to be enormously influenced by their friends and school heroes. Children are affected by what the other children are eating, by what they are served at friends' houses, and by the meals served at the school cafeteria (even if they bring their own lunch). School lunches, by law, have to supply one-third of the child's basic daily nutrients. But, at the same time, they rarely reflect what most nutritionists would call an optimum diet. Cost and convenience are often more important factors than nutrition. Finally, and perhaps most significant, is the subculture of hanging out at local candy stores, supermarkets, and liquor stores that sell junk food. Sometimes vending machines are even located within the school itself. Children are drawn into the habit of candy-store eating because of social needs as well as a valid need for food.

The second external factor that influences a child's nutritional habits is "eating out." Nowadays a significant amount of the average family's

What foods TV ads sell to children

Cereals (3 to 1 sugared)	25%
Candy and sweets	25%
Snacks	8%
Fast foods	10%
Miscellaneous foods	32%

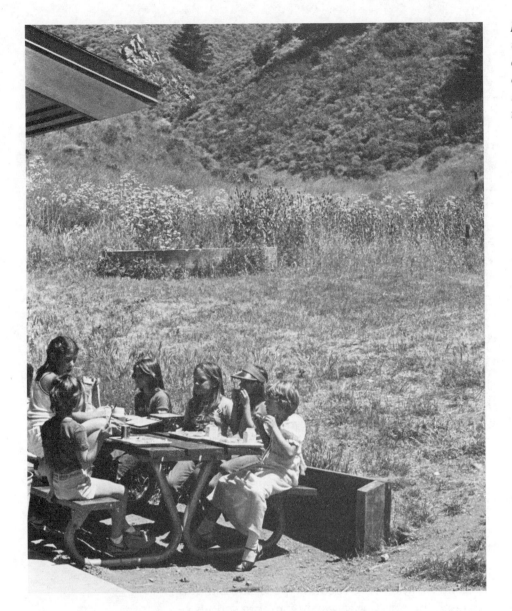

Parents need to be aware of what school lunches serve, and should recommend changes if the lunches are high in sugar, starch, or additives.

meals consist of eating food prepared outside the home. Eating out represents fun for the family and a respite for a tired homemaker. Much of the fare unfortunately consists of fast foods that are high in carbohydrates, animal fats, sugars, and salt. The family's pleasure in eating out definitely conditions children to food habits that probably don't exist in the home.

A third major factor that influences many children's food habits is television. It is estimated that the average child watches 25 hours of television a week—more than one full day. Fifteen percent of this time is filled with commercials, and, of this, 70 percent are commercials for foods: 2 hours and 45 minutes! Children begin watching television virtually before they can talk. It has been shown that pre-schoolers don't make any distinction between the commercials and the programs, and believe the commercials are "true." The commercials almost exclusively link goodness of a food to taste factors with words like "sweetness, chocolatey, and richness." [4]

Food values of some fast foods

Food	Calories	Protein (grams)	Carbo-hydrate (grams)	Fat (grams)	Sodium (milli-grams)
Recommended Daily Allowance, child 4–14 years	1300–2700	30–46	50–100	15–25	500
Big Mac	540	26	39	31	962
Kentucky Fried Chicken (original)	830	52	56	46	2285
Pizza Hut ½ of 10″ pie	560	31	68	18	—
Taco Bell taco	186	15	14	8	79
Burger King french fries	214	3	28	10	5
McDonald's chocolate shake	364	11	60	9	324

Nutrition and childhood illness

A major new concept in childhood nutrition is that the eating patterns children establish when they are young can contribute significantly to their illness patterns. Diet is related to two types of illness in children. The first type is illness that they contract as children, the second type is illness that they contract as adults. In general the adult diseases are far more serious, but the childhood illnesses, though not usually life threatening, should not be minimized. These concerns are so serious that the Surgeon General, the Department of Health and Human Services (formerly Health, Education and Welfare), and the U.S. Senate Select Committee on Nutrition, as well as the American Academy of Pediatrics, have all issued specific dietary guidelines that they believe can have a major impact on the health of the country.

The illnesses most immediately affecting ostensibly well-nourished children are obesity and dental caries. In this culture, 50 percent of all 3-year-olds already have tooth decay. By 12 years of age, the figure has risen to 90 percent! In fact, tooth decay is so common we tend to take it for granted. But, in tribal cultures that eat no sugar there is almost no tooth decay. There is nothing magic about this. When sugar was rationed in Norway during World War II the number of cavities dropped strikingly,

Preventing cavities

Avoid "sweet" tasting foods—sugar, honey, molasses, sweetened and dried fruits.

Forbid between-meal snacks sweetened with sugar.

Only allow sugar-sweetened food to be eaten after meals if at all, once or at most twice a day.

Substitute carbohydrates such as breads, corn, and so on for sugar-sweetened foods.

Encourage eating of raw fibrous vegetables and fruits that need chewing. These foods increase saliva flow and clean the teeth.

Use some form of internal fluoride (tablets or vitamins) until the child is 13 years old.

Use a fluoride oral rinse from 6 to 18 years (0.5 fluoride rinse).

Adapted from Nizel, A. E., "Preventing Dental Caries: The Nutritional Factors," *Pediatric Clinics of North America* 24:141 (1977).

then went back up after the war when rationing ended. In our society it is estimated that 75 percent of all cavities could be prevented.[5] The incidence of tooth decay, both on an individual and a group level, rises in direct proportion to the amount of sugar consumed.

In a long-term institutional study it was found that if sugar was eaten between meals, the number of cavities resulting was greater than if larger amounts of sugar were taken at meals. A healthy diet, high in calcium, protein, fluoride, and vitamins C, A, and D, also lowers cavities by strengthening the tooth enamel. Parents who tend to dismiss these facts casually would do well to consider the high cost of dental work in terms of time, money, and emotional stress.

Another result of childhood eating habits is obesity. In many Western countries childhood obesity is a significant problem. Approximately 10 percent of all children in the U.S. are considered medically obese. Eighty percent of obese children remain overweight as adults; 30 percent of overweight adults were obese as children. This pattern of obesity frequently begins at a very early age—half of all obese children were overweight before the age of six. Moreover, babies overweight at six months are ten pounds heavier on the average at the age of five.[6] This is not to say that all fat infants remain overweight, or that all heavy adults were overweight as children, but obesity in childhood should not be dismissed simply as a stage the child will grow out of eventually.

The causes of obesity are complex and not completely understood. At some point, obese people must take in more calories than they use. There are many theories as to why people do this—genetic, hormonal, and psychological. Certainly nutritional habits and availability of different foods play a major role. Obesity in early infancy has been linked to bottle-feed-

Dealing with childhood obesity

Make the child aware of his or her food intake.

Encourage the child's inner control and responsibility.

Rid the house of junk food.

Provide low calorie snacks such as carrots, celery, unbuttered popcorn.

Give small portions.

Limit second servings and desserts.

Encourage the child's own decision making.

Serve a balanced diet of healthy foods.

Encourage exercise (walks, hikes).

Encourage stair climbing and walking or biking.

Restrict television viewing, which is sedentary and exposes the child to many food commercials.

Involve the child in physical activities during the summer.

Sweet foods are the cause of obesity and dental caries.

Thiebaud, Wayne. Pie Counter. 1963. Oil on canvas. 30 × 36". Collection, Whitney Museum of American Art, New York. Larry Aldrich Foundation Fund. Photograph by Geoffrey Clements.

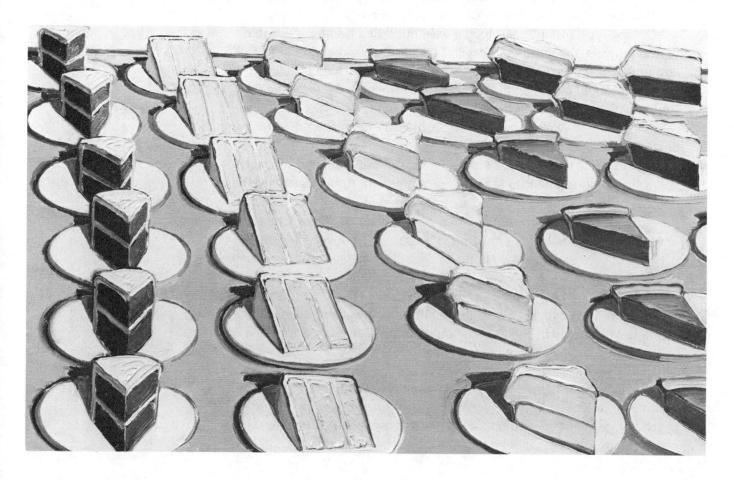

ing as opposed to breast-feeding, early feeding of solid foods, forcing a baby to finish a bottle or plate, and regular feeding of high-carbohydrate baby foods and desserts. Development of obesity in school-age children is linked to diets containing high amounts of starchy, fried foods, soda pop, and candy; high television viewing and lack of exercise; and stressful events such as moving, losing friends, or the mother starting work.

Obesity in school-age children has both physical and psychosocial problems associated with it. As researcher C. G. Neumann puts it: "It has been well-documented that these children have a poor self-image and express feelings of inferiority and rejection. They encounter teasing, ridicule, and are often left out of games, activities, and athletics, and thus become increasingly more inactive. In response they withdraw and indulge in antisocial behavior, and school performance may deteriorate. A vicious cycle is set into motion whereby the increasing frustration and isolation results in even greater withdrawal, and as a substitute for acceptance and activity, eating is resorted to for gratification and solace."[7]

In addition to psychosocial problems, obesity can cause problems with physical health. Actuarial statistics from major insurance companies show that adults who are overweight have significantly lower life expectancies than those with average weights. Adult obesity predisposes a person to heart disease, diabetes, arthritis, and gastrointestinal cancer. In view of this, most parents will want to make sure their children maintain a reasonable weight and, more than that, develop healthy eating habits. Attention to diet is especially important in families that have a tendency toward heaviness. Junk foods should be minimized or eliminated and sugar and starch intake drastically lowered. Such changes benefit *all* members of a family, not just those who are overweight.

How childhood nutrition affects adult illness

In a striking new trend, nutritionists and physicians are beginning to seriously consider the long-range health effects of eating certain kinds of foods. In the nineteenth century, nutrition was concerned with the results of gross deficiencies, such as severe lack of vitamin C causing scurvy. Now nutrition is concerned with how general patterns of eating are related to the kinds of illness that are currently prevalent. Unlike scurvy, today's major illnesses—heart disease, diabetes, arthritis, cancer—cannot be ascribed to a single cause. This makes it very difficult to accurately assess the importance of any one nutritional factor, because it is almost impossible to isolate one factor from the rest of a person's life.

The inability to separate nutritional habits from other life patterns has been the major stumbling block in nutritional research and has rightfully

Increased chance of death due to obesity in men 20% overweight

Cause of death	Percent increased risk of death
Heart disease	18–28%
Stroke	10–16%
Cancer	0–5%
Diabetes	100%
Digestive diseases	25–68%
All causes	20%

How mortality increases with increases in weight

Percent overweight	Percent increased risk of death
–20%	0–10%
–10%	–10–0%
10%	7–13%
20%	10–25%
30%	30–42%
40%	36–67%
50%	50–100%

cast doubt on the validity of many, if not all, nutritional studies. For example, researchers can study two groups of people, one group that eats a high-cholesterol-and-fat diet, and one that eats a low-cholesterol-and-fat diet. They may find that the high-cholesterol-and-fat group has much more heart disease than the other group. But the obvious conclusion is not valid unless the researchers have matched the group for other factors such as stress, genetic background, salt intake, smoking, exercise, and so on.

Virtually all nutritionists have their own *beliefs* about nutrition, but *facts* are relatively scarce. A striking example of this is provided by the 1979 Department of Health, Education and Welfare (HEW) study on nutritional recommendations for the United States. The American Academy of Nutrition met to review all the food research in relation to health. The fact that health planners ascribed such importance to nutrition was a holistic landmark. Unfortunately, the nutritionists could not reach a consensus based on the research at hand. A majority did agree on five general recommendations, although they admitted that only two were supported by evidence, and it was not conclusive. In fact, there were even studies that supported the opposite view.

The Academy's purpose was to assess the role of nutrition in relation to the major killers of our society, heart disease and cancer. The Academy recommended that people (1) *decrease cholesterol,* (2) *decrease saturated fats,* (3) *decrease refined and processed sugars,* (4) *increase vegetables, fruits, and grains,* (5) *decrease alcohol and eliminate smoking.* The Academy stated its recommendations as based on links and associations rather than on causes, and as applying to large populations rather than to any one individual.

The strongest evidence from studies indicates that high-fat, high-cholesterol diets are linked with atherosclerosis. Atherosclerosis is a disease in which fatty plaques build up in arteries causing high blood pressure and/or reducing blood flow. When blood flow is drastically reduced to the heart or brain, a heart attack or stroke occurs. During World War II in Western Europe, when intake of fats and cholesterol decreased drastically, heart attacks and strokes decreased proportionately. Groups with diets that happen to be low in fats and cholesterol—like the Mormons and the Maori Indians of the South Pacific—also show lower rates of atherosclerosis. In addition, studies indicate that if these same people adopt a more "Western" diet, their rates of all forms of heart disease go up. Research animals who are fed high cholesterol and fat also develop high blood levels of lipids and cholesterol, as well as plaques on artery walls. When people have a high blood level of lipids and cholesterol, they are more likely to have heart attacks. By changing their diet, they can lower their lipid and cholesterol levels dramatically. But despite all this evidence, there are also studies showing that certain groups of people, such as the Eskimo and Navaho Indians, have high-cholesterol diets and little or no heart disease. And there are many individuals with high-cholesterol-and-fat diets, and high blood levels, who never develop heart disease.

National health recommendations and diet goals

Eat only enough calories to meet body needs (fewer if overweight).

Eat less saturated fat and cholesterol.

Eat less salt.

Eat less sugar.

Eat more whole grains, cereals, fruits, and vegetables.

Eat more fish, poultry, beans, peas.

Eat less red meat.

Check to see what's in processed foods.

From the Surgeon General's Report *Healthy People*, 1980.

Studies such as these notwithstanding, the healthiest thing on a statistical basis is to lower the intake of fats and cholesterol. It is now believed by most nutritionists that if children are raised with such a diet they will decrease their chances of contracting heart disease both from lower levels of fat and cholesterol in the blood during childhood and from better life-long dietary habits.

Another example of how food can affect adult health is high blood pressure (hypertension) caused by a high intake of salt. Medical researchers now believe that 10 to 20 percent of all people are genetically susceptible to developing high blood pressure on a high-salt diet. These people retain more salt than necessary, which, in turn, causes them to retain more fluids, raising their blood pressure. There is no way to identify these genetically susceptible people until they develop the disease. But if they eat a low-salt diet they will never develop it. Compared to people of other cultures, Americans consume large amounts of salt. By the age of 18, 10 percent of the population already has high blood pressure. By decreasing the use of salt, parents can prevent children from developing high blood pressure when they are grown.

Other nutritional trends—special diets

In recent years a number of people interested in nutrition have suggested several highly specialized diets. The proponents of each particular diet tend to believe in it completely, basing their faith on personal experience and reports from patients rather than on studies. Each school of dietary thought has elaborate regimens for curing a wide variety of illnesses, and the books about these diets characteristically are written in an evangelical style. Almost all the special diets are based on the belief that *all* illness is caused by nutritional factors and that it can be cured by adherence to the diet.

This one-cause, one-disease model does not reflect current holistic thinking. Moreover, none of the diets is supported by hard research—that is, by controlled studies. Health professionals working with these diets impart their strong belief in their diet to their patients. The patients, in turn, must consciously choose to undertake the particular regimen and then work to follow it. In other words, the followers show real motivation and attention. In terms of attitudes as related to healing, it is no wonder that people often report good results from following the diet. Animal studies have shown that if the people feeding an animal believe they are feeding nutritious food, the animals are healthier than if the keepers believe the food is not nutritious. In order to prove whether the nutrient itself is causing the change, a controlled double-blind study must be conducted in which two groups, unbeknownst to all, are fed a diet with and without the nutrient. Up to now, none of the unusual diets has stood up to these rigorous tests.

Currently there are several popular special diets that involve either eating large amounts of or entirely avoiding particular kinds of food. These include no wheat, no homogenized milk, high amounts of meat and vegetables, and high amounts of vitamin C or E or magnesium.

Each of these diets is based on a theory. For example, the no-wheat diet holds that man has been a meat-eater for most of his existence on earth and has not truly evolved to eat grains. The basic theory behind the megavitamin diet is that people are presently in abnormal biochemical states due to poor nutrition and stress, and they need massive amounts of vitamins to counter these problems. Megavitamin advocates believe that taking high doses of various vitamins will cure behavior problems, anxiety, tension, schizophrenia, alcoholism, sexual dysfunctions, aging, and almost all physical illnesses.

The megavitamin school covers a broad range of regimens. Proponents vary as to which vitamins they prescribe and which foods they recommend. And another tenet of megavitamin theory is biochemical individuality, that is, that every person's body requires different amounts of each nutrient. Patients arrive at the correct dosage by taking larger and larger amounts until they feel best. Some of the vitamin doses suggested are so high that it is impossible to get the nutrients through natural sources. The classic examples of this are vitamin C and the B vitamin niacin. The suggested C-dose of 30,000 milligrams per day is the equivalent of 600 oranges and must be taken as powdered ascorbic acid. This is so much acid that it has to be taken in small amounts at least four times a day and may have to be buffered to prevent high stomach acidity. The suggested niacin dose of 3,000 to 5,000 milligrams per day can have significant side effects including nausea and flushing. To get this much niacin naturally would require eating up to 500 chicken breasts or up to 15 cups of fortified Torula yeast.

As of 1978 most major nutritional organizations were strongly against megavitamin therapy and warned of its dangers. They expressed concern that vitamins in these doses could be toxic, functioning more as drugs than food. For example, high doses of niacin result in skin reddening, itching, increased heart rate, low blood sugar, liver damage, and increased excretion of uric acid. Obviously niacin in such high doses changes the body's whole physiochemistry. The American Society of Clinical Nutrition, in its journal, also expressed concern that people taking megavitamins might tend to neglect their real food intake. And they point out that no combination of vitamins supplies all the nutrients contained in real food. The Society goes on to say that megavitamin therapy "is not a wise practice in terms of either nutrition or health."[8] The American Academy of Pediatrics' Committee on Nutrition also warns of the dangers of megavitamin therapy and says that "Megavitamin therapy is not justified on the basis of documented clinical results."[9] Many of the special diets such as the megavitamin are based on sound nutritional theories that have been taken to extremes. No nutritionist would question the need for vitamins; what is at question is the amount.

Toward an optimum diet

Since our bodies are made up of the molecules we eat, it is simply common sense to feed our bodies the "best" molecules we can. Our bodies have evolved through millions of years on planet Earth to efficiently make use of the foods nature provides. The body has complex and

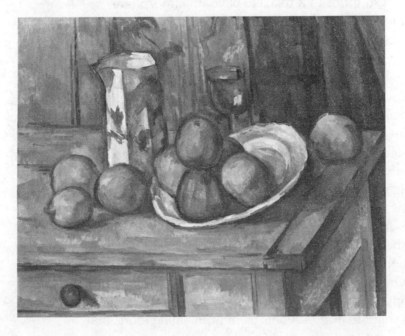

The basic rule for an optimum diet is to eat foods that are high in essential nutrients.

Cezanne, Paul. Still Life. c. 1900. Oil on canvas. 18 × 21⅝". National Gallery of Art, Washington. Gift of the W. Averell Harriman Foundation in memory of Marie N. Harriman.

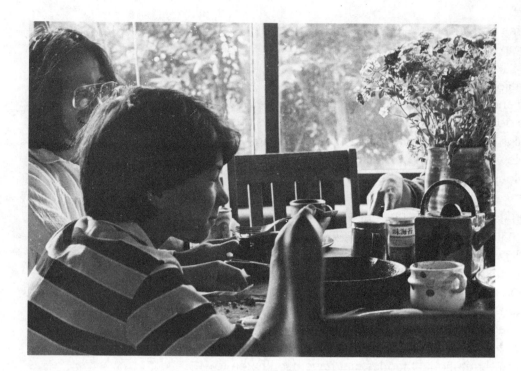

A relaxed mealtime, free of stress, fosters the maximum absorption of nutrients from food.

beautiful mechanisms for extracting all the necessary food value from the plants and animals around us. Rather than becoming trapped by the pros and cons of all the conflicting nutritional fads, each family needs to design a diet they feel good about and enjoy, that also meets reasonable nutritional requirements. History has shown that there are as many ways of getting a good diet as there are cultures and life-styles. The purpose of food should be to sustain us and keep us healthy, not to cure all problems. Children naturally learn to enjoy a healthy diet if they are served a wide variety of simple, fresh foods in a relaxed, pleasant atmosphere.

The majority of nutritionists and doctors currently recommend a number of general principles that are helpful in evaluating a family's diet. The basic rule is to eat foods that are high in such essential nutrients as proteins, carbohydrates, fats, vitamins, and minerals. This means eating fruits, vegetables, grains, dairy products, and meats. Nutritionists agree that an adequate diet *can* be designed without meat and meat products. The important point, for vegetarians and meat-eaters alike, is that they eat a balanced diet and a diet that is not high in nutritionally *empty foods*.

Quite simply, the major problem in most Western diets is that a large portion of many people's calories come from foods that do not contain many proteins, vitamins, or minerals. Such "antinutrients" actually *require* vitamins to metabolize, rather than provide them. In this way they undermine the body rather than build it up. Antinutrients basically fall into two groups—*very sweet foods* that contain sugar, honey, or syrups, and *highly refined foods*, which lose most of their nutritive value in processing. Every mouthful of empty food that children eat not only depletes nutrients, it fills up the children and prevents them from eating foods that will sustain them. If a third of children's diets are antinutrients—which is all too frequently the case in this country—they probably get only half the food value of a good diet. Even if they then take a daily vitamin or eat vitamin-enriched foods, they are still getting back only a few of the nutrients present in unprocessed foods. Processing of any kind not only lessens or removes essential vitamins, it also changes the texture and particle size of food. Highly processed foods, like many highly cooked foods, are virtually devoid of fiber, or roughage. Such roughage is an important aid to digestion and elimination and may play a role in preventing cancers of the gastrointestinal system.

A second general rule is to decrease fatty foods, especially saturated fats and high-cholesterol foods. Despite the debate over cholesterol and fat as a *cause* of heart disease and cancer, most nutritionists agree that it is a good idea to change our eating habits with regard to these foods. They recommend reducing the total amount of fat consumed from all sources. They especially suggest decreasing saturated fats, including animal fats, lard, hydrogenated oils, and olive oil.

A third basic rule is to avoid food colorings, artificial flavors, preservatives, and other chemicals, such as pesticides that are sprayed on foods. In general, the more chemicals a food contains, the more refined and nutritionally empty it is likely to be. Moreover, many of these chemicals are suspected of being, or have been proved to be, carcinogenic (see Chapter 3).

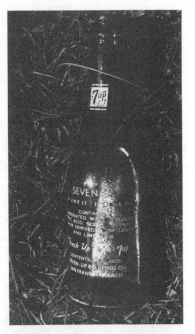
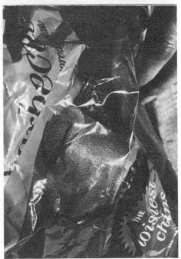

Many children overindulge in soft drinks and snack foods that are low in essential nutrients and high in sugar or salt.

Guide for reducing fat in your family's diet

Use low-fat milk instead of regular milk.

Use ice milk instead of ice cream.

Use uncreamed cottage cheese instead of creamed.

Use skim milk cheeses.

Trim fat from meat before cooking or eating.

Trim skin from poultry.

Avoid processed meats, luncheon meats, cold cuts, hot dogs, sausage, hamburger.

Use lean hamburger.

Substitute vegetable shortening and margarine for lard and butter.

Avoid saturated oils like olive oil.

Eat more fish and poultry, less red meat.

Safety of common food additives

Avoid

All artificial colorings.
Orange B (hot dogs)—causes cancer in animals.
Red #40 (soda, candy)—causes cancer in mice.
Red #3 (cherries, candy)—may cause cancer.

BHT (cereals, potato chips)—may cause cancer.

Saccharin (soda, diet foods, toothpaste)—causes cancer in animals.

Sodium nitrite (bacon, ham, luncheon meats)—can be chemically transformed into cancer-causing nitrosamines, especially in fried bacon.

Caution

Artificial flavoring (soda, candy, gum, breakfast cereals)—may cause hyperactivity in children.

BHA (cereals, chips)—needs testing.

Gums (ice cream, beverages)—poorly tested, probably safe.

Monosodium glutamate (soups, sauces, Chinese food)—damages brain cells in mice. Causes headache and burning in head, neck, and arms in some people.

Propyl gallate (soups)—poorly tested.

Sodium bisulfite (wine, grape juice, dried fruits)—destroys vitamin B-1. Probably safe.

Safe

Alginate—seaweed gel.
Alpha tocopherol—vitamin E.
Ascorbic acid—vitamin C.
Beta carotene—vitamin A.
Calcium propionate—preservative.
Calcium stearoyl lactylate—dough conditioner.
Carrageenen—seaweed thickener.
Citric acid—natural flavoring.
EDTA—impurity trapper.
Ferrous gluconate—iron.
Gelatin—animal thickener.
Glycerin—natural fat.

Lactic acid—natural acidifier.
Lecithin—natural thickener.
Polysorbate 60, 65, 80—synthetic emulsifier.
Sodium benzoate—preservative.
Potassium sorbate—natural preservative from berries.
Vanillin—synthetic flavoring.

Adapted from *Malignant Neglect* The Environmental Defense Fund by J. H. Highland and R. H. Boyle (New York: Knopf, 1979).

These simple guidelines seem like common sense and few people would disagree with them, but, paradoxically, their implementation requires major dietary changes for most Western families. A nutritionist has found that the average 6- or 8-year-old American child needs to change his or her diet in the following way to meet 1979 HEW guidelines: increase milk by 12 percent, decrease eggs by 12 percent, decrease meat by 22 percent, increase vegetables by 22 percent, increase citrus fruits by 23 percent, increase whole grains by 76 percent, increase whole-grain breads by 48 percent, decrease fats by 42 percent, and decrease sugar by 62 percent. Basically the average family needs to eat *more* fruits, vegetables, whole grains, poultry, and fish, and *less* red meats, oils, fats, eggs, sugar, and salt.[10]

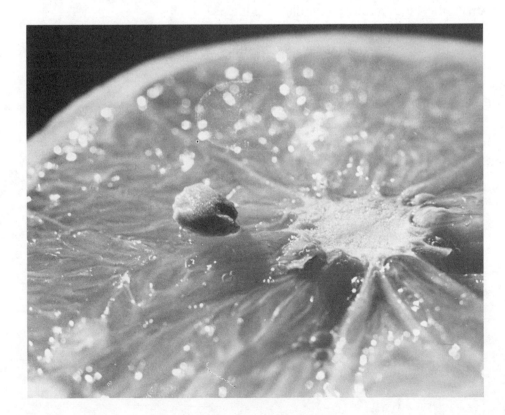

The U.S. Surgeon General's Report suggests that most Americans will be healthier if they eat more fruits, vegetables, and whole grains.

Guide for reducing salt in your family's diet

Use fresh foods, which have their own flavors.

Use herbs and spices for seasoning.

Avoid bacon, bologna, salami, corned beef, sausage, hot dogs, sardines, anchovies, lox.

Avoid sauerkraut and olives; they are prepared in brine.

Avoid snack foods like crackers, pretzels, potato chips.

Avoid soups, bouillon cubes, some peanut butters, catsup, chili sauce.

Avoid "onion salt" and "garlic salt."

Avoid salting foods while cooking.

Avoid salting foods at the table.

In addition to the nutrients children get, the social situation surrounding food consumption is very important. Studies show that children's emotional states can radically affect which nutrients are absorbed and how much of them. A famous nutritional study was done on children in two orphanages after World War II. Both orphanages had enriched diets; one orphanage had a stern matron, the other a warm, friendly one. It was found that the children with the friendly matron consistently grew much faster.[11] A more recent study done on American families found that "mealtime criticism about nonfood-related activities reduced the levels of food consumption and adversely affected intakes of vitamins A and C in 9- to 11-year-old children."[12] Our appetite is controlled by the hypothalamus, which is affected by stress. It is therefore not unreasonable to conclude that a relaxed mealtime, free of stress and confusion, will foster not only the ideal intake of nutrients, but the maximum absorption as well.

Chapter 3

Chemicals

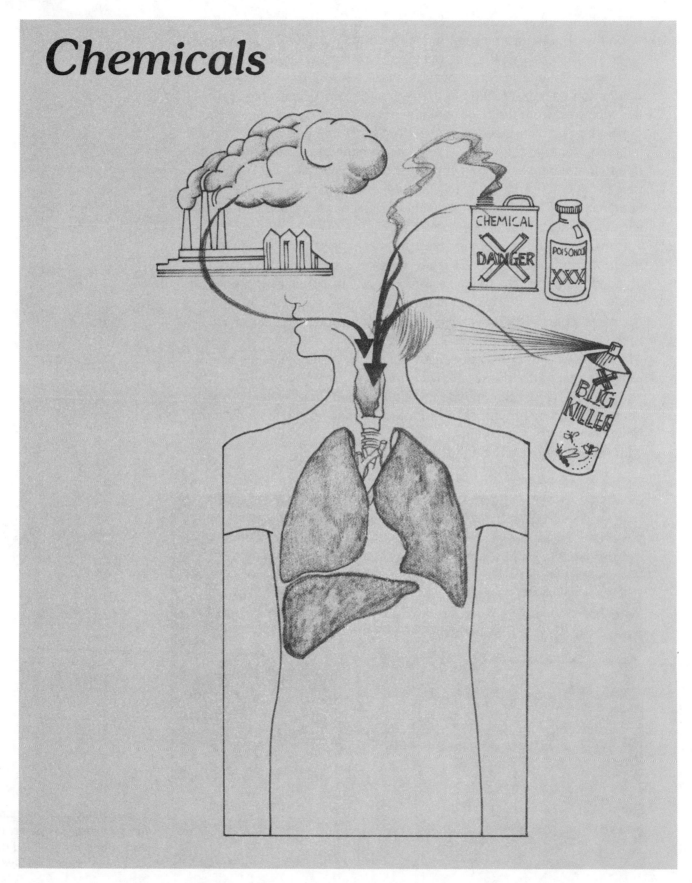

The chemical environment

All substances that children ingest or come into contact with have effects upon their bodies. Some substances are vital to growth and maintenance; some substances aren't useful, but aren't harmful; and some are actually harmful or potentially dangerous. Essentially we exist in a "soup" of matter and energy. We tend to think of our bodies as being discrete entities separated from the outside world and protected by our skin. In fact, our bodies are giant sieves that strain out some elements of the surrounding matter/energy soup and allow other elements to pass through. This dynamic straining or filtering effect proceeds at a micro level. We cannot perceive it at a normal sensory level; we can only visualize it with our imaginations. This picture is verified by scientific research carried out with extraordinarily powerful new tools.

Preventive medicine of the 1800s found dangers in the outside world in the form of microorganisms, such as tuberculosis and smallpox, that invaded the body. The identification of these small organisms cannot be made with the naked eye and only became possible with the invention of the microscope. New preventive medicine is focusing on things much, much smaller than microorganisms: It is focusing on the chemical environment. This is of utmost importance because in the last fifty years man has radically altered the chemical environment by creating a number of new compounds never seen in nature. Up until World War II, one million chemicals had been synthesized; since then an additional three million have been synthesized. Of these four million, around 50,000 are in use, with several thousand being used daily by many people.[1]

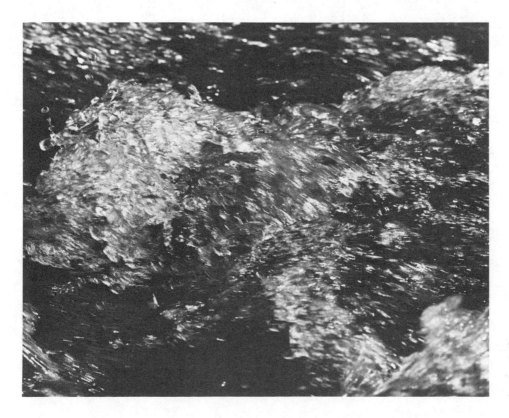

Scientists now believe that there is virtually no water on earth that is not polluted with some man-made chemical.

Due to the production, use, and disposal of chemicals, there are now hundreds of man-made chemicals that are widely dispersed in our air, water, and soil. There is virtually no living cell on earth, plant or animal, that does not have detectable levels of synthesized chemicals. Testing has only begun, but experts like John Higginson believe "there is probably no such thing as pure water or air, nor food composed only of harmless nutrients. There are few parts of the general environment where trace amounts of polycyclic aromatic hydrocarbons, nitrosamines or other toxic chemicals cannot be demonstrated with appropriate technology."[2]

Chemicals and cancer

Conservative, responsible researchers presently estimate that 60 to 90 percent of all cancers in man are related to environmental influences.[3] Most adults have been raised to believe that the cause of cancer is unknown, or genetic, or viral, or an effect of aging—that is, that nothing can be done to prevent it, and that medical research will eventually find a single "cure" for it. Although these assumptions about cancer causes are sometimes true, in the last ten years scientists have come to realize that most cancers are caused by exposure to chemicals in the environment. This idea is less than ten years old. It is almost totally accepted by researchers in cancer, but it is still known by very few lay people and voiced by too few doctors. Industries, and in particular chemical companies, have tended to suppress pertinent data and argue that just being *alive* makes one susceptible to cancer.

Cancer researchers now take an opposing view: They believe that there are, indeed, certain groups of chemicals that cause cancer and that the chances of getting cancer can be markedly reduced by lessening exposure to these chemicals.

The discovery that 60 to 90 percent of cancers are environmentally caused came from several lines of research. First, it has been known since the 1700s that coal tars caused scrotal cancer in chimney sweeps and snuff caused nasal cancer. In the 1800s, skin cancers were recorded among workers in the paraffin industry, and bladder cancer in the aniline dye industries. More recently it has been determined that several kinds of cancer are strongly associated with cigarette smoking, and other cancers are associated with industrial exposure to asbestos and vinyl chloride. Out of these observations came the first animal studies in which control groups were compared to groups that were deliberately exposed to suspected carcinogens. Since the 1940s, animal studies have shown that hundreds of chemicals, the majority of them man-made, consistently produce a variety of cancers.

Surprisingly enough, the major discovery linking cancer with environmental chemicals came from epidemiological studies, made possible by

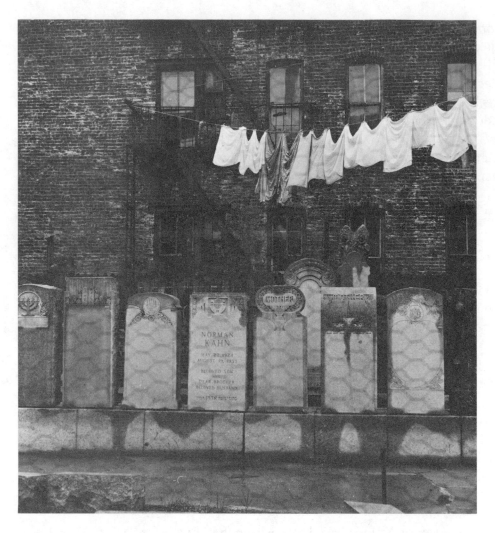

It is estimated that 60 to 90 percent of all cancers are caused by man-made chemicals.

the advent of computer technology in the 1970s. When large groups of people all over the world were studied, it was found that there is tremendous variation in the incidence of specific tumors in different populations. Worldwide, rates for specific cancers varied by a factor of three to several hundred. Within the U.S. alone, cancer rates for different populations varied by a factor of 8 to 40.

Scientists assumed that the lowest level recorded for any particular tumor was the result of spontaneous changes in cells, possibly caused by natural mutation. Any incidence above the baseline figures was assumed to be caused by environmental agents. This theory was substantiated by the finding that when a number of people moved from one area to another, their risk of cancer would change from the area of origin to the place where they moved.

Some of the chemicals that cause these differences in incidence have been specifically identified. The chemicals responsible for 30 to 40 percent of human cancers are now well known. The most important of these are tobacco products which cause lung cancers, high amounts of alcohol

The National Cancer Institute has put together its incidence data in the form of maps. These maps draw a striking picture of higher incidences of cancer in industrial areas.

Mortality of all kinds of cancer in white males, by county, 1950–1969 Age-adjusted rate

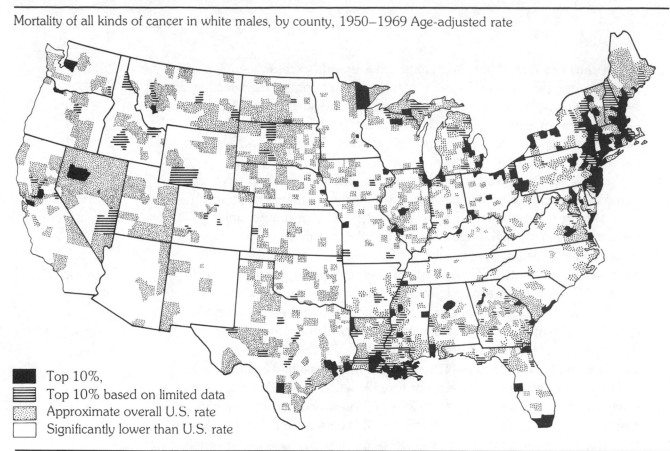

■ Top 10%,
≡ Top 10% based on limited data
∴ Approximate overall U.S. rate
□ Significantly lower than U.S. rate

Mortality of all kinds of cancer in white females, by county, 1950–1969 Age-adjusted rates

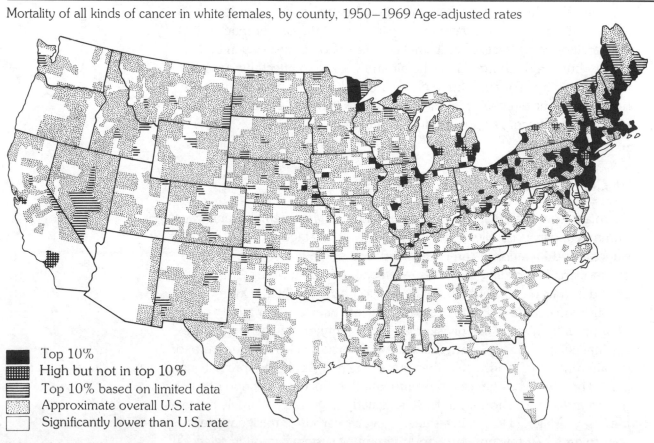

■ Top 10%
▦ High but not in top 10%
≡ Top 10% based on limited data
∴ Approximate overall U.S. rate
□ Significantly lower than U.S. rate

Adapted from Atlas of Cancer Mortality for U.S. Counties: 1950–1969, DHEW Publication #75–780.

which cause cancer of the esophagus and liver, and excessive sunlight which causes skin cancer. In some nonindustrial countries, high incidences of cancers were found to be due to natural carcinogens. For example, cancer of the mouth in Asia (which represents 35 percent of all Asian cancers, as opposed to 1 percent of all cancers in North America) is caused by chewing betel nuts with tobacco leaves and lime juice.

Recently the National Cancer Institute has put together its U.S. cancer death and incidence data in the form of state and county maps for each kind of tumor in men and women. These cancer maps draw a striking picture of distinctly higher cancer rates in industrial areas, particularly near petrochemical plants. Specifically, in areas where there are chemical-manufacturing plants, there are high incidences of lung, bladder, and liver cancers. Communities around petroleum industries have high incidences of lung, nasal, and skin cancers. Areas around furniture-making factories also show elevated rates of nasal cancer. The cancer death rates for the five highest states, all in the industrial Northeast, are 45 percent greater than the five lowest states, which are in the rural West and South.

The newly compiled cancer maps actually reflect the habit patterns and environmental exposure of people 20 to 40 years ago because cancers are generally very slow to develop. In the last 20 years there has been a very significant increase in cancer rates—10 percent in men and 20 percent in women. And these increases are not due to better diagnosis or longer life span. One of the most frightening implications of the cancer maps is that the carcinogenic effects of industrial chemicals do not just stay in the factory but are discharged into the air and water and affect the surrounding community. Today, a huge number of industrial chemicals enter our homes—either directly or indirectly. The effects of these chemicals will undoubtedly become apparent in the future.

How chemicals cause cancer

Scientists now have a fairly good idea of how environmental agents cause human cancer. Basically, it is thought to be a two-stage process. The first stage, called *initiation*, "can be effected by a single dose of the carcinogen," according to cancer researcher Elizabeth Miller. "[It] is considered to be completed rapidly and to be irreversible." During initiation the molecules within the exposed cell are altered. After a long period of apparently normal cell division, a tiny minority of the offspring of the original cell fail to mature due to some unknown block in their maturation or differentiation. These cells then live in the host as altered, premalignant cells. The second stage, called *promotion*, "occurs over a period of weeks and months, and is found, at least in its early stages, to be largely reversible," says Miller.[4] During this stage, a few cancerous or malignant cells start to grow. At this point the body's immune system can often select out these cells and render them harmless.

The chemicals responsible for the two stages aren't cancer-causing *until* the body breaks them down. These cancer-causing metabolites are deficient in electrons and they seek to bind with atoms that have easily shared electrons. DNA, RNA, and other proteins in the cell nucleus have within their structure nitrogen and oxygen atoms, which are "rich" in electrons. It is DNA that contains the code by which proteins are synthesized and cells are replicated. The code is in the form of a template that has four different bases. Each base is involved in manufacturing different amino acids. When a carcinogenic chemical binds with the DNA it actually alters the genetic program of the cell and produces a cell whose ability to replicate or differentiate is altered. This alteration is thought to be the basic mechanism that causes normal cells to become cancerous.

Remarkably, the body has special enzymes that cut out these altered base-groups, as well as other enzymes that can reinstate the correct groups and seal them off. This repair process probably involves an inborn homeostatic healing mechanism that prevents most abnormal cells from turning into tumors.

If this homeostatic process fails, the body's immune system provides a second line of defense. Lymphocytes recognize the altered proteins in the surface of tumor cells and move in to destroy them. Thus, when the body is functioning optimally, it can repair or eliminate tumor cells that are starting to form. When the body is under stress and its immune system is not functioning well, its ability to protect itself is lowered.

Carcinogens cause cancer by slipping into the DNA in the nucleus of a cell. This alters the genetic information and causes the cell to produce abnormal cells.

A personal cancer plan for families

What then can a family do to lessen the chances of any member developing cancer? Obviously, the healthier we are, the better our natural defenses can work. This means reducing stress and optimizing diet and exercise. At the same time, of course, we can lessen the work of the body by making every effort to reduce exposure to carcinogenic materials.

One of the foremost cancer researchers, Dr. John Higginson, director of the International Agency for Research on Cancer, has suggested that people develop a *personal cancer plan.* "Some degree of personal activity is not only possible but essential to produce any significant decrease in cancer incidence," says Higginson. "The development of a disciplined personal cancer plan, through modification of lifestyle, represents the individual's responsibility. If he does not do so, because of age or lack of will-power, he should at least insure that his children have the opportunity to do so. No one should rely on some future community action as an excuse for avoiding personal action now for himself or his family." Dr. Higginson goes on to say that "many neoplasms [cancers] will eventually be prevented. . . . In the immediate future, however, the greatest benefits will depend on personal action, whereby an individual controls his personal environment and that of his family." Some people will wonder why such

A personal cancer plan

Most important: Stop smoking (40% of all cancers).

Avoid heavy alcohol drinking (5% of all cancers).

Avoid heavy exposure to sunlight in summer.

Avoid X-rays.

Avoid animal fats and decrease red meats (carcinogens accumulate as you go up the food chain).

Wash fruits and vegetables before eating.

Avoid organ meats, especially liver.

Avoid foods high in preservatives, chemicals, or colorings, especially red dye #40 and saccharin.

Beware of your drinking water; use a filter if necessary.

If possible do not live near a chemical plant, refinery, asbestos plant, or waste-disposal site.

Educate yourself if you work with any chemicals.

Avoid pesticides and chemicals at home.

Avoid drugs if not absolutely necessary, especially Flagyl, Griseofulvin, Lindane (Kwell), and estrogen.

Avoid cosmetic products with warning labels.

Adapted from *The Politics of Cancer* by S. Epstein (Garden City, New York: Anchor Press/Doubleday, 1979).

information is not more widely disseminated by health professionals. Dr. Higginson suggests that "unfortunately, until now there is little evidence either in medical school, among doctors, or among public health workers, that they practice such control of their own lives and are therefore that much less capable of advising others."[5]

Working out a personal cancer plan involves gathering information, observing your own life, and setting up personal risk/benefit ratios. Above all, it involves reducing exposure to known carcinogens whenever possible. It must be kept in mind, however, that it is virtually impossible to eliminate exposure to all carcinogenic chemicals. On the one hand, many man-made chemicals, as we have said, have spread through the food chain and water cycles to come in contact with virtually every living cell. On the other hand, there are natural carcinogens like sunlight, cosmic rays, fungi, and nitrites that are part of our existence on earth. Man has coexisted with them for thousands of years. The point is not to become so depressed as to do nothing or so frightened as to become phobic. All this accomplishes, quite literally, is to lower the effectiveness of your immune system. Also, it's important to remember that exposure to chemicals does not cause cancer on a simple one-to-one basis. Only a small percentage of people exposed do eventually develop cancer.

But we must realize we can lower our risk of cancer by about 50 percent. Every time you eliminate a carcinogen from your life you are taking a positive step. Furthermore, many carcinogens interact with each other and *multiply,* rather than merely *add* to, the risks of exposure. For example, an asbestos worker who smokes has four times greater chance of developing lung cancer than a heavy smoker, and 35 times greater chance than an asbestos worker who does not smoke. Thus, when you avoid any one carcinogen, you may be avoiding multiplied synergistic effects with another carcinogen.

Statistical studies show that the effects of carcinogens are both time- and dose-dependent. That is, the *more* a person is exposed, and the *longer* a person is exposed, the greater his chances of developing cancer. Conversely, the more people can reduce or stop exposure, the less risk they run. This information becomes especially significant when one realizes that children are developing future lifelong habits and that the average child spends almost 20 years being exposed to family styles of chemical ingestion.

Although there is no universally agreed-upon personal cancer plan, several eminent researchers in the field have suggested guidelines. The most sweeping are described by Dr. Samuel S. Epstein, in an excellent, alarming book, *The Politics of Cancer.* Similar suggestions are outlined in the book *Malignant Neglect* by the Environmental Defense Fund. The major points they suggest are agreed upon by virtually all researchers studying carcinogenic hazards in environmental medicine.

Smoking and cancer

The most significant single act in a personal cancer plan is to stop smoking and educate your children about the real dangers of smoking. It is estimated that in men smoking accounts for nearly 40 percent of all cancers and 90 percent of lung cancer.[6] Cancer specialist Samuel S. Epstein says, "Smokers develop lung cancer at about thirty times the rate of non-smokers, and about one out of ten smokers of a pack or more a day will develop lung cancer. Smoking also increases risks of cancer of the larynx, esophagus, mouth, and bladder,"[7] as well as pancreas, kidney, and liver. And smoking greatly intensifies the effects of some carcinogens such as alcohol, asbestos, and other industrial chemicals.

There is no question that smoking during pregnancy causes low-birth-weight babies who are much more likely to die or have troubles at birth. Spontaneous abortion and prematurity rates are much greater among

Deaths from smoking

Kind of cancer	Deaths in 1974	Deaths due to smoking	Percent of deaths due to smoking
Lung	78,873	63,966	81%
Larynx	3,262	2,150	66%
Mouth	7,968	4,494	56%
Esophagus	6,652	3,998	60%
Bladder	9,397	2,819	30%
Pancreas	17,376	5,213	30%
Kidney	7,073	2,122	30%
Total	130,601	84,762	65%

smoking women, and these rates are proportional to how much the mother smokes. But the most alarming new evidence is that the carcinogens nicotine and benzo[a]pyrene cross the placenta and enter the fetus during developmental times that are particularly sensitive.

Smoking not only affects smokers, it also affects people around them. "Secondhand" or "sidestream" smoke has high concentrations of carbon monoxide, nitrogen oxides, tar, and nicotine. It is estimated that 10 percent of the population is actually allergic to cigarette smoke, and that they have increased rates of eye and throat irritation and respiratory illness. One study has shown that in a closed room or car, the burning of one pack of cigarettes results in nitrosamine carcinogen levels ten times higher than the inhaled smoke itself, and significant levels of tar and carbon monoxide. Just being in a room with smokers is the equivalent of smoking one cigarette in terms of carbon monoxide. Nonsmoking adults in smoky rooms have twice as much carbon monoxide in their blood as normal. That amount is sufficient to bring on chest pains in heart patients with angina. Such levels of carbon monoxide result in decreased vigilance, altered time discrimination and estimation, changes in perceptual ability, decreased visual acuity, decreased ability to do arithmetic and reading tasks, and changes in sleep patterns and irritability.

In spite of such information, cigarette sales increase 1 to 2 percent annually. During the years from 1964 to 1970, the Surgeon General presented public health messages about the dangers of smoking in rebuttal to cigarette advertisements on TV and radio. Cigarette smoking declined during this period. As of 1970, the tobacco industry switched all advertisements to newspapers and magazines where the rule of equal time does not exist. Since then cigarette smoking has again been on the increase. By far the greatest rise recently has been among teen-agers and preteens, especially girls. By 1977, 27 percent of all teenage girls and 25 percent of all preteen girls were smoking.

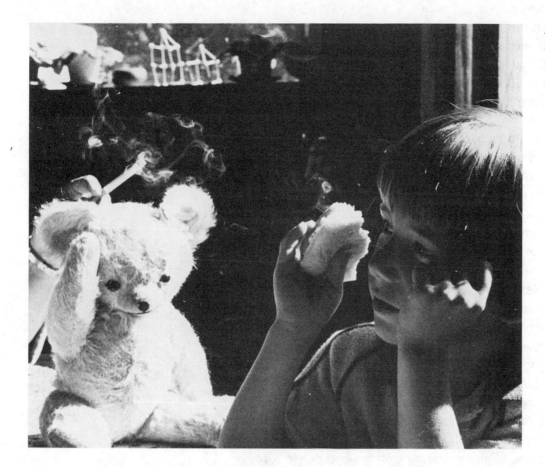

It is estimated that smoking accounts for 90 percent of all lung cancers and 40 percent of all other cancers.

Studies show that children of smokers are more likely to smoke. This is not surprising when one considers what significant role models parents are. Moreover, the antismoking announcements on TV show that education and public pressure against smoking can be effective. Of college graduates who smoked, half have quit. Obviously, the idea of reducing their chances of cancer by 40 percent was enough motivation to help them make the admittedly difficult choice to give up smoking.

Alcohol and cancer

Alcohol is not a primary carcinogen, but it has an important effect on increasing the cancer rate. As opposed to other chemicals, it is not clear how alcohol contributes to cancer development. Possibly it is other chemicals in alcoholic beverages. A variety of carcinogens such as nitrosamines, alkaloids, and asbestos are found in some alcoholic drinks. Heavy drinking in conjunction with smoking may account for 75 percent of cancers of the mouth and 5 percent of all other cancers. Heavy drinking alone, especially of hard liquor, increases the risk of cancer of the mouth, throat, esophagus, larynx, and liver. Cancer maps show that the highest incidence of esophageal cancer occurs in the Calvados brandy area of France.

Sunlight, radiation, and cancer

People are exposed to natural forms of radiation as well as to man-made forms such as X-rays. Sources of natural radiation include cosmic rays, naturally decaying radioactive substances, and even body constituents such as potassium that emit radiation normally. The average person receives 130 units (millirems) per year from such sources. The Environmental Protection Agency estimates that the average person also receives another 100 to 200 units from man-made sources, *largely* from medical X-rays, but also from radioactive medicines, "fallout" from nuclear tests in the atmosphere, and from the use of nuclear fuel.

All forms of radiation cause damage to the DNA in cells in proportion to the amount and length of exposure. There appears to be no threshold amount below which damage is not seen. Any amount of radiation will result in a certain number of malignant tumors per population per year. As with other chemical carcinogens, the results of radiation may not be apparent for decades. Natural background radiation plus man-made radiation is currently thought to be responsible for 2 to 3 percent of all cancers.

In the past, X-rays were used to *treat* as well as diagnose a number of conditions. These treatments involved much higher amounts of radiation than those used in diagnostic X-rays. For example, children were given X-ray treatments for enlargement of the thymus gland, which is a part of the lymph system. Children thus treated showed an increased likelihood of developing cancer of the thyroid gland. In addition to radiotherapy, atomic fallout in Japan and pelvimetry in pregnancy have been associated with increased cancer rates. Children whose mothers had pelvic X-rays while pregnant are one and one-half to two times more at risk of developing leukemia or some other malignancy by the age of sixteen. Fortunately, cancer in this age group is rare and the chances of any one child developing cancer following prenatal X-rays remains very low.

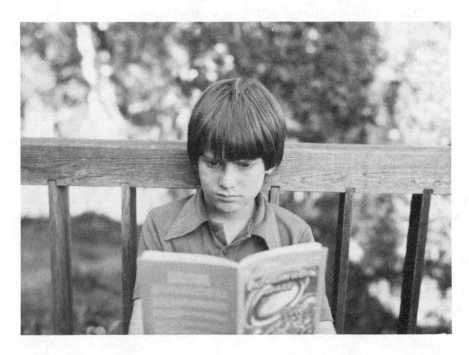

There are natural carcinogens like sunlight that are part of our existence on earth, but we can limit our exposure to them.

Because of the definite increase in the risk of cancer from all forms of radiation, many doctors, including Samuel S. Epstein, now advise people to "avoid unnecessary X-rays like the plague."[8] Some cancer researchers are much more adamant about this than the average doctor or dentist. They advise against all X-rays that are not absolutely necessary. This includes routine or repeat chest or full-mouth X-rays, routine mammography in women under 50, and chiropractic full-body X-rays.

The radiation in sunlight is the major cause of skin cancer and is related to increased occurrence of melanomas in melanoma-prone individuals. The incidence of skin cancer is much higher among light-skinned people who live in southern latitudes and among people who work out-of-doors. Because of this, cancer researchers advise against excessive exposure to tropical sun and against sunburning.

Diet and cancer

The relationship between diet and cancer is by no means fully agreed upon or clearly understood by nutrition and cancer experts. But numerous carcinogens are undoubtedly in the foods we eat. The question is not whether they will cause cancer, but rather, how many cancers they will cause.

Scientists now postulate that diet affects cancer in several ways: First, many foods contain carcinogens; second, different foods can change intestinal bacteria, which in turn metabolize some foods into carcinogens; third, diet can change people's immune capability and thus their response to the development of new tumor cells.

In addition to specific carcinogens in food, there is evidence that obesity, overeating, and high meat and fat consumption are associated with higher incidences of many tumors, including breast and colon. Both meat and plant fats seem to promote the growth of tumors by themselves. Moreover, any carcinogens consumed by animals tend to accumulate in their fat in high amounts. At this point most meat from animals is contaminated with hormones and antibiotics given to the animals themselves, and with pesticides and fungicides contained in their feed.

Because of the ways carcinogens are distributed in foods—either intentionally or by accident—cancer researchers are making new suggestions about what constitutes a healthy diet. They recommend a decrease in red meats and animal fats and an increase in whole grains, fresh fruits, and vegetables. (Interestingly enough, these first recommendations of cancer researchers closely parallel those suggestions made by general nutritionists to prevent other illnesses such as heart disease and obesity.) Cancer specialists also suggest avoiding organ meats because they concentrate feed additives. They recommend thoroughly washing fruits and vegetables —some even suggest using soap. Range-fed animal meat generally has

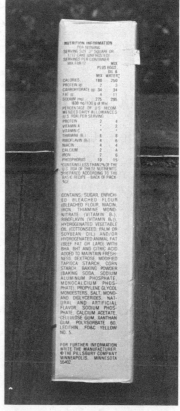

Many preservatives and food additives have been shown to cause cancer in laboratory animals.

fewer carcinogens than feedlot meat, and deep-water ocean fish are less contaminated than fresh-water fish. Cancer experts also recommend avoiding junk foods and highly processed foods that are high in preservatives, colorings, and additives. At this point a number of carcinogens, generally weaker ones, are still being legally used in food. Possibly the most widespread are Red Dye #40 and saccharin. In a 1979 report from the U.S. Academy of Science it was noted that "saccharin ingestion presents a predicted cancer risk to humans."[9]

In one year the average American eats nine pounds of chemical additives. According to the Food and Drug Administration (FDA), some children eat as much as a quarter of a pound of coal tar dyes each year. By the time a child is 12, he or she will have eaten between 1 and 3 pounds of coal tar dyes. At the current consumption rate, a child will consume a third of a pound of Red Dye #40 in his or her lifetime. In 1976, 7 million pounds of saccharin were used in foods—three-quarters of it in diet sodas. Most was eaten by teen-agers. One hundred quadrillion molecules (10^{17}) of acrylenitrile, a carcinogenic plastic, found their way into each bottle of Coca-Cola from early types of plastic.

These facts are very depressing. A family's best defense is to become conscientious label readers and learn to buy foods that contain a minimum of additives. These changes are especially important for nursing mothers because these same carcinogens become concentrated in the fat

Drinking water and cancer

Presently there are literally hundreds of carcinogens in the drinking water of almost every city in the country. This is not surprising when one considers that the water comes from rivers or wells that are heavily polluted by improper chemical disposal. Since the quality of bottled water varies spectacularly, a number of cancer researchers suggest installing a household activated-charcoal filtering system.

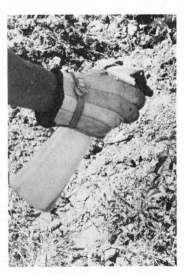

Industrial chemicals and cancer

This category includes carcinogens that are airborne, waterborne, or improperly disposed of. Not only are chemical workers themselves at greater risk, so are their families and even people who live in the vicinity of these plants. The Environmental Protection Agency (EPA) is researching one area after another in regard to the health of citizens living near chemical manufacturing plants or disposal sites. Samuel S. Epstein says, "If you can possibly avoid it, do not live close to a chemical plant, refinery, asbestos plant, or metal mining, processing or smelting plant, or hazardous

A number of paint removers, solvents, and pesticides used around the home contain known cancer-causing agents.

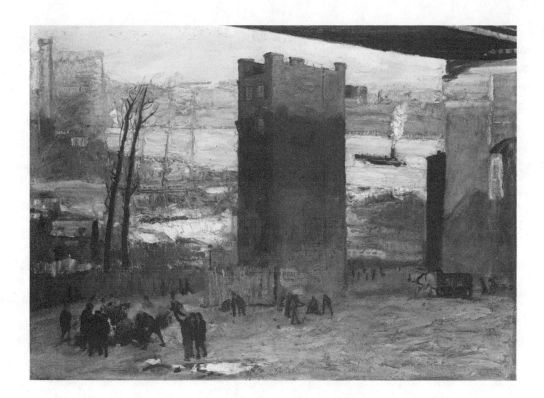

Air pollution from industry and automobiles is a serious problem that causes illness and makes all lung diseases worse.

Bellows, George. The Lone Tenement. *19th–20th cent. Oil on canvas. 36⅛ × 48⅛". National Gallery of Art, Washington. Gift of Chester Dale, 1962.*

waste disposal site, even if claimed to be well managed."[10] He also advises against living near major highways because of the air pollutants produced by cars.

Consumer products and cancer

Many of the products people confidently buy for home use are proven carcinogens. These include many pesticides, cleaning agents, paints, home building materials, cosmetics, drugs, and even chemically treated clothing. Fifteen percent of the total U.S. pesticide sales are to homeowners to kill bugs, weeds, and rodents in and out of the house. Some of these are such potent carcinogens that they are banned from industrial use. The National Academy of Sciences states that the U.S. citizen encounters the highest concentration of pesticides on his own lawn and around his house. "Suburban lawns and gardens receive the heaviest application of pesticides including dieldrin of any land areas in the U.S."[11] Studies have shown that animals absorb pesticides merely by lying on treated ground. Consider what this means for children playing in the grass.

This brings up the point that dangerous chemicals can be absorbed through the skin as well as inhaled or ingested in food or water. For example, studies in the mid-seventies showed that children wearing nightwear treated with the flame-retardant Tris had measurable levels of Tris metabolites in their urine.

Cancer-causing chemicals commonly found in the home

Aerosols, pesticides (chlordane, heptachlor)

Cleaning agents and paint solvents (carbon tetrachloride, benzene)

Paints, welding gases, sawdust (use masks when doing hobby or art projects).

Protecting the family from carcinogenic consumer products involves ridding the house of known carcinogens wherever possible. When carcinogenic products cannot be avoided, proper safety procedures such as using respirators and gloves and allowing adequate ventilation become of utmost importance. Children should never be allowed to help in the use of these chemicals.

Chapter 4

Exercise

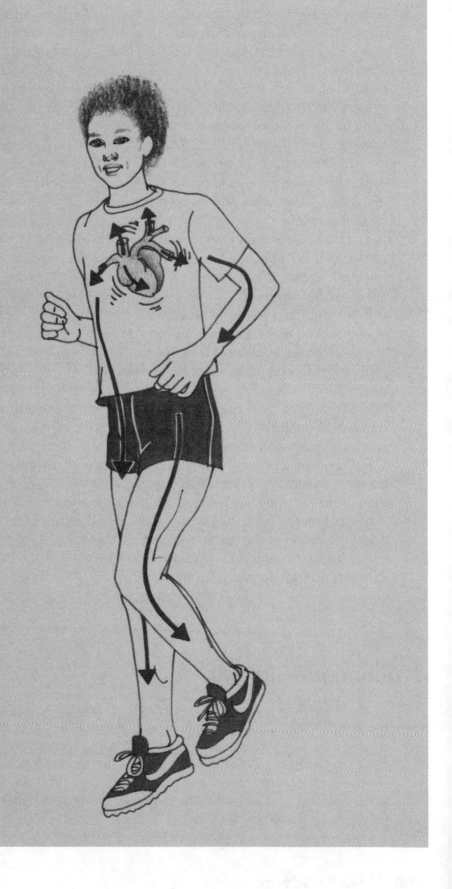

Energy is movement

Living is inextricably bound up with the health and functioning of our bodies. Death itself is defined as the cessation of cellular metabolism. The mind—that is, our consciousness—is associated with the brain, which in turn is connected through the nervous system to all the cells in our body. For all practical, if not philosophical, purposes, mind and body must be thought of as parts of one whole. One way to describe their relationship is to say that mind and body reflect each other: Every thought held in the mind is reflected by changes in the body, such as slight muscle tension; likewise, every movement in the body is registered in the brain, in the form of nerve impulses. Some scientists feel that the mind has an image of the body that serves as a template for the body's growth, and, furthermore, that sensations from the body affect the thoughts that go to make up that template.

The body is constant energy, change, and movement of physical substances. When energy is applied to the body in particular patterns, we call this *exercise*. When exercise is balanced, physical and mental health are most likely to result.

If the preceding sounds a bit abstract, it is meant to be, for the mind/ body problem is not the kind of issue that can be definitively resolved by scientists or philosophers. The confusion about mind and body has a profound effect on people's attitudes toward their bodies and on doctors' methods of healing. Entire healing systems in both traditional Western and holistic medicine have been based on underlying theories that mind and body are separate and that one or the other is primal and can be the only source of effective healing.

Rather than espouse the view that the mind is all there is and the body is only a dream, *or* the view that atoms and molecules are all there is and there is no separate mind or soul, we see body and mind as one whole. What that means from the point of view of health is that just as thoughts affect the health of the body, the health of the body affects one's frame of mind; positive thoughts produce a healing physiology; and balanced exercise produces an even state of mind.

Training physiology

Exercise involves contracting and relaxing muscles in a regular pattern. All muscles have the ability to contract and relax to a certain extent. The degree to which a muscle can contract (its *strength*), and the ability for it to relax (its *flexibility*), depend on how much that muscle is normally used. A muscle develops an appropriate muscle-fiber size and blood supply to accommodate its level of activity; the more activity, the larger fibers and more blood-borne oxygen it needs. If the increased activity is repeated on a regular basis, the muscle responds by increasing its size and circulation.

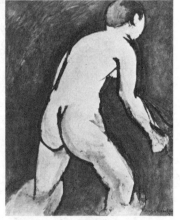

The healthy body is constant energy, change, and movement.

Matisse, Henri. Bather. 1909, summer. Oil on canvas. 36½ × 29⅛". Collection, The Museum of Modern Art, New York. Gift of Abby Aldrich Rockefeller.

If muscles are suddenly required to do much more than they are accustomed to, they simply cannot comply. But all muscles are capable of doing a *little* more than normal. If they are frequently required, over a period of time, to do a little extra, this increase will become the normal workload for that muscle, as the muscle's size and blood supply increase. Essentially this is what we call *athletic training.*

Serious athletes, after years of training, may reach the maximum muscle development achievable over time. It is not necessary for everyone to achieve maximum levels, but there are minimum levels below which health suffers and people are more likely to develop illness. Lack of exercise is probably not a sole cause of illness, but is certainly an important contributing factor.

Exercise physiologists have delineated a number of physiological processes that are enhanced by exercise. We've already mentioned increased blood supply and muscle-fiber size. The other changes can be divided into three categories: (1) changes within the muscle itself, (2) changes within the body's oxygen supply system, and (3) changes within the nervous system, which controls the muscle.

When a muscle contracts, two proteins within the muscle fibers slide past each other, causing it to shorten. This process requires energy. Energy is produced within the muscle cells when glucose combines with oxygen. Carbon dioxide and lactic acid are the waste products of this chemical reaction. As exercise continues the sympathetic nervous system sends messages to the arterioles—tiny arteries leading to the muscle fibers. This results in dilating, or widening, the arterioles and increasing the blood supply to the muscles in response to an oxygen need in the muscle cells. Meanwhile the veins in the muscle are squeezed by the muscular contraction, causing increased amounts of oxygen-poor blood to return to the heart. The heart pumps harder and faster in response to the increased volume of blood coming back to it. In turn, this increased pumping sends more blood to the lungs, where it takes up new oxygen in the alveoli and gives off carbon dioxide. To increase this oxygen supply, a person breathes deeper and faster. The maximum amount of oxygen a person can take in per minute under heavy work is called the *maximal aerobic power.* It is a key factor in determining the amount of muscle work someone can do in a prolonged situation.[1]

Maximal aerobic power is also the exercise factor most directly related to a person's health. In simple terms it represents how efficiently the heart, lungs, and blood vessels can work. The amazing thing about aerobic power is how profoundly it is influenced by exercise. With graduated exercise, the heart muscle itself becomes more powerful and thus works more efficiently; that is, a strong heart can pump more blood with each stroke or beat. So it beats fewer times a minute to do the same work. Over a lifetime this added efficiency is probably a major factor in preventing heart disease.

Initially, muscles have enough oxygen to contract for a short period.

Exercise and training—
Physiological changes

Heart volume increases.

Heart capillaries increase in number.

Blood volume increases.

Heart rate decreases.

Stroke volume of heart increases.

Oxygen uptake with work increases.

Strength of bones and ligaments increases.

Muscle size increases.

Capillaries in muscle increase.

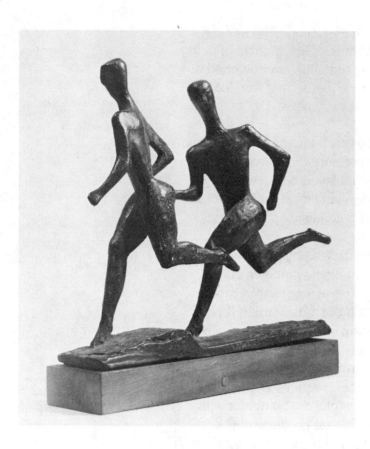

When muscles need to contract for several minutes, they need more oxygen from the heart and lungs. Thus aerobic power is increased only when strenuous exercise regularly lasts more than a few minutes and is gradually increased over time. In fact, leading exercise physiologists now say that in order for people to increase their aerobic power they have to engage in 12 to 20 minutes of exercise vigorous enough to raise their pulse to a sustained rate of approximately 150 beats per minute during the exercise.[2]

In addition to building up muscle and blood supply, training also helps to create learned pathways in the nervous system. These circuits play a part in developing agility, balance, coordination, and reaction time. These skills can only be learned and perfected with practice. They are important feedback circuits that help children move and orient themselves in space at all times, not just when they are exercising. Many of these learned neuromuscular acts are required for more complicated maneuvers. For example, balance precedes balance-while-running, which precedes catching-a-ball-while-running. Everyone is conscious of the amazing neuromuscular learning that takes place in babies between birth and two years. But this motor learning does not end with walking. It continues through the teen-age years of rapid growth and body changes, and can even be continued into adulthood. Such neuromuscular circuits are thought to be important for intellectual and emotional development as well.

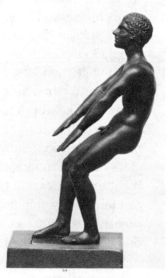

Training helps create learned neuromuscular circuits for agility, balance, and coordination.

Greek. Youth Finishing a Jump. 5th cent. B.C. Bronze. Height: 8⅛". The Metropolitan Museum of Art, New York. Rogers Fund, 1908.

How exercise affects growth

No one questions the necessity of good nutrition in relation to optimum growth, but few people realize how important exercise is to growth. In recent years many physiologists have come to believe that exercise plays a crucial role in stimulating and directing growth and development.

As children grow, their genetic potential is shaped by their environment. We've described how gradually increasing exercise causes growth of muscle tissue and blood vessels. So it is not surprising that during childhood, when growth is fairly continuous, regular exercise will maximize the genetic potential. All tissues of the body grow in proportion to the load put on them. Bones, for example, actually develop structural bracing lines as a result of forces continuously exerted on them. Current studies indicate that bone length and density, muscle size and strength, muscle flexibility (ability to stretch), leanness (muscle-to-fat ratio), and aerobic power all increase with exercise in childhood. This means that children who exercise regularly will be stronger, more flexible, thinner, have greater aerobic power, and have larger muscles and bones than similar children who do not exercise regularly.

Moreover, the Canadian exercise physiologist Dr. D. A. Bailey says that there are indications that these "functional changes are a result of training during youth persisting into the adult years."[3] One study compared two groups of men who both led sedentary adult lives. One group had been athletes as children, the other hadn't. The childhood athletes had an average of one-third better maximum aerobic power. Were both of these groups to undertake training as adults, the nonathletes could never catch up.[4]

In light of the lifelong benefits to be derived from regular exercise, it is astonishing to find that the physical fitness levels of most children are very low. A Canadian study by Bailey showed that "for the ordinary Canadian child (not the athlete or exceptionally skilled, but the ordinary boy), physical fitness as expressed by aerobic power factoring out size, seems to be a decreasing function of age from the time we put him behind a desk in our schools."[5] A similar statement could be made about the average American child. In countries where physical education is emphasized in the elementary schools, the opposite appears true.

Taking all the exercise data into consideration, UNESCO recommends that growing children receive between a third and a sixth of their total educational time in physical activity. Not only has it been demonstrated that exercise positively affects physical growth, but studies are showing that exercise also affects emotional and intellectual functioning and development. A remarkable study was undertaken in a primary school in Vanves, a suburb of Paris. The French Ministry of Education, in 1951, revised the schedule of several classes so that one-third of the students' time was devoted to physical education. As compared with carefully matched control classes following the regular schedule, the one-third P.E. classes showed striking differences. The Ministry's report stated that they had "better performances academically and less susceptibility to stress.

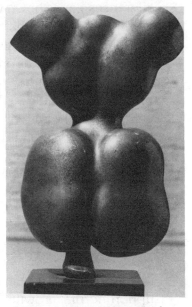

Exercise stimulates muscle growth.

Lachaise, Gaston. Torso. 1930. Bronze. 11½ × 7 × 2¼". Collection, Whitney Museum of American Art, New York. Purchase. Photograph by Geoffrey Clements.

Differences have shown up markedly in intellectual development. We would not conclude that those taking physical education are more intelligent, but the tools of intelligence are much keener. As the physical education pupils have fewer problems, their minds are more open, and they receive more from their teachers."[6] Additionally, P.E. pupils were found to mature more quickly, be more independent, be more social and less aggressive, have better motor development and balance, and better physical and mental health. This study certainly supports the concept that mind and body are part of a whole and that if one part is neglected, the development of the whole will suffer.

How exercise affects health

Not only is a "certain minimum of physical activity . . . necessary to support normal growth"[7] and intellectual development, but it is now strongly believed that "the importance of physical activity in terms of preventive medicine and positive health is clear," according to Dr. Bailey.[8] For many years doctors have *intuitively* believed that exercise was important in lowering the likelihood of all kinds of blood vessel disease, including heart attacks, strokes, angina, and hypertension. Physiologically, exercise requires a good blood supply to both the heart and skeletal muscles, so the connection between exercise and health seemed obvious.

A growing number of studies show that exercise does, indeed, prevent heart disease. The first of these studies was done in England twenty years ago by Dr. J. N. Morris. He found that men whose work was physically active had half the heart attacks of ones whose jobs were sedentary. In addition he found that the type of heart disease suffered by the active people was much less serious and they tended to recover much more quickly. The basic theory that emerged from this research was that exercise conveys a "protection" and, conversely, that inactivity makes people more prone to all the forms of blood vessel disease.

More recent studies have corroborated Morris's work. In 1977, Ralph Paffenbarger studied 17,000 college alumni and found that exercise protected them against heart disease even if they were subject to other high-risk factors such as smoking, high blood pressure, or a family history of heart disease.

Another famous research project called the Framingham study (1967) found that of 5,127 men and women in a Boston suburb, "the most sedentary were particularly liable to fatal heart attacks" and "those who were most sedentary had a five-fold greater mortality from coronary heart disease than those who . . . were presumably the most active."[9] People who had a history of high physical activity also tended to have lower weights, greater lung capacities, and slower pulse rates, indicating that exercise had radically altered their heart and lung physiology.

Exercise and health

Exercise helps prevent heart disease by building collateral vessels and by improving the condition of the heart muscle.

Exercise may lower blood pressure.

Exercise helps people control their weight.

Exercise tends to decrease depression and help people relax.

Exercise helps people with emphysema.

Exercise helps some diabetics reduce their need for insulin.

Animal studies have shed light on the mechanism by which exercise protects against heart disease. A classic study examined two groups of dogs: One group was run on a treadmill and the other had no exercise. On autopsy it was found that the dogs who exercised had developed more blood vessels to the heart. Doctors call such blood vessels "collaterals." As a result of exercise, collaterals are found to develop to both the heart and skeletal muscles. Such collaterals are of extreme importance because even if some blood vessels become blocked, as in the case of a heart attack, the collaterals will still carry blood to that area, thereby preventing the muscle cells from dying.

Other studies indicate that in addition to developing collaterals, exercise lowers blood pressure, modifies people's reactions to stress, lowers blood lipids (cholesterol), and tends to prevent obesity. By increasing stroke volume and thereby lowering heart rate, the whole cardiovascular system is made more efficient. This added capacity means that people in good cardiovascular condition are in much less danger of potentially overstressing themselves even when they are doing very strenuous work.

It is very difficult to isolate the effects of exercise from all the other factors in people's lives that affect their chances of heart disease. A number of other factors including stress, smoking, obesity, nutrition, genetic predisposition, and other illness (for example, emphysema or diabetes) play a part in the development of heart disease. It may be years before it is known exactly what role exercise plays in relation to these other factors, but currently it is believed to be vital enough to encourage everyone to increase his or her level of activity. This is especially important for children because they are still young enough to be able to radically alter their health and development for the better.

Parents are exercise models for their children

Children learn their basic exercise patterns primarily from their parents. Just as children learn lifelong food habits from their parents, they also learn and are conditioned to lifelong exercise habits. The culture that we live in has become basically a sedentary one. Most adults rely on cars, buses, and trains for transportation, they work at jobs requiring minimal physical activity, and few have active recreational pursuits. All too commonly, children are bused to and from school, spend hours sitting at desks, and go home to watch television, take music lessons, or study for several more hours. Even children who appear to be active may not be getting sufficient aerobic activity or good practice in motor-coordination skills.

Generally speaking, physically active parents have physically active children. This is probably due to children's desire to emulate their parents, as well as the parents channeling the children into such activities. Elementary school children love doing physical activities with their parents. They enjoy the attention, physical release, and time shared. This sharing forms a nonverbal bond and helps to promote other kinds of close ties. And for many children special instruction and encouragement are important when they are trying to master the skills required by a new sport. A child's memories of a parent who will play catch, hike, or shoot baskets will persist throughout a lifetime.

Beyond learning and doing the sport, shared exercise provides children with an unconscious picture of how adults spend their time. If the parents' activities are totally sedentary, the child will develop an inner model and will likely grow up pursuing basically nonathletic activities. If questioned, most inactive adults will realize that their own parents did not exercise regularly and generally preferred to read, listen to music, or putter around

Evaluate your home exercise habits

Do you run, walk, bike, swim? How many times per week?

Do you play racketball, handball, squash, basketball, tennis, and so on?

Do you take hikes or walks?

Do you garden or build?

Does your child do any of the above activities alone or with you?

Does your child play soccer, basketball, tennis, and so on?

Do you or your children watch TV on weekends and in the afternoon?

Do you read or do paperwork on weekends and evenings?

in the house. Too few parents realize that their exercise patterns affect not only their own health, but also directly and indirectly the health of their children.

Dr. Kenneth Cooper has written at length on how to exercise for aerobic capacity. He designed the fitness program used by both the American and Canadian armed forces. The program begins with a brief, accurate test to rate aerobic fitness. Cooper's test involves running and walking "as far as you comfortably can in 12 minutes. If you get winded, slow down a while until you get your breath back. Then run again for a stretch. The idea is to cover the greatest distance you can in those 12 minutes." [10] The results of this test correlate accurately with fitness levels based on oxygen consumption measured by sophisticated laboratory equipment.

Cooper has designed carefully graduated 10- to 16-week programs for all the common types of aerobic exercise. These include running, swimming, bicycling, walking, stationary running, handball, squash, and basketball. The basic training theory is to do a little more each week than your previous exercise level until you develop a reasonable level of fitness. Once attained, this level can be kept up by running 1.5 miles in under 12 minutes 4 times a week, by swimming 1,000 yards in under 25 minutes 4 times a week, bicycling 8 miles in under 30 minutes 4 times a week, or

Dr. Kenneth Cooper's fitness test

Cover the greatest distance you comfortably can in 12 minutes by running or walking. If you get winded, slow down till you catch your breath. (Dr. Cooper says if you're over 30 years old and presently get no exercise, start a limited exercise program before you attempt the test.)

Physical condition	Men under 30 (miles)	Men 30–39, and Women under 38 (miles)	Men 40–49, and Women 30–39 (miles)	Women 40–49 (miles)
Excellent	1.75+	1.65	1.55	1.45
Good	1.5–1.75	1.4–1.64	1.3–1.54	1.15–1.44
Fair	1.25–1.49	1.15–1.39	1.05–1.29	.95–1.14
Poor	1.00–1.24	.95–1.14	.89–1.04	.75–.94
Very poor	less than 1.00	less than .95	less than .85	less than .75

Exercise advice

Get in shape slowly, and train over a long period of time.

Do five minutes of warm-up exercises: stretches, sit-ups, walking in place.

Don't exhaust yourself: avoid extreme fatigue, trouble breathing, dizziness, or nausea.

Do five minutes of cool-down exercises when you finish: walking out and stretching exercises.

Exercise regularly, three to five times a week.

Amount of exercise needed to maintain good aerobic condition after you build up to fitness

Type of exercise	Frequency	Distance	Time
Walking	3 times per wk.	4 miles	48–58 min.
	5 times per wk.	3 miles	36–43 min.
Running	3 times per wk.	2 miles	13–16 min.
	5 times per wk.	1.5 miles	12–15 min.
Biking	3 times per wk.	8 miles	24–32 min.
	5 times per wk.	6 miles	18–24 min.
Swimming	3 times per wk.	1000 yards	16–25 min.
	4 times per wk.	800 yards	13–20 min.

walking 4 miles in less than an hour 4 times a week. Dr. Cooper advises everyone to progress slowly, to exercise at least 3 times a week (and *not* 7), to warm up for 5- to 8 minutes first, to cool down slowly for 5 minutes, and to avoid straining and pushing to fatigue.

Cooper has not yet published exact figures on the times and distances that are applicable for young children. But he suggests that the same kinds of aerobic exercises are good for kids. Like adults, children should build up gradually and should never exhaust themselves. For children under six, Cooper advises exercises designed for agility and coordination, rather than aerobics. He believes that children over ten can follow adult exercise schedules (see Aerobic exercise in Chapter 7). Aerobic conditioning in childhood is especially important because its effects will last a lifetime even if the child eventually leads a more sedentary life as an adult.

Exercise in the school

Schools can and should provide good physical exercise training for children. Elementary schools have widely differing physical education programs, many of which, unfortunately, are sadly inadequate. Too little time is devoted to P.E., and the program itself does not provide much training in either aerobics or flexibility. United States schools devote *less* time to physical education than the schools of most other countries. East Germany, Japan, and the Scandinavian countries devote 50-minute periods to P.E. 3 to 4 times a week, and they concentrate on exercise designed to promote flexibility and aerobic training. American programs frequently devote most of the time to a few competitive sports like football and baseball. Competitive sports tend to benefit a small number of children—only a few top athletes play. Late maturers and small children especially tend to be left out, and often they are the ones who need the training most. Moreover, most of the players' time in baseball and football is spent watching. Even the play itself does not last long and does not promote aerobic power or flexibility, although it does promote eye-hand coordination and balance. Another drawback of these particular sports is that the kind of eye-hand coordination they require does not develop fully until an average of ten years. So if baseball, for instance, is the mainstay of the P.E. program, then most of the children up to fourth grade will not be able to participate very successfully.

A good P.E. program in elementary school should ideally have 3 to 4 periods a week of 45 to 60 minutes of planned activities that stimulate aerobic power, flexibility, motor coordination (in proper maturational sequence), balance, and relaxation.

Parents can evaluate their child's P.E. program and judge what it offers. Often great improvement can be made simply by making the faculty or

Many schools do not provide enough aerobic exercise to make all children physically fit.

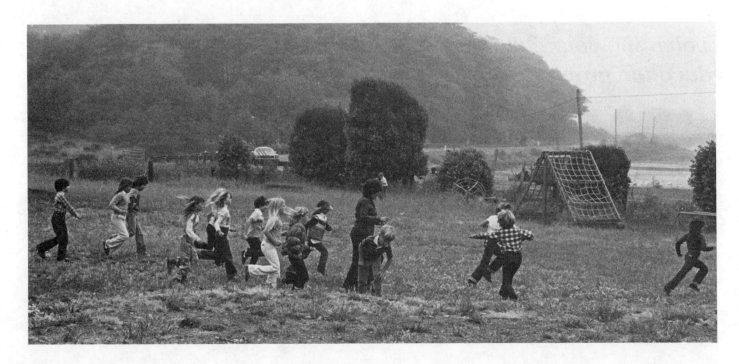

Average hours of physical education around the world

East Germany	Four 45-minute periods/week
West Germany	Three 45-minute periods/week
Japan	Three 45-minute periods/week, grades 1–6 Three 50-minute periods/week, grades 7–12
Denmark	Two 50-minute periods/week, grades 1–4 Three 50-minute periods/week, grades 5–12
Your children's school	?

PTA aware of shortcomings in the program. Parents can also substitute for gaps in the school program with extracurricular activities like tumbling, dancing, swimming, biking, running, and so on.

For children who are interested in competitive sports, there are after-school soccer clubs and baseball Little Leagues that can devote more time and attention to training than can be done in a school period. But parents should make sure such competitive programs don't engender excessive emotional stress. In some Little Leagues the adults become very involved in the competition at the expense of the children. The American Academy of Pediatrics has cautioned against the exploitation of children that is sometimes involved in these league sports.[11]

Evaluating your children's school's physical education program

How much time is spent in exercise?

What physical education training do teachers have in the elementary school?

Does the program progress from grade to grade?

Do they teach skills that can be used as adults?

Do they emphasize competition or participation?

Can small or late-maturing children do well?

Are aerobic skills taught, as well as strength and flexibility?

In addition to aerobic exercise, body movement is important to the growth and development of children.[12] Programmed courses in body movement train maturing neuromuscular circuits between the brain and specific muscles. Like an infant's standing and walking, older motor skills are stimulated and perfected by frequent practice at appropriate ages. Just as with standing and walking, there is great variability in the age at which these older skills develop. There are several basic categories of motor development in elementary school-age children: *balance, total body coordination, eye-hand coordination, small-muscle coordination, flexibility, strength,* and *agility*.

Some of these skills are naturally stimulated by kids' normal activities like bike riding, tree climbing, and playing catch. Some are stimulated by good playground equipment like balance beams and monkey bars. Still other skills require specific instruction by parent or teacher. These include all the various stretching activities taught in yoga, dance, or body movement classes, relaxation, and certain balance skills.[13,14,15]

Exercise and the mind

Both body movement skills and aerobics help to integrate the child's body and mind. Adults who exercise find that their activities can produce an altered state of consciousness similar to meditation. In this state they feel sensations of detachment from their body, slowing of time, heightened focus and attention, merger with the world around them, and freedom and enjoyment. Moving the body in space somehow profoundly affects thoughts in the mind.

Health benefits of common sports

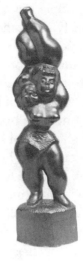
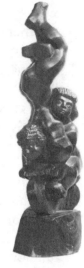

Sport	Aerobic training	Flexibility	Balance
Soccer	Excellent	Good	Good
Basketball	Good	Good	Good
Baseball	Poor	Good	Good
Gymnastics	Poor	Excellent	Excellent
Biking (long distance)	Excellent	Good	Good
Swimming (long distance)	Excellent	Good	Poor

Balance is a crucial skill learned in childhood.

Top:
Gross, Chaim. Handlebar Riders. *1935. Lignum vitae. 41¼″ high, at base 10½ × 11½″. Collection, The Museum of Modern Art, New York. Gift of A. Conger Goodyear.*

Bottom:
Gross, Chaim. Acrobatic Dancers. *1942. Ebony. 40½ × 10½ × 7″. Collection, Whitney Museum of American Art, New York. Purchase. Photograph by Geoffrey Clements.*

Many people have found that when they picture a physical activity in their mind (visualization), they improve when they actually do it. For example, people who imagine throwing basketball free throws improve their free throw scores; people who imagine themselves floating feel that it is easier to run. Clearly, optimum usage of mind or body involves stimulating the energies of both and forging a connection between them.

The connection between the central nervous system and the muscles of the body should not be neglected during childhood. Physical activity creates circuits that help us develop so we function as a whole. Scientists now know that the two lobes of the cerebrum serve different functions. In almost everyone (including most left-hand people), the left brain is involved with verbal, analytic-mathematical, and time-oriented thought, the right brain with images, orientation in space, body image, and grasping whole concepts from parts. The right brain is also crucially involved with dreaming and creative thought. Dance and yoga positions seem to stimulate characteristic right-brain thought. Optimum health surely involves training both sides of the brain. Since schools tend to concentrate so heavily on left-brain, academic skills, it is doubly important that parents see that their children pursue body learning, which stimulates the right brain.

Early man led a balanced life of exercise and thought. The rigors of an outdoor life guaranteed everyone adequate exercise. In fact, the human body evolved to be active. D. A. Bailey, a children's fitness expert, says that the industrial age no longer spontaneously satisfies the biological need for physical activity.[16] "Children today are entering a post-industrial society characterized by sedentary living patterns, emotional stress, poor dietary habits and lack of physical activities," says Dr. Bailey.[17] It is important for the health of their children that parents see that balanced physical exercise becomes integral to their lives.

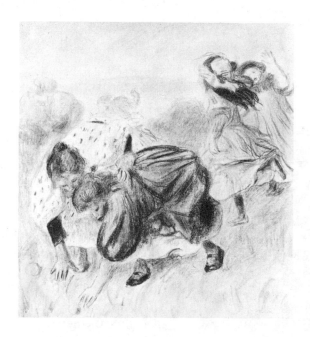

The right side of the brain is involved with orientation in space and body image.

Renoir, Pierre-Auguste. Children Playing Ball. *1900. Color lithograph. 23⁹/₁₆ × 20¼". Collection, The Museum of Modern Art, New York. Lillie P. Bliss Collection.*

How the body works— for children

I focus on the pleasure,
Something I can treasure.
Can you picture that?
Really nothin' to it,
Anyone can do it.

—Paul Williams and
Kenny Ascher,
"Can You Picture That,"
The Muppet Movie

Chapter 5

Anatomy
and
Physiology

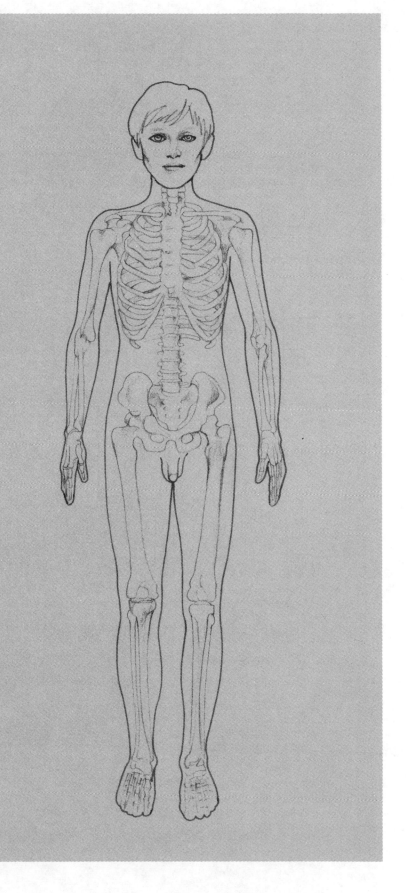

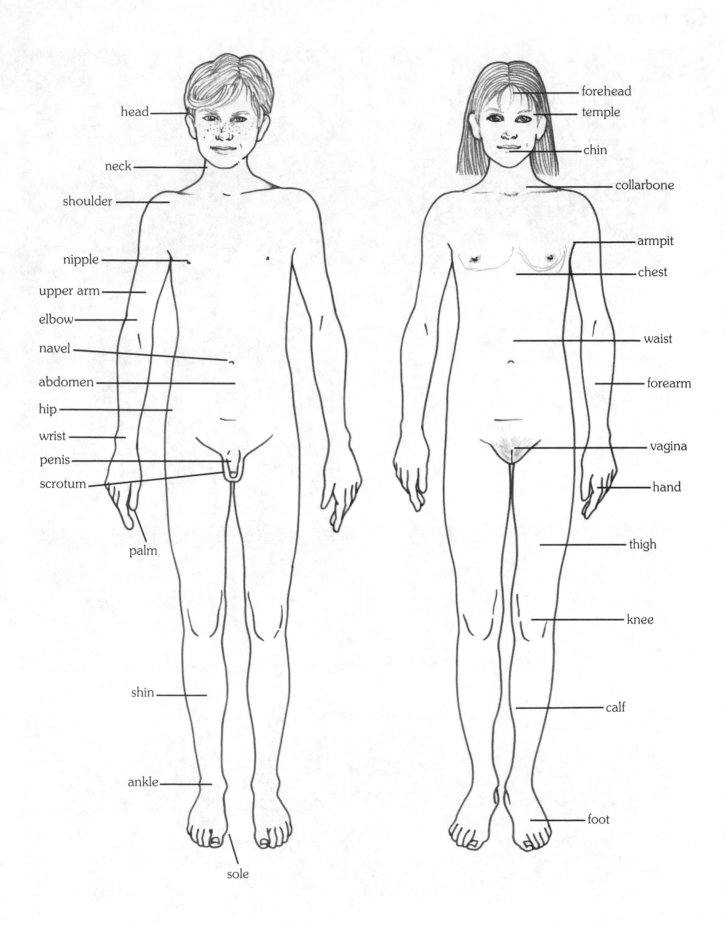

head

neck

shoulder

nipple

upper arm

elbow

navel

abdomen

hip

wrist

penis

scrotum

palm

shin

ankle

sole

forehead

temple

chin

collarbone

armpit

chest

waist

forearm

vagina

hand

thigh

knee

calf

foot

External body

The body plan   Human beings are miraculous, complex creatures. Although the human body is special in many ways, it has much in common with that of other animals.

Like many other creatures in the animal kingdom, humans have a backbone that is central to the design of their body. This backbone is actually a stack of small bones with hollow centers through which a large nerve runs. Animals with this kind of backbone are called *vertebrates.* Like other vertebrates, humans have a head that contains a brain and pairs of organs for seeing, hearing, and smelling. If a line is passed down a vertebrate's body from top to bottom, the right and left sides are symmetrical; that is, they are alike or balanced: there is an arm on each side and a leg on each side, as well as an *eye* and an *ear.* Vertebrates' bodies have a basic plan that is made up of tubes within tubes: The main part of the body forms the outer tube; inside, the digestive system is a tube and the blood vessels are tubes. All vertebrates also

Like all vertebrates, human beings have a head, a backbone, and two matching sides of the body. Like all mammals, they breathe air, have warm bodies, grow hair, and nurse their young.

have a heart to pump the blood through these vessels.

Humans are a special kind of vertebrate called *mammals.* All mammals have certain things in common that make them different from other kinds of vertebrates. Like other mammals, humans have warm bodies, they breathe air, and they have hair. In mammals, the body tube is divided inside into two parts. The chest contains the heart and lungs, while the abdomen contains the digestive system and other organs. One of the most unusual things about mammals is the way their young are born. Rather than hatching eggs, the young develop completely inside the mother. After they are born, they are fed milk from the mother's mammary glands, the breasts.

Humans belong to a special group of mammals called *primates.* Monkeys and apes are other primates. All primates have hands and feet that are specially able to grasp and hold things. Unlike other primates, humans walk standing up. To make this possible, the backbone has become curved and the feet have developed curves called arches. Humans take a longer time to grow than most primates, which means they spend a long time learning from their parents. Humans also have a very large brain and the ability to talk. This has led to languages with many

words, the ability to teach and pass on complicated ideas, and ways of writing down these ideas.

Like all animals, humans have bodies that are able to take in air and food to grow and make energy; that can repair many kinds of injuries and protect themselves against illness. The body does these things automatically to keep in balance and stay alive. The ability to grow, stay alive, and stay healthy has been called the wisdom of the body. We think that the more kids know about how the organs of the body work, the more they will take care of, love, and help their own bodies.

Growth chart

Time	Growth in inches per year
Before birth	20″
1st year	10″
2nd year	5″
3rd and 4th years	3″–4″
Age 5 until puberty	2″–3″

Seasonal growth

You grow taller in spring than fall.

You grow fatter in fall than spring.

Growth There are two big things that influence growth: what you are born with and what happens to you. All children have basic information in their cells (see page 210) that comes from both their parents. This information is carried on protein chains called chromosomes. It determines what their skin, eyes, and hair look like and how big they can grow. Once children start to grow, they are affected by what they eat, what kind of exercise they get, and how healthy they are.

Children grow following a sequence, or pattern, that is the same for all kids. What varies from one child to another is *when* they grow, how *fast* they grow, and how *big* they grow. But all kids go through the same basic growth steps—that's what's automatic. Babies grow very quickly right before they are born and in the first two years. By two, most babies have grown more than 30 inches and gained 25 to 35 pounds. There's no other time when children grow quite so fast. From 2 to 5 years, growth slows down in both height and weight. From 5 to 9 kids grow steadily, but gain fewer inches and pounds per year. After this steady, slow growth comes another spurt.

Somewhere between 9 and 12 in girls and 11 and 14 in boys, children suddenly grow a lot taller in about a year or two. They also gain a lot in weight, but over a little longer time. This second big growth period is called the *adolescent growth spurt*. Following this big spurt, growth slows down and then stops at about 16 in girls and 20 in boys.

At the same time that children are growing in height and weight, the shape of their bodies is also changing. Change in shape or proportion follows a general pattern, too. Before birth, a baby's head grows faster than any other part of its body. A baby's head is much bigger in comparison to its body than an adult's. From birth to one year, a baby's body grows most from the shoulders to the legs. Then from one year until the adolescent growth spurt, most growth is in the legs, so the mid point of the body drops from the belly button to the middle of the legs.

In the adolescent spurt the mid part of the body again grows the fastest. Boys gain most in muscle and bone—especially in their shoulders. Girls gain more in fat—especially around their hips. Boys end up weighing more because muscle and bone are heavier than fat.

Up until 8 or 9, boys and girls grow at about the same rate. Since girls generally begin their growth spurt several years before boys, they tend to be bigger than

Boys' and girls' average heights and weights by age

	Boys					
	Smaller than average *		*Average*		*Bigger than average* †	
Age (years)	**Weight (pounds)**	*Height (inches)*	**Weight (pounds)**	*Height (inches)*	**Weight (pounds)**	*Height (inches)*
5	**37**	42	**42**	44	**50**	46
6	**41**	44	**48**	46	**56**	49
7	**46**	46	**54**	49	**64**	51
8	**51**	49	**60**	51	**73**	54
9	**56**	51	**66**	53	**81**	56
10	**61**	52	**72**	55	**90**	58
11	**66**	54	**78**	57	**99**	60
12	**72**	56	**84**	59	**110**	62

* 10% are smaller.   † the biggest 10%.

External body games

Human beings are symmetrical; that is, their right and left sides look alike. To see this, try holding a mirror against the middle of a friend, with one edge touching him or her and the other edge pointing straight out. The mirror will reflect the half it's pointed toward, and when you look in the mirror it will seem as though you're looking at the whole person. The face is especially fun to try. You may even be able to see the slight differences between the two sides.

Look at animals that live around you or at the zoo. Which ones are vertebrates? That is, which ones have a backbone? Which ones have arms and legs, as well as a backbone? Which of these animals not only has a back-bone, but has a warm body and hair? These are mammals. Which of these animals also has nails and thumbs that can squeeze things? These are primates.

See how fast you grow. Mark your height on a chart or wall and measure yourself every few months. Weigh yourself at the same time. This is especially fun when kids begin to spurt up between the ages of 9 and 14. If you can, compare your growth now with a record of how fast you grew when you were a baby. If your teacher is interested, try this with your whole class.

See how body proportions change as you grow. Measure a baby and see which part is longest—the legs, the trunk, or the head. Also, measure around the baby's head and tummy, and compare those figures. Now make the same measurements on a four-year-old, yourself, and on one of your parents. Compare all the measurements.

Figure out which body shape you have. Are you thin and wiry, big boned and muscular, or round and soft? Which shape are your friends?

Girls

Smaller than average*		Average		Bigger than average†	
Weight (pounds)	Height (inches)	**Weight (pounds)**	Height (inches)	**Weight (pounds)**	Height (inches)
36	41	**41**	43	**48**	45
40	44	**47**	46	**54**	48
45	46	**52**	48	**61**	51
49	48	**58**	50	**70**	53
53	50	**64**	52	**79**	55
57	52	**70**	55	**90**	58
63	54	**79**	57	**100**	60
70	56	**88**	60	**112**	63

* 10% are smaller.   † the biggest 10%.

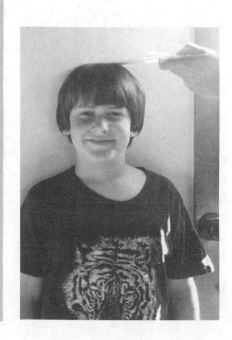

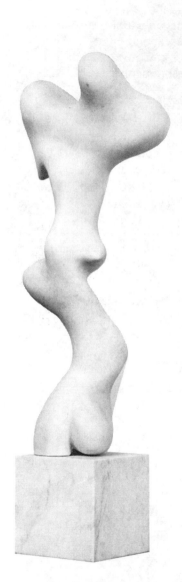

Growth is a steady upward movement, with one spurt in the first year and another in the teenage years.

Arp, Jean. Growth. *1938. Marble. Height: 39½". Collection, The Solomon R. Guggenheim Museum, New York. Photograph by Robert E. Mates.*

boys on the average between the ages of 9 and 12 or 13. When boys begin their spurt around 12 to 14 years, they catch up and become bigger than girls, on the average. Even though this is the general pattern, an early-growing boy may start the growth spurt ahead of a late-growing girl. Boys or girls who start to get their adolescent growth spurt early tend to stop growing sooner. So early-growing kids may be the biggest for a while, then later-growing kids may grow taller or bigger.

Body shapes People come in three basic body shapes or types. These types apply to boys and girls as well as to men and women. Some people fit a body type perfectly, but many are a mixture. One shape is called *ectomorph.* These people are thin and wiry. They have a long neck, a flat chest and belly, small bones, and long arms and legs. A second shape is called *mesomorph.* These people are very muscular and big-boned. They have broad shoulders and a wide chest. The third basic shape is *endomorph.* Their bodies look round and soft. They have large heads, short necks, and short arms and legs. Unless people are *very* thin or *very* overweight, all the shapes are healthy. No one shape is better than another; they are just different.

Cells

Every organ, every muscle or bone, every part of the body, is made up of cells. Cells are the building blocks of the body. But unlike building blocks, cells are *alive.* They can take in food, digest it, give off waste products, and make new cells.

Cells come in different sizes and shapes, and they do different jobs. But all the cells in the body do have some things in common. They all have the same basic parts and are made up of the same chemicals. And they all are so small that they can only be seen under a microscope.

Every cell is covered by a *membrane,* which, like skin, keeps all the cell's parts inside. The cell membrane is made up of fat and protein and has many tiny holes in it called *pores.* Chemicals enter the cell in several ways. Some substances, like water, salt, and minerals, simply dissolve or pass through the tiny holes in the cell membrane. And some, like sugar, are actively carried across the cell membrane by special chemicals. Yet others, like proteins, are sucked in by the cell membrane.

The inside of the cell is filled with *cytoplasm,* a syrupy liquid made of protein, minerals, sugar, and fat. In the midst of the cytoplasm is a large, double-walled body called the *nucleus.* The

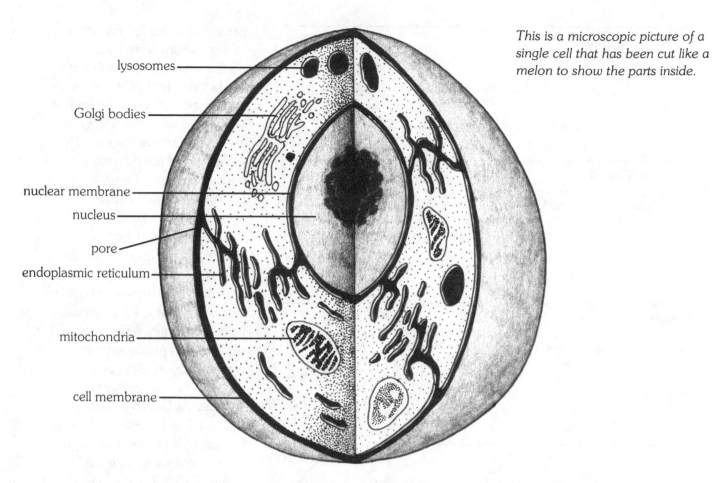

lysosomes

Golgi bodies

nuclear membrane

nucleus

pore

endoplasmic reticulum

mitochondria

cell membrane

This is a microscopic picture of a single cell that has been cut like a melon to show the parts inside.

nucleus is the control center, or "brain," that directs the cell's activities. The nucleus is surrounded by two layers of cell membrane and is made up of a special protein. This protein contains codes for creating more cells like itself and other proteins. The proteins it makes are related to the particular job that the cell does. For example, a stomach cell will make digestive *enzymes,* which help the body to break down food.

There are a number of cell parts, or structures, in the cytoplasm around the nucleus. These cell parts are called *organelles,* which means little organs. All the organelles are built out of cell membrane, but they look different and each does a different job. *Mitochondria* are bean-shaped energy factories that contain many little shelves lined with enzymes. These enzymes take digested food, combine it with oxygen, and make carbon dioxide and ATP. ATP is a chemical that releases energy when it is broken down. Cells use this energy (1) when they move, like muscle cells, (2) when they make proteins for growth or digestion, and (3) when they carry or pump things across the cell membrane.

Other kinds of organelles are little fluid-filled sacs called *lysosomes.* The fluid in them contains powerful digestive enzymes that would dissolve the cell itself if they weren't walled in. The lysosomes digest any bacteria the cell eats. They also digest injured or broken parts of the cell itself. When the cell dies, the lysosome wall bursts and the fluid digests the entire cell. This is a kind of self-destruct mechanism that gets rid of damaged cells so new ones can take their places.

The *endoplasmic reticulum* is a network of tubes or canals that starts from the membrane of the nucleus and goes all over the cell. This network is the cell's factory where

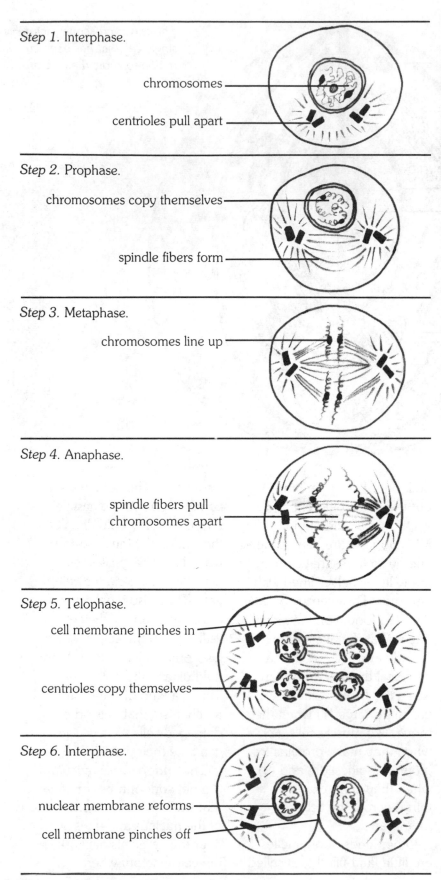

Step 1. Interphase.

chromosomes

centrioles pull apart

Step 2. Prophase.

chromosomes copy themselves

spindle fibers form

Step 3. Metaphase.

chromosomes line up

Step 4. Anaphase.

spindle fibers pull chromosomes apart

Step 5. Telophase.

cell membrane pinches in

centrioles copy themselves

Step 6. Interphase.

nuclear membrane reforms

cell membrane pinches off

proteins are made according to instructions from the nucleus. The *Golgi bodies* are the place where proteins are "wrapped," stored, and finally shipped to all parts of the cell and even outside the cell. The Golgi bodies are actually the ends of some of the endoplasmic reticulum canals.

Cell division All cells are capable of making other cells exactly like themselves. They are constantly replacing themselves because each one only lives a short time. They also replace or reproduce themselves as the body grows bigger. The way cells make new cells is by *cell division,* or *mitosis.* The nucleus of the cell contains information on what the cell does and how it's made. This information is stored on chains of protein molecules that contain deoxyribonucleic acid (DNA). They are called genes. The order in which the molecules are arranged tells the cell which proteins to make. When a cell divides, the protein chains make a copy of themselves. Then these chains pull apart and the cell splits in half. The result is two identical cells.

Cell division always follows the same steps, but it is really

Cells make new cells by dividing in half. The material in the nucleus copies itself, so each new cell has exactly the same information. This is how it looks under a microscope.

one continuous process. First, the *centrioles,* two pairs of tubes outside the nucleus, move apart. As they move apart, tiny microtubes called *spindle fibers* grow between them. Meanwhile, the protein chains of DNA in the nucleus called *chromosomes* tighten

Cell games

Carefully tape a piece of coffee-filter paper across the middle of a bowl. Fill both sides with water. Sprinkle a teaspoon of salt into the water on *one* side and gently stir it around. Taste the water on that side. Wait a few minutes and taste the water on the other side. The salt has passed through the filter. This is how cells take in food and let out waste products. Now try the same experiment with bread crumbs. Do they pass through the filter?

Make a rough model of a cell. Fill a plastic bag half full of gelatin (mix one package of unflavored gelatin with two cups of water, following directions; then whip it before it sets). Put a plum into the gel. This is the cell's nucleus. Then add green grapes to represent the mitochondria, and tiny canned peas to represent the lysosomes. Finally, add little pieces of cooked spaghetti to represent the cell's tubes and canals (see drawing).
To show cell division, add another plum and then squeeze the bag in half, splitting the contents and putting one "nucleus" on each side.

into cords and begin to duplicate themselves. Next the centrioles reach opposite sides of the cell and the membrane around the nucleus disappears. Then the spindle fibers attach to the chromosomes, and the matching chromosomes line up across the center of the cell. The spindle fibers move further apart, pulling the matching pairs of chromosomes to opposite sides of the cell. The cell membrane begins to pinch inward across the middle of the cell. The centrioles make copies of themselves and a new nuclear membrane forms around the newly separated chromosomes. Finally, the cell membrane pinches through, leaving two separate cells, each with its own complete membrane. The spindles now disappear and the chromosomes become uncoiled again.

The skin

The skin covers the whole body. It is a barrier, or "wall," that protects the muscles and organs underneath.
Although the skin does a good job of protecting the body, there are some things that it lets in. Many chemicals, some of which aren't good for you, can pass through the skin in small amounts and get into the blood. The skin marks the end of the body, but it doesn't totally separate the body from what's outside.
The upper layer of the skin,

Substances that pass through the skin

Water

Some chemicals in soaps, sprays and hand lotions

Skin creams

Sunlight

Paint solvents and pesticides

the *epidermis,* constantly makes new cells. These cells flatten and become hard as they move up and newer cells are made underneath. By the time they reach the top, they have died and are like dry scales. These flaky cells fall off day by day as people rub, brush, and scratch their skin.
In the bottom of the epidermis there are special cells called *melanocytes.* They make a dark substance called *melanin,* which protects the skin from the ultraviolet rays of the sun. The more the skin is exposed to the sun, the more melanin is made. This is why people get a tan when they spend time in the sun. Melanin determines the basic color of the skin as well. Black people, Indians, Orientals, and whites all have the same number of melanocytes, but they produce different amounts of melanin depending on the information the cells were given from the parents.

This drawing is an imaginary cube that shows what is under the skin from two sides. It's like cutting a square out of a layer cake to see the inside. This kind of drawing is called a three-dimensional cross section and is many times larger than real life.

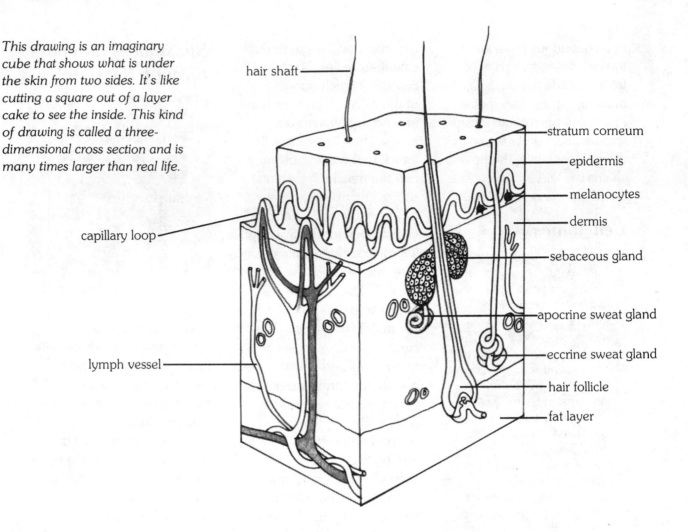

hair shaft

stratum corneum

epidermis

melanocytes

dermis

sebaceous gland

apocrine sweat gland

eccrine sweat gland

hair follicle

fat layer

capillary loop

lymph vessel

Fingernails and toenails are special areas in which the top skin layer turns into a hard, clear plate. The plate looks pink because of the blood vessels underneath. Under the flap of skin in the nail root, there are special cells that constantly grow outward. As these cells are pushed out, they die, dry out, and become hard. Because there are no nerves in the nails and the cells are dead, it doesn't hurt to cut them.

Like hair, nails are made of cells that have turned to keratin, a special protein. If a nail comes off in an accident, a new one will grow out from the root in about six months.

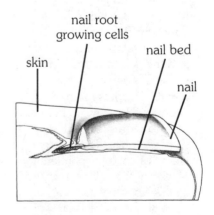

nail root

growing cells

skin

nail bed

nail

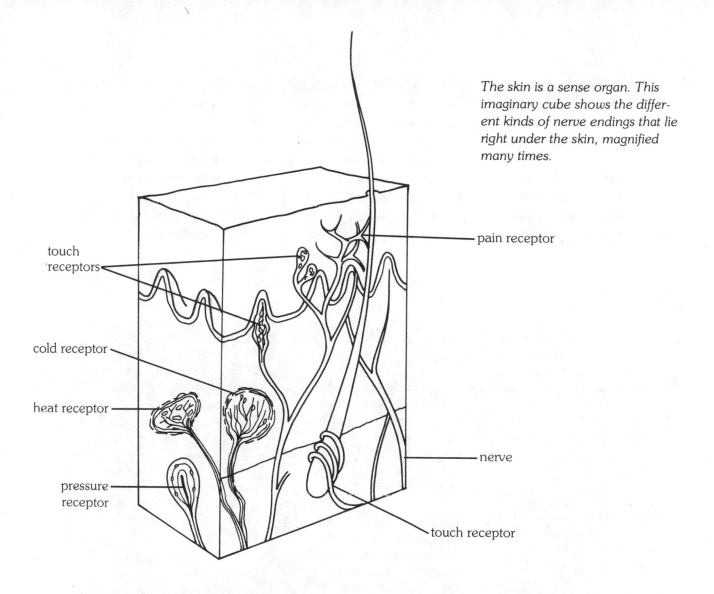

The skin is a sense organ. This imaginary cube shows the different kinds of nerve endings that lie right under the skin, magnified many times.

touch receptors

cold receptor

heat receptor

pressure receptor

pain receptor

nerve

touch receptor

The second layer of the skin is called the *dermis*. It is made of another kind of cell that is slightly elastic, or stretchy. In this layer there are tiny blood vessels, nerves, oil glands, sweat glands, and hair follicles. The little nerve endings signal information to the brain about temperature, pain, and pressure, or touch. The tiny blood vessels bring food to the cells of the dermis and epidermis. Even more important, they help to regulate the body's temperature. When these tiny vessels are full of blood the skin looks pink and flushed.

This is what happens when someone blushes. When there is little blood in the vessels, a person looks pale.

Every hair is made in special places called *follicles*. Each follicle is made up of cells from the top skin layer (epidermis) that have grown down into the dermis. Just like the top layer of skin, hair follicles keep making new cells. The cells are pushed up through the follicle in a long skinny line and dry out and die as they grow out. So hair is actually just a special kind of skin cell.

The oil-making glands produce a fatty substance called *sebum,* which keeps out water and keeps body fluids in. These glands produce the waxy covering on newborn babies. For many years after that, the oil glands don't produce much. They become very active for a time when the reproductive glands start to mature (see Puberty, 216 to 220). Boys generally make more sebum than girls, and people in hot climates make more than people in cold climates.

Underneath the dermis there is a layer of fat cells. Fat

provides a cushion against bumps and, like insulation, it helps to hold in body heat. Also, fat stores food energy.

Skin messages Like the eyes or ears, the skin is a sense organ that sends the brain information about the outside world. In the skin are "feeler" nerves with several different kinds of special endings. These endings are called *receptors* because they receive information. *Pain receptors* lie in the top layer of skin, the epidermis. They send messages only when they are poked by something sharp or hard. *Touch receptors* are in the top of the skin and in the hair shafts. They are set off by even the tiniest touch. *Pressure receptors* lie in the deepest layer of skin, so they react only when the skin is pushed hard. Two other receptors in

Skin games

On a dry day, scratch firmly along your arm with your fingernails. If you look closely you will see little dry flakes of skin where you scratched. This is the top layer of skin, which is dead. It is continually being replaced by new cells from underneath.

Look for little dark brown birthmarks or moles on your body. This is the color of melanin made by the pigment cells in your skin.

Compare a tanned area of your body with an area that has been covered. The tanned area has more melanin to protect your body from the sun's ultraviolet rays.

With clean hands, rub your index finger alongside your nose on a hot day. Then rub your finger on a thin piece of paper. The oil made by little glands under the skin will leave a shiny mark. Compare the mark with a tiny bit of butter or margarine rubbed on the paper. Now sprinkle a drop of water on the marks and see what happens. This is how oil helps to protect your skin.

Put a slightly damp sponge in a saucer of grape juice. Put another sponge in some sand. The juice will pass through the sponge, but the sand won't. Your skin works in a similar way.

Blindfold a friend. Then touch the friend in different places with a feather (light touch), a pencil eraser (pressure), and a metal spoon dipped in icy and then hot water (cold and hot). See if your friend can tell when, where, and with what he or she is being touched.

You can test for pain receptors on your own body by pricking yourself with a pin. If you press very gently you'll feel pressure but no pain. The pain receptors lie deeper under the skin. This is why you can stick pins under the skin on your fingertips without feeling any pain.

Wet the inside of your arm with water. Swing your arm back and forth. How does the wet part of your arm feel? On a hot day when you sweat, your skin cools by evaporation.

Look closely at the skin on your arm the next time you're cold and get goose bumps. What happens to the hairs on your arm? Where are the hairs in relation to the goose bumps?

Find out where your sweat glands are. Run around on a hot day and see which parts of your body perspire or sweat first.

On a hot day, lick the skin of your forearm. What does it taste like? Your skin "excretes" or releases salt when you sweat.

Stretch a rubber band and let one end go. What happens? Now pull up a pinch of skin between two fingers. Watch closely as you let go. What happens? Like the rubber band, your skin has great elasticity. It can stretch and return to its original shape.

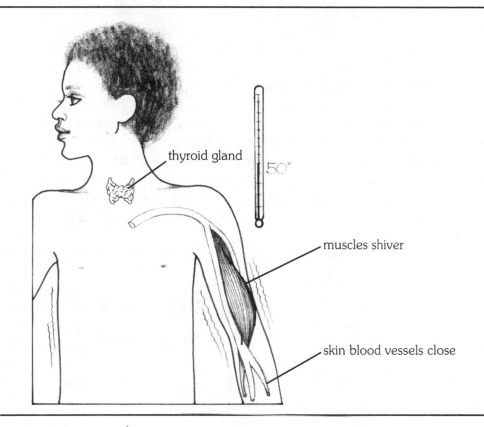

thyroid gland

50°

muscles shiver

skin blood vessels close

When it's cold, blood vessels in the skin squeeze down and send most of the blood away from the skin. Then you shiver and the thyroid tells the body to burn more food to make heat.

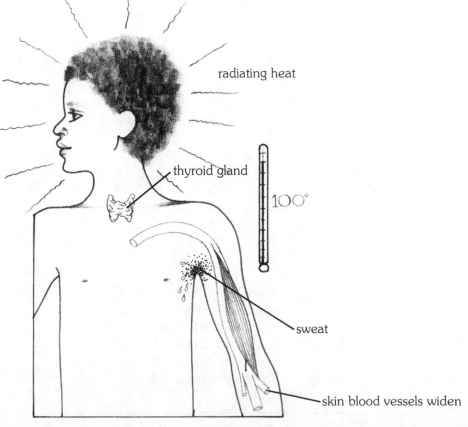

radiating heat

thyroid gland

100°

sweat

skin blood vessels widen

When it's hot, blood goes to the skin and gives off heat. You sweat and the thyroid gland tells the body to burn less food.

the middle layer react to heat or cold. All these receptors help people to sense danger and feel pleasure.

Temperature regulation

Deep in the brain, in the *hypothalamus*, there are nerves that measure the temperature of nearby blood and act like a thermostat. When the blood is slightly cool the thermostat sends messages along the nerves, telling the body to get warmer. Blood vessels in the skin squeeze down sending most of the blood deep into the body, below the layer of skin fat that helps to hold in heat. Chemicals called *hormones* from the thyroid and the adrenal glands tell cells to take in more food and produce more heat. Muscle cells are given messages to tense, then stretch very quickly. This is what causes shivering, which actually makes heat. Also tiny muscles make the body's hairs stand up, causing "goose-bumps." In furry animals this helps to trap warm air next to the skin. For people, goose-bumps don't help to warm them much.

When the body's thermostat finds the blood too warm, it sends out messages to cool off. Blood vessels in the skin widen, bringing more blood to the surface of the body. The skin becomes like a radiator and gives off heat into the air. Chemicals from the adrenal

and thyroid glands tell cells to rest and stop making heat. If the body is still hot, signals are sent to the sweat glands to pump out water. As the water evaporates into the air, the body is cooled.

Normal body temperature is *said* to be 98.6°F. (37°C.). But temperature can vary for many reasons. Body temperature is higher in warm weather, in the afternoon, and after exercise. When people have a fever their thermostat doesn't tell their body to cool down as it normally does. The thermostat is actually reset by chemicals released by the bacteria or virus that are making the people sick, telling them to get even hotter. Thus, even though they have a fever, people shiver and have

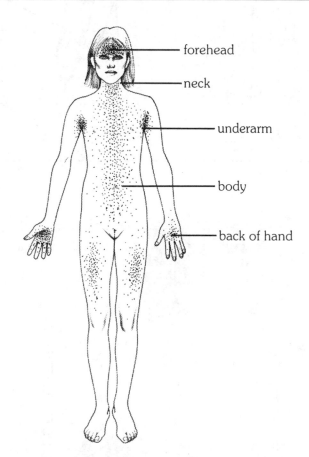

forehead

neck

underarm

body

back of hand

When it's hot, eccrine glands release sweat—first on the fore-head, next on the neck, and then on the back and chest. In very hot weather, sweat will appear wherever there are dots in this drawing.

chills. When the body goes above the thermostat setting, the people begin to sweat.

Sweat glands There are two basic types of sweat glands: *eccrine* and *apocrine*. Eccrine glands are found all over the body. Some work when it's hot to cool the body by evaporation; others work when people are nervous or excited.

Little cells in the bottom of the glands send tiny drops of salt water up tubes that open on the surface of the skin. When eccrine sweat dries on the skin it mixes with sebum from the oil glands and forms an invisible acid covering that protects the body by killing bacteria.

The apocrine sweat glands don't start to work until people are 10 to 16 years old and their reproductive organs begin working. These very large sweat glands work when people are nervous or excited. This sweat has fat in it and when it is digested by bacteria living on the skin, it produces a strong odor. Among animals this kind of odor may be important to attracting members of the opposite sex.

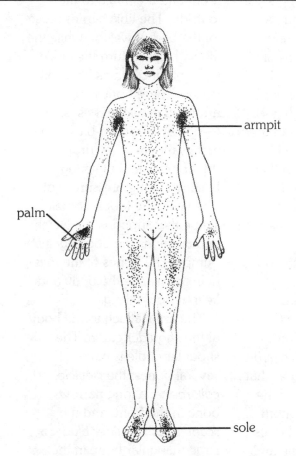

When people are excited or upset, other eccrine glands release sweat, first on the palms of the hands and soles of the feet, and then wherever there are dots in this drawing.

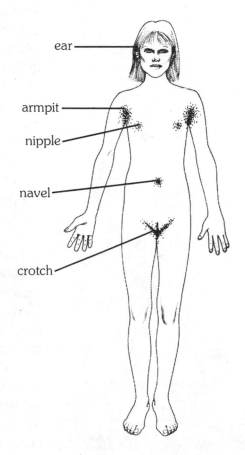

Apocrine sweat glands are located around the armpits, crotch, and nipples. They only work in adults when they are nervous or excited.

The skeleton

There are 206 bones inside the body. These bones hold up the body, give it shape, and protect the soft organs inside. Bones also make it possible for us to move when muscles pull on them like big levers. Many people don't realize it, but bones are alive. Throughout childhood the bones are growing and changing shape. But even after growth stops, bones remain alive, constantly making new cells and replacing old ones.

Not only do bones act as a frame for the body, they make all the cells in the blood. They also store calcium, a mineral that is very important for sending messages along the nerves and for tightening or contracting muscle cells.

All the bones together are called the *skeleton*. The skeleton has two parts. One part is the *axial*, or central, *skeleton*, which is made up of the skull, the backbone, and the ribs. The second part is the *appendicular skeleton*, which is made up of the bones of the arms and legs, and the hips and shoulders to which they are attached. The word "appendicular" comes from the Latin word for "something which is tacked on."

The legs attach to the body with bones called the *hipbones*, or *pelvic girdle*. Girdle comes from the Old English word for "go around, or encircle." The pelvic girdle is made up of two bones that hook on to each side of the big flat bone at the bottom of the backbone. These bones curve around in a circle and join at the front, making a kind of basket that holds and protects the organs in the belly. The bottom of the basket is open. (This opening is bigger in women than in men, which allows a baby to pass through when it is born.) In the sides of the basket are hollow bowls called sockets, to which the legs are attached. The legs have one big bone, the *femur*, that runs from the hip to the knee. At the top of this bone is a ball that is shaped to fit perfectly in the hip socket. This joint allows the leg to swing back and forth for walking.

Between the knee and the foot are two bones, the *tibia* in front and the *fibula* to the outside. The tibia carries most of the body's weight, while the fibula helps to turn the ankle.

The foot contains 26 small bones. These bones are arranged in two arches, side-to-side and front-to-back. The arches move—they drop under pressure but spring back when the pressure is off. They give the foot a domelike shape that supports the weight and cushions the body against bumps. The bones of the toes help to balance the body and keep it from falling.

The arms attach to the body at the *shoulder girdle*. The shoulder girdle is made of several bones: the *clavicle*, or *collarbone*, a long narrow bone in the front, and the *scapula*, or *shoulder blade*, a large triangular bone in the back.

The shoulder blade does not attach directly to the spine or ribs in the back, but is loosely connected to the body by muscles. This means that it moves freely in almost all directions. The end of the

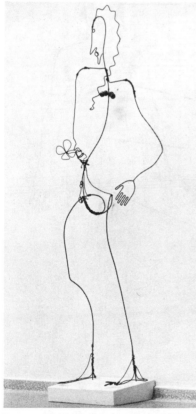

Bones hold up the body and allow it to move when they are pulled on by muscles.

Calder, Alexander. Spring. 1929. Wire and wood. 94½ × 36 × 19½". Collection, The Solomon R. Guggenheim Museum, New York. Gift of the artist, 1965.

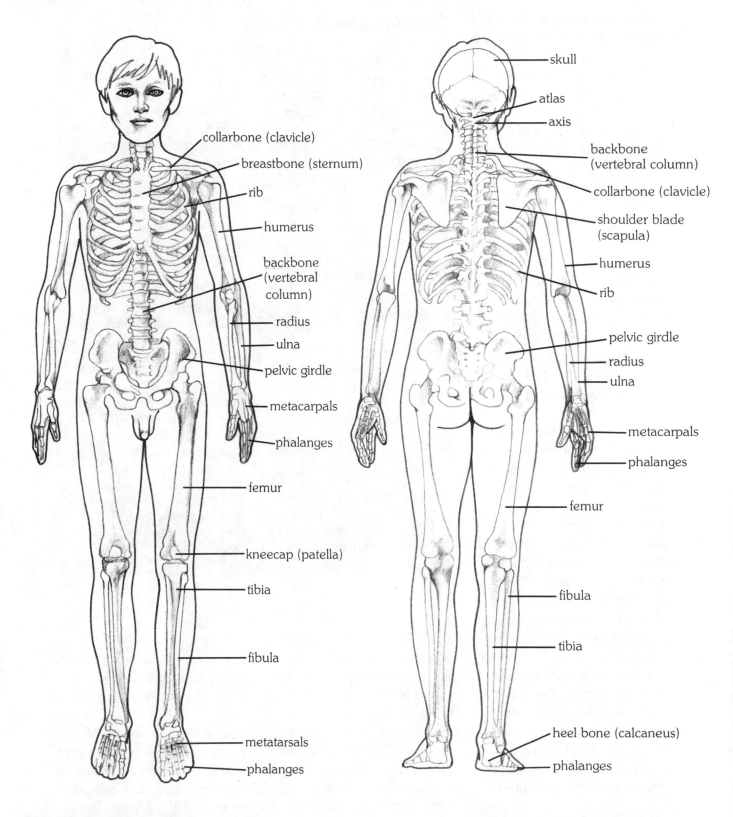

collarbone (clavicle)

breastbone (sternum)

rib

humerus

backbone
(vertebral
column)

radius

ulna

pelvic girdle

metacarpals

phalanges

femur

kneecap (patella)

tibia

fibula

metatarsals

phalanges

skull

atlas

axis

backbone
(vertebral column)

collarbone (clavicle)

shoulder blade
(scapula)

humerus

rib

pelvic girdle

radius

ulna

metacarpals

phalanges

femur

fibula

tibia

heel bone (calcaneus)

phalanges

*There are 206 bones in the
human skeleton. This shows the
skeleton from the front.*

*This shows the skeleton from the
back. The bones are alive. They
make blood and store minerals.*

collarbone is connected to the *breastbone,* or *sternum,* in the middle of the chest. The collarbone runs across the shoulder and touches the shoulder blade on the "bump" at the edge of the shoulder. Below this bump is a very shallow hole or socket. This is where the arm attaches.

The upper arm has one big bone, the *humerus,* that goes from the elbow to the shoulder blade. At the top of the humerus is a ball-shaped bump that rests loosely in the socket. It is held there by a circle of muscles. The shallowness of this socket lets the arm move in a wider circle than the leg.

Like the lower leg, the lower arm has two bones. The bones go from the elbow to the wrist. The *radius* runs down the arm to the thumb. The *ulna* begins with the bump of the elbow and ends with a small bump at the wrist, above the little finger. The ulna supports the forearm. The radius can cross over it, making it possible to turn your hand over.

The hand has 27 bones. They are arranged so that the hand can grasp, cup, and pinch. Without all these bones, the hand would not be able to make as many tiny different motions as it does.

Axial skeleton   The *axial,* or central, *skeleton* is made up of the bones of the skull, back,

Skeleton games

See how many different bones you can feel in your body. Feel your skull, your jaw, your backbone, your collarbone, your hips, and your arms and legs. Take a deep breath and try to count all your ribs. How many bones can you feel in your upper arms? Your forearms? In your thighs? In your calves? How many *separate* bones can you count in your hands and your feet?

Make footprints in wet sand. Which ways do your feet curve?

Get an uncooked chicken leg. Dissect or cut open the joint between the leg and the thigh. Notice the gristly white bands called ligaments that hold the bones together. Move the joint to see how it works. Then break it open to look at the capsule inside. See the shiny cartilage on the ends of the bones, which makes them slide more easily.

Ask the butcher to saw a long bone in half and another crossways. Notice the fat and the blood vessels in the marrow cavity. Look for lines of force, and compact and spongy bone (see drawing, page 142). Try and peel off the covering (periosteum) of the bone.

Boil a chicken bone in vinegar for several hours. This will dissolve the calcium out of the bone and leave only the collagen-fiber framework. Feel the bone. Is it still hard?

Make a model of your backbone. For the vertebrae, string big wooden beads tightly on a piece of fairly heavy wire. In between the beads put rubber washers (or foam rubber) to act like the discs. See how the rubber washers get squeezed as you bend the wire.

and ribs. The skull is made up of a number of bones, many of which have become knit or joined together. Eight of the bones form the large dome that surrounds and protects the brain. The joints between these bones are called *sutures* because they look as if they were sewn together. The skull bones are not joined at birth, which means it's possible for the bones to overlap slightly as a baby is being born. The bones join or fuse after several years, making a stronger protective container for the brain.

The face is made up of 14 more bones. They join in such a way as to leave openings for the eyes, nose, and ears. The nose itself is not bone, but is made up mostly of rubbery material called cartilage. The *lower jawbone,* called the

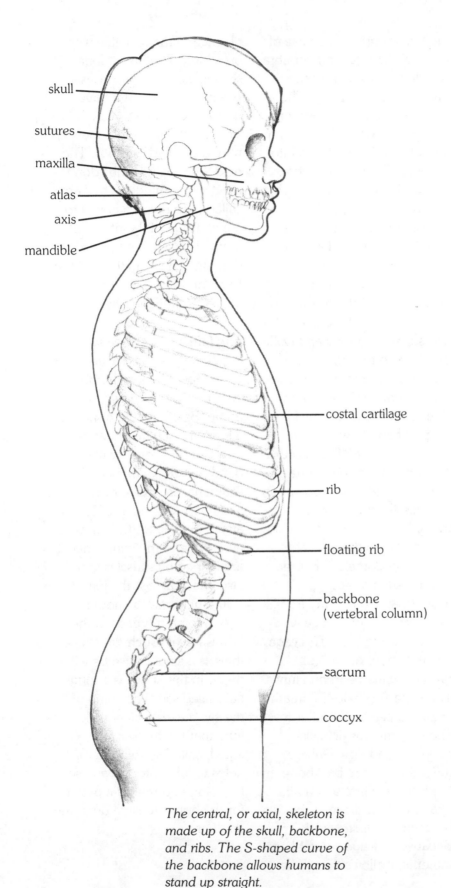

skull

sutures

maxilla

atlas

axis

mandible

costal cartilage

rib

floating rib

backbone
(vertebral column)

sacrum

coccyx

The central, or axial, skeleton is made up of the skull, backbone, and ribs. The S-shaped curve of the backbone allows humans to stand up straight.

mandible, is the only movable part of the skull. It attaches on either side of the head in front of the ears.

The bottom of the skull has a large hole through which the spinal cord joins the brain (see page 184–89). On either side of this hole are two bony knobs that fit into shallow cups in the top of the backbone.

The *backbone,* or *vertebral column,* is a strong, bendable rod that supports the skull and protects the spinal cord. The backbone is made up of 33 bumpy bones that stack neatly, one on top of another, in a slight S-shaped curve. At birth, the curve has a simple C-shape. As a baby learns to hold up its head, the top of the column bends backward. As the baby learns to walk, the bottom also bends backward.

Between every two verte-brae is a tough, shiny pad of cartilage with fluid in the center. These pads are called *disks,* and their job is to cush-ion bumps to the brain and spinal cord. Vertebrae all have the same basic butterfly shape with a hole in the middle through which the spinal cord runs. Different vertebrae have somewhat different shapes depending on what they do. The ones in the neck are specially shaped to hold up the skull. The top vertebra is named the *atlas* after the Greek god who held up the heavens on his head. The atlas is a ring with shallow cups on either side that fit over

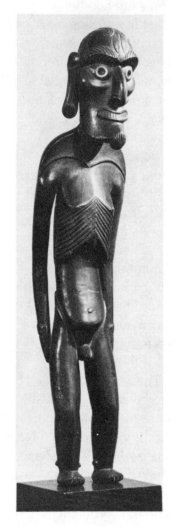

The ribs protect the heart and lungs and help in breathing.

Easter Island. Figure. 19th–20th cent. Wood. Height: 17⅞". The Metropolitan Museum of Art, New York. The Michael C. Rockefeller Memorial Collection of Primitive Art, Bequest of Nelson A. Rockefeller, 1979.

the two bumps at the base of the skull. The second vertebra is called the *axis*, from the Latin word for turning. The axis acts like the axle around which a car wheel turns. It has a long part that sticks up into the ring of the first vertebra. The skull and the first vertebra turn around this part.

The vertebrae in the chest area have special places to which the ribs attach. The ones in the lower back are very large in order to support the body's weight and take the pressure of standing and walking. The bottom nine vertebrae are fused into two bones: the *sacrum* and the *coccyx*. The sacrum is a flat, shield-shaped bone to which the hipbones attach. The coccyx is a little arrow-shaped bone at the tip of the spinal column. In animals like the cat, there are many bones in the coccyx and they make up the tail.

The ribs come off the side of the vertebrae, curve around, and join in the front. This forms an oval cage with the ribs as the bars. This cage has the important job of protecting the heart and lungs. The cage also helps in breathing. As a person breathes in and out, the ribs actually move up and down where they hinge to the backbone. In the front, the first seven ribs attach with cartilage to the breastbone, or *sternum*. Because cartilage is a rubbery material, it allows the whole

rib cage to move a little with breathing. The breastbone shields the chest and consists of several bones that have grown together and fused. The ribs that attach to the sternum are called *true ribs*. The next three pairs of ribs don't meet in the middle. They are called *false ribs*. They join to the cartilage of the ribs above them. The last two pairs of ribs don't attach to anything in the front, and are shorter. They are called *floating ribs*.

The joints   The area where two bones meet is called a *joint*. Most joints in the body are built so that they can move. Basically, the bones at a joint are held together and steadied by strong, white bands called *ligaments*. The ligaments are made of collagen fibers (see page 141) that attach directly to the bones on either side of the joint. They are helped by muscles that also attach across the joint from one bone to another.

At a joint, the ends of the bones never touch directly— there is a small space between them. In this space is a tough, fluid-filled sac. The lining of the sac makes a clear yellow fluid that fills the sac. This liquid, called *synovial fluid*, helps to lubricate or "grease" the joint, and makes it easier for the bones to slide over one another.

Types of joints

Type	Place	Movement
Hinge	Elbow, ankle	Bends in one direction only
Pivot	Skull	Rotates
Gliding	Wrist	Slides up and down
Ball and socket	Hip, shoulder	Moves all directions in a circle
Saddle	Thumb	Bends in two directions

between muscles and make them slide over one another more easily.

Different joints have different types of movements. The kind of movement a joint can make is determined by the shape of the bones and the location of the muscles and ligaments that hold the bones together. Some joints bend like a hinge, some turn like an axle, some swivel like a ball and socket.

The ends of the bones themselves are covered with a layer of shiny, slippery cartilage, which also makes for smoother sliding. In some joints there are separate cartilage pads that cushion the joint and make it steadier. Joints that receive tremendous pressure have a number of other little fluid-filled sacs called *bursae*, which also help to reduce friction and make movement easier. Bursae are found under the skin at the elbow and knee and help the skin to slide over the joint. Other bursae are found

Growth and anatomy of a long bone Bones are made up of long protein ropes called *collagen fibers*. Crystals of calcium are stuck to these fibers. The fibers make the bones strong; the calcium makes them hard. This framework is laced with many

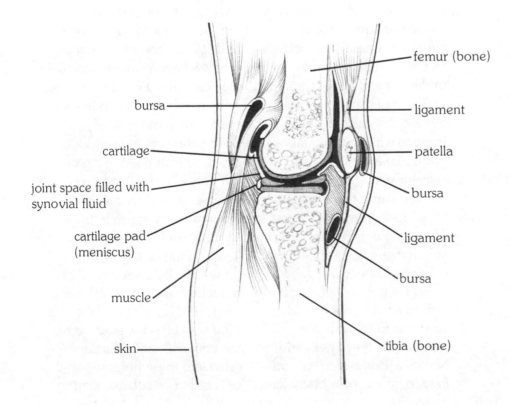

femur (bone)
bursa
ligament
cartilage
patella
joint space filled with synovial fluid
bursa
cartilage pad (meniscus)
ligament
muscle
bursa
skin
tibia (bone)

This drawing shows the inside of the knee joint. Joints are the places where two bones meet. Fluid and cartilage cushion the bones so they can move over one another easily.

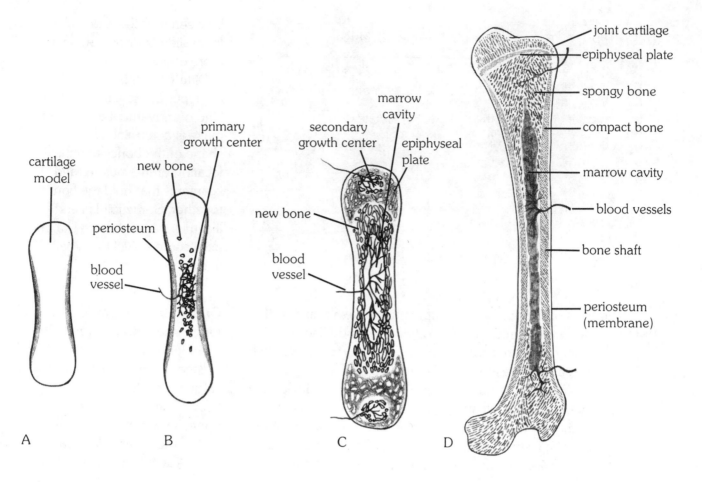

joint cartilage

epiphyseal plate

spongy bone

compact bone

marrow cavity

blood vessels

bone shaft

periosteum (membrane)

marrow cavity

secondary growth center

epiphyseal plate

new bone

blood vessel

primary growth center

new bone

periosteum

blood vessel

cartilage model

A

B

C

D

A. Bones begin growing as rubbery cartilage.

B. The cartilage starts turning to bone in the middle.

C. The bone gets longer as new growth centers form at the ends of the bones.

D. The bone stops growing when all the cartilage inside has turned to bone.

tunnels. In spongy bone the tunnels are quite big; in compact bone the tunnels are so tiny they can be seen only under a microscope. Caught in this mesh of tunnels are live bone cells, which become trapped while making the bony framework. The bone cells have long tubes that reach out into the tiny tunnels to get food from blood vessels. Throughout the bone, live cells that are not trapped continue to build.

Bones start developing long before a baby is born and continue to grow until a person is in his or her early twenties. Bones start as *cartilage,* a very solid rubbery kind

of connective tissue. The cartilage serves as a rough model and framework for the bones that will later form. Only cartilage can grow as fast as a baby needs to grow; bone is made much more slowly.

The cartilage framework is replaced with bone in a gradual process. The first step is when tiny hard crystals of calcium start to form in the cartilage and make it hard. Then, in the center of long bones, the cartilage cells that made the original model start to die and leave little holes. Tiny new blood vessels from the covering of the cartilage grow into these holes. Special cells called *osteoblasts* start to make hard bone. Other cells called *osteoclasts* dissolve the solid bone making more little tunnels through it so that more blood vessels can come in, bringing food to the osteoblasts. What forms is a material that looks like a sponge but is made hard by the calcium crystals.

As this spongy bone replaces the cartilage, the osteoclasts dissolve a big hollow space in the center of the bone. This hollow is called the *marrow cavity*. It helps to lighten the bones and becomes a place where blood cells are made and blood vessels bring food to the bone cells.

Meanwhile, in the midsection of the bone, osteoblasts in the bone covering begin to make layer upon layer of bone around the outside. This makes the bone thicker. Unlike the spongy bone, this *compact bone* is firmly packed and has only microscopic tunnels through it. It is the compact bone which makes bones strong.

About the time that a hollow marrow cavity starts to form in the middle of the bones, new growth centers appear at the ends. They are called *secondary growth centers*. Here, the same bone-forming process occurs: Cartilage cells begin to die, osteoblasts come in and lay down bone, and osteoclasts make tunnels through this bone so that blood vessels can grow in.

In this way new spongy bone is made near the ends of the bones, too.

Dissolving old bone frees up calcium, which is then used in the work of muscles and nerves, as well as in building new bone elsewhere. This process of dissolving and rebuilding goes on for a person's whole life. If it stopped, the bones would become brittle and break. The rebuilding of the bones can make them even stronger. As more force is put on a particular bone, the osteoblasts make it thicker. The harder people exercise or work, the bigger and stronger their bones become.

The growing bone has a large area of spongy and compact bone in the middle and in small areas at both tips. In between are flat areas of cartilage. These areas are called *epiphyseal plates* or *growth plates*. They are what cause the bone to grow longer. The cartilage cells in the plates divide rapidly and make new cells. The new cartilage cells toward the middle of the bone die and are replaced by bone cells.

Ages when bone growth-centers fuse

Bone growth stops when growth centers at the ends of bones fuse with the middle. The list shows the *average* age when this happens.

Joint	Growth	Boys' age (years)	Girls' age (years)
Elbow	starts (upper arm)	13	11
	finishes (forearm)	15	13
Ankle	starts (big toe)	14	13
	finishes (leg)	16	14
Wrist	starts (fingers)	15	13
	finishes (forearm)	18	16
Knee	starts	15	14
	finishes	18	16
Hip	starts (leg joint)	16	14
	finishes (pelvis)	after 18	18
Shoulder	starts	16	14
	finishes	after 18	18

The new cartilage cells toward the tip keep dividing. In this way the cartilage plates leave hard bone behind them and move outward as the bone grows longer.

This process of bone growth goes on for years. When the bone reaches its full size, the cartilage cells in the plates stop dividing, die, and are replaced by hard bone. At this point the spongy bone growing in the center reaches the spongy bone at the tips. This is called *fusion*. Now all the cartilage cells have been replaced by bone cells and the bone is solid and can't grow anymore.

In the tibia bone in the lower leg, bone starts to replace the cartilage in the middle before a baby is even born. The secondary growth centers appear at the ends by the age of two, first at the top near the knee, then at the bottom near the ankle. The growth plates cause the bone to slowly grow longer for more than 15 years. In the tibia the growth plate by the ankle stops dividing and fuses at about 17, the plate at the knee by about 20. All the long bones of the arms and legs have a secondary growth center at either end. But the exact time when these centers appear and when they fuse is different for each bone. Most secondary growth centers appear in the first or second year, but some not till the fifth or even twelfth year. Just as teeth tend to appear in a set order, the secondary growth centers tend to appear in a fixed pattern. Like teeth, the exact age that any one of the centers appears varies slightly from one child to another.

The teeth

Humans, like most mammals, get two sets of teeth. (Sharks get four!) The first set of human teeth are called *baby*, or *deciduous*, teeth because they fall out during childhood. The second set are called *permanent* teeth because, if

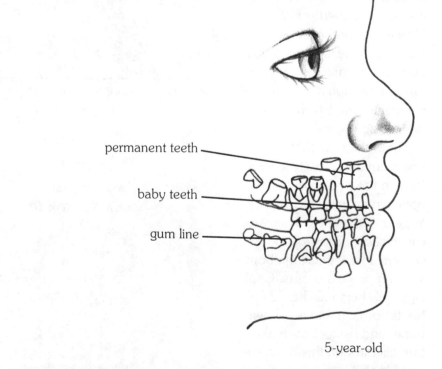

permanent teeth

baby teeth

gum line

5-year-old

The permanent teeth are starting to form in the jaw before the baby teeth fall out. As the jaw grows and the baby teeth are lost, the permanent teeth move into position.

Eruption chart for permanent teeth

This table gives the *average* age of eruption (in years). Some children's teeth come in earlier, some later.

Teeth	Upper jaw	Lower jaw
Central incisors	7–8	6–7
Lateral incisors	8–9	7–8
Cuspids (canines)	11–12	9–11
1st premolars	10–11	10–12
2nd premolars	10–12	11–13
1st molars	5½–7	5½–7
2nd molars	12–14	12–13
3rd molars	17–30	17–30

they are well cared for, they will last a lifetime.

The first teeth start to form long before babies are born. While teeth are forming they are completely below the gum and cannot be seen, but they do show up on an X-ray. The hard part on the outside of a tooth, the *enamel,* is completely formed before the tooth comes through the gum or *erupts.* The *dentine,* the living part inside, keeps growing for years after the tooth has come in. The age at which children's teeth come through the gum can vary by months, even years. Some children tend to get their teeth earlier than others.

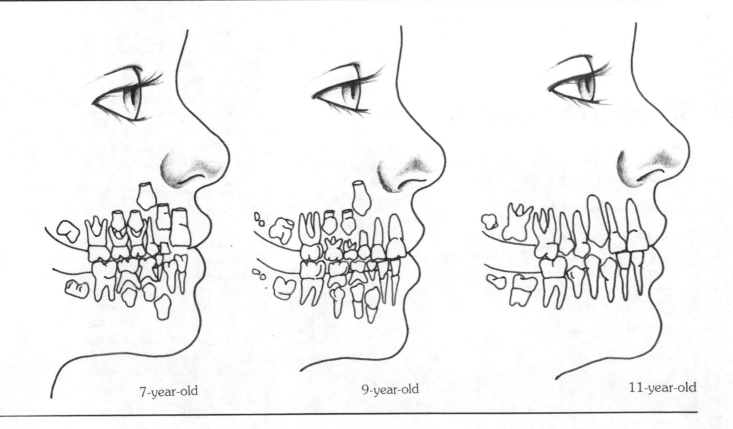

7-year-old   9-year-old   11-year-old

There are 20 baby teeth and 32 permanent ones. Dentists have special names for each tooth. The front teeth are called *incisors*. They are narrow and sharp and are made for tearing or biting through food. There are four incisors, two on the top and two on the bottom. On each side of the incisors there is a long, sharp, pointed tooth called a *cuspid*. Cuspids are also called the *eye teeth*, or the *canines*, because they look like a dog's teeth.

Behind the canines are *bicuspids* or *pre-molars*. They have two points, or cusps, and are rather flat. These do not occur in the baby teeth, only in the permanent set. The bicuspids' job is to grind up food, making it easier to digest.

Behind the bicuspids are the *molars*. They are large flat teeth with small points on them. These teeth are perfectly shaped to crush food into tiny pieces. In the baby teeth there are two molars on the back of each jaw; in the permanent set there are three molars. The third pair of molars is known as the *wisdom teeth* because they come in when a person is grown-up. But they are sometimes missing altogether.

Teeth tend to come through the gum in the same sequence in all kids. The sequence is slightly different for baby teeth and permanent teeth. The first grown-up teeth to come in are the first molars. They are sometimes called the *six-year molars* because they usually come in between five and

Shedding chart for baby teeth

This table shows the average age of losing baby teeth (in years). Some children lose their teeth earlier, some later.

Teeth	Upper jaw	Lower jaw
Central incisors	7–8	6–7
Lateral incisors	8–9	7–8
Cuspids (canines)	11–12	9–11
1st molars	9–11	10–12
2nd molars	9–12	11–13

Tooth games

Look at an old tooth you have lost. You can see the crown, the neck, and the beginning of the roots.

Make a mold of your teeth. The simplest way is to press a clean piece of Silly Putty or clay against your upper teeth and another against your lower teeth. If you want to make a real model, pour plaster of Paris into these molds. After it hardens, peel off the clay or Silly Putty.

Put an old tooth in a glass of soda pop. Take the tooth out and look at it two or three times a week. What happens to the tooth after several weeks?

Eat a bite of the following foods: a raw carrot, a piece of meat, a cracker, a piece of sticky candy, a nut, a raw apple, a piece of cheese, a piece of celery, a graham cracker. Which teeth do you use to eat each food? Do you start chewing with some teeth and then switch to others? Which foods stick to your teeth? Which foods get caught between your teeth? Which foods naturally clean your teeth?

Check how well you brush your teeth. Brush as usual. Then chew up a colored disclosing tablet you get from your dentist. Now look carefully in the mirror to see if the color has stuck to any plaque on your teeth that you missed with the brush.

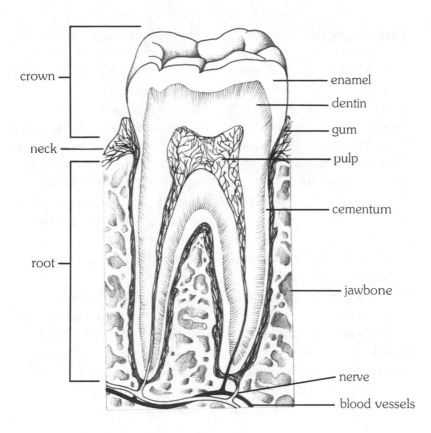

crown

neck

root

enamel
dentin
gum
pulp
cementum
jawbone
nerve
blood vessels

The inside of a tooth is alive and contains blood vessels and a nerve. Most of the tooth is under the gum and is cemented to the jawbone.

seven. The permanent molars don't replace baby teeth; they come in behind the baby molars as the jaw grows longer. All the permanent teeth toward the front replace baby teeth as they fall out. As the permanent teeth push toward the surface they actually dissolve or erode the roots of the baby teeth.

Including the wisdom teeth, there are teeth forming from before birth until a person is over 20. The permanent teeth actually start forming by about three months.

Tooth structure   Dentists divide a tooth into three areas: the crown, the neck, and the

root. The *crown* is the part of the tooth you can see above the gum. The *root*—the part that attaches the tooth to the jawbone—is below the gum. The *neck* is the area at the gumline where the root and crown meet.

Every tooth is made up of several layers. The crown is covered with *enamel*. Enamel is composed of tiny crystals of calcium stuck in a mesh of tiny hairlike fibers. These crystals are the hardest part of the tooth. In fact, they are the hardest thing in the body. The mesh is made of a special protein, similar to that in hair, that is very hard to dissolve.

Enamel buildup on all but

the wisdom teeth is finished by about eight years of age. This is why good nutrition, and especially enough calcium, is so important in the early years. During this same period, fluoride in drinking water will also be absorbed by tooth enamel and make it harder.

Most of the rest of the tooth is made of *dentine*. It lies beneath the enamel. The dentine is composed of calcium crystals embedded in a different kind of mesh than the enamel. The fiber in this mesh is made of the leathery protein called collagen. Calcium crystals make the dentine hard; the collagen makes the tooth strong so it won't break. Bones are also made of collagen and calcium, but have nerves and blood vessels running through them (see page 141).

In the center of the tooth is the *pulp*. It is made of a nerve and blood vessels in a tube. The pulp brings food and oxygen to the cells in the dentine.

The tooth fits into a tight hole, or socket, in the jawbone. The covering of the lower tooth holds it in this socket. It is called *cementum*. The cementum actually has fibers of collagen that run out into the bone.

The pulp, the dentine, and the cementum are living tissues. The calcium in them is constantly renewed by the body. Only the enamel is not renewed once it is formed. Cavities are a disease of the teeth in which the enamel is dissolved by enzymes and acid made by bacteria (see page 310). The bacteria live in food stuck to the teeth, and they especially like sugar. Since the enamel is made before the teeth come in and cannot be remade, it is very important for kids to take good care of their teeth.

Muscles give the body shape.

Michelangelo. Studies for the Libyan Sibyl. 15th–16th cent. Red chalk on paper. 11⅜ × 8⅜". The Metropolitan Museum of Art, New York. Purchase, 1924, Joseph Pulitzer Bequest.

The muscles

Almost half the body is made of muscle. In fact, there are over 400 muscles in the body. Muscles are the parts of the body that make things move. They do this by alternately contracting and getting shorter, then relaxing and getting longer. The name *muscle* comes from the Latin word for tiny mouse, because some muscles look like a mouse under the skin when they move.

There are three types of muscles in the body. Under a microscope the cells in each kind look different, but they all move or contract. The first two kinds of muscle work without a person thinking about them. They are the *cardiac* muscle of the heart and the *smooth* muscles of the digestive system and the blood vessels. The third kind are the *skeletal* muscles. They are the muscles that move the body when people decide to move. They are called skeletal muscles because all but a few are attached at each end to bones in the skeleton.

Each skeletal muscle is made up of thousands of elastic fibers that are like rubber bands. A number of these fibers join to make a *bundle*. A number of bundles join to make up a single muscle. Each

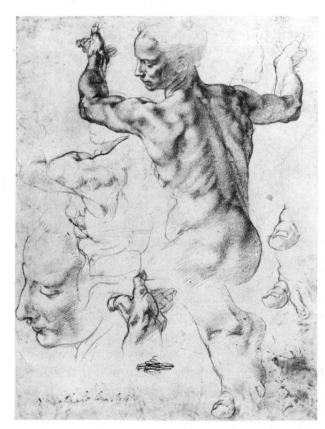

muscle is wrapped in a tough, white, shiny covering called a *sheath*. And every muscle has many nerve endings attached to it. These nerves bring the messages from the brain telling the muscle bundles when to contract, or shorten, and when to relax, or lengthen.

When people lift something light, a few muscle fibers tighten. When people lift something heavy, a lot of muscle bundles tighten. But each fiber can only squeeze for less than a second. In order for someone to carry something heavy for a long distance, groups of muscle fibers must tighten one after another.

Inside the muscle are many blood vessels. They bring food to the muscle, which gives the fibers the energy to contract. They also take away the waste products that are left after the food has been used up in the muscle fibers. The process is somewhat like running a car: gas is put in, the car burns it to move, and exhaust comes out.

When a muscle uses up all the food and oxygen brought in by the blood, it starts to lose its power. The muscle rests when it stops contracting. New food and oxygen are brought in and the waste products (carbon dioxide and lactic acid) are taken away. If the waste is not taken away, the muscle sends messages to the brain that it is tired. Finally, the muscle will start to hurt or ache.

Everyone has the same number of muscles and almost the same number of fibers in a particular muscle. But some people are stronger than others. This is because they use their muscles more. The more muscles are used, the bigger the fibers get and the bigger the blood vessels in the muscle become. If muscles are not used, they will become weak and flabby and actually shrink. This is called *atrophy-*

ing. It can happen when people have an arm or leg in a cast for a very long time.

As kids grow and use their muscles, the muscle fibers become longer and wider. Muscles grow very fast when children are babies, then grow more slowly for a long time. As kids start to reach adolescence, their muscles again start to grow very rapidly. In boys, muscles are usually growing fast at the same time

A count of the muscles of the body

Face	17
Hand (each)	19
Eye	6
Neck	14
Back	20
Abdomen	9
Foot (each)	17
Forearm	19
Chest	6

Muscles in unusual places

Pupil of the eye
Tongue
Heart
Stomach

There are many layers of muscle under the skin. Muscles make the body move.

Tchelitchew, Pavel. The Cave of Sleep: Series of 18 gouache designs for the ballet. 1941. Unproduced. Costume design, gouache. 14 × 11". Collection, The Museum of Modern Art, New York. Gift of the artist.

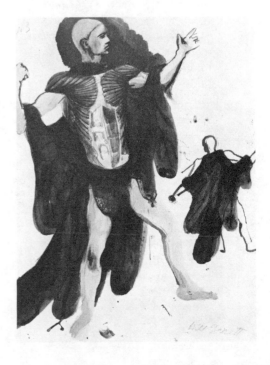

This drawing shows the topmost layer of muscles in the front of the body. Muscles generally act in groups, bending and lifting parts of the body.

Muscle games

Get a whole chicken leg. First remove the skin. Watch the muscles move when you bend the leg. Try pulling a muscle to see what *it* moves. Notice where the tendons attach the muscle to bone.

Try feeling your own tendons. Turn your head and feel the tendon that sticks out in front at the bottom of your neck. Bend up your foot and feel your Achilles tendon at the back of your leg just above the heel. Feel the two hamstring tendons on either side of the back of your knee. Raise your big toe and feel the tendon on top that pulls it up. Make your hand into a claw and see tendons on the underside of your wrist and on the back of your hand. Wiggle your fingers and watch the tendons move in the back of your hand.

Try feeling your muscles. Move any part of your body. Try to figure out what muscle or muscles contract to make that movement. The muscles that are doing the work will feel hard (see page 251). Use the muscle drawings to help you. For example, put your hand on your cheek. Feel what happens when you chew.

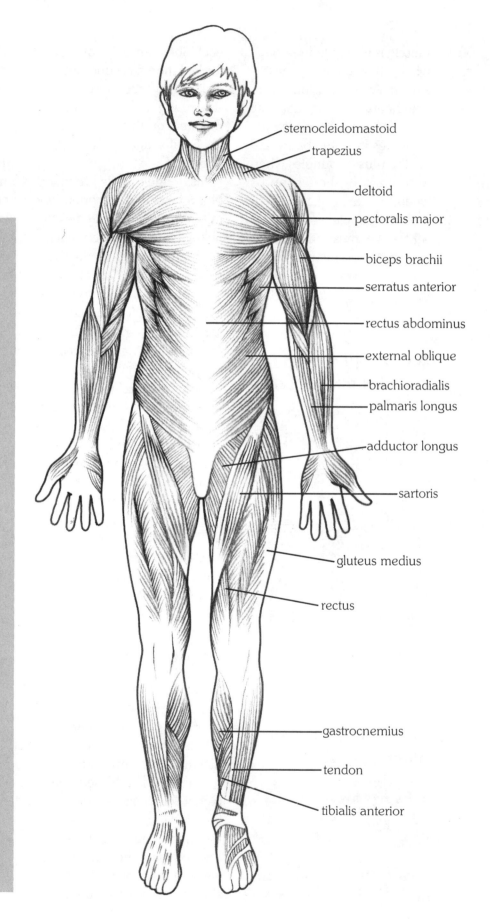

- sternocleidomastoid
- trapezius
- deltoid
- pectoralis major
- biceps brachii
- serratus anterior
- rectus abdominus
- external oblique
- brachioradialis
- palmaris longus
- adductor longus
- sartoris
- gluteus medius
- rectus
- gastrocnemius
- tendon
- tibialis anterior

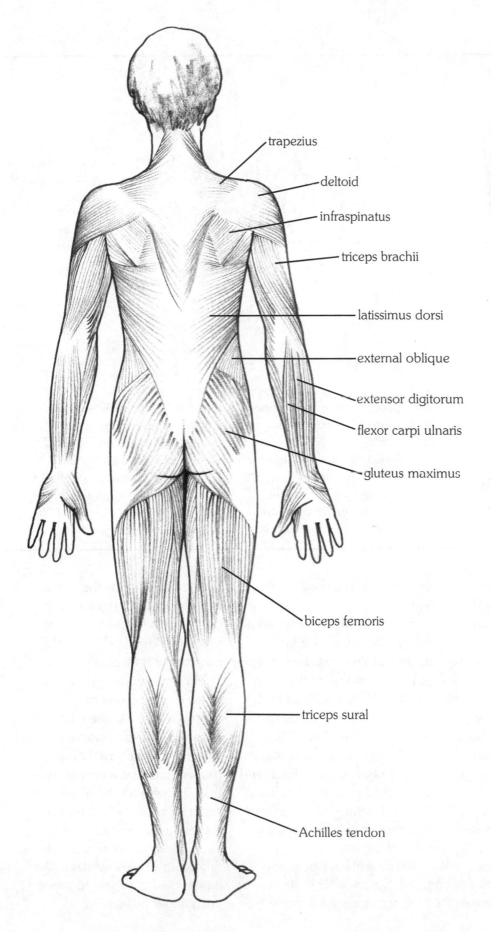

trapezius

deltoid

infraspinatus

triceps brachii

latissimus dorsi

external oblique

extensor digitorum

flexor carpi ulnaris

gluteus maximus

biceps femoris

triceps sural

Achilles tendon

This drawing shows the top layer of muscles in the back of the body. Muscles end in narrow bands or wide sheets of tough white connective tissue that attaches to bones. The narrow bands are called tendons. Sometimes they are long. Long tendons act like a rope and help the muscle pull a bone that is far away.

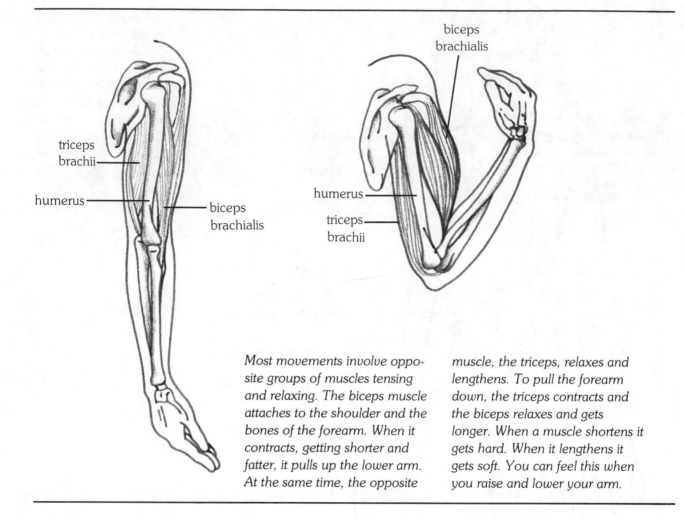

triceps
brachii

humerus

biceps
brachialis

biceps
brachialis

humerus

triceps
brachii

Most movements involve opposite groups of muscles tensing and relaxing. The biceps muscle attaches to the shoulder and the bones of the forearm. When it contracts, getting shorter and fatter, it pulls up the lower arm. At the same time, the opposite muscle, the triceps, relaxes and lengthens. To pull the forearm down, the triceps contracts and the biceps relaxes and gets longer. When a muscle shortens it gets hard. When it lengthens it gets soft. You can feel this when you raise and lower your arm.

as the body is spurting up in height. Girls' muscle growth tends to come 6 months *after* their height has spurted.

Kids don't reach their maximum muscle strength until several years after their muscles have stopped growing. Up to the age of 11, boys are not much stronger than girls. In fact, a big girl is likely to be stronger than a small boy. But between 10 and 16, boys generally become quite a bit stronger than girls, especially in the arms and chest. This growth is tied up with the development of the reproductive organs (see pages 210 to 220).

Every skeletal muscle has a fat middle, called the *belly,* and two thin ends. The ends join the covering of the bone to which they are attached with tough, shiny bands of tissue called *tendons.* The attachment is so strong that it almost *never* breaks. Each end is attached to a different bone. When the muscle contracts or shortens, it pulls one bone toward the other.

Muscles always pull, never push. So, in order to work they are arranged in pairs:

One muscle bends the arm or leg, the other straightens it; one muscle turns the arm or leg toward the body, and the other turns it away.

Most movements require more than one pair of muscles; they require whole groups of muscles working together. The more different movements that a part of the body can make, the more separate muscles that part of the body has. For example, each hand has more than 19 different muscles, which make it possible for people to move each finger by itself.

Your face muscles

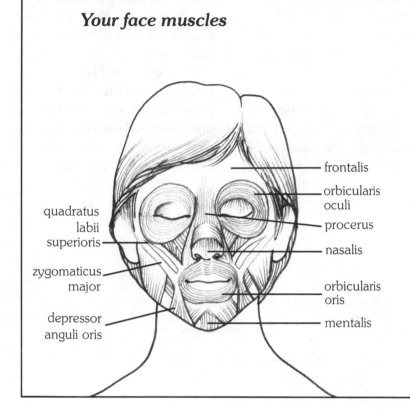

quadratus labii superioris

zygomaticus major

depressor anguli oris

frontalis

orbicularis oculi

procerus

nasalis

orbicularis oris

mentalis

The muscles of the face make it possible for people to show a huge number of expressions, ranging from joy to sadness. They also enable people to chew their food and make certain sounds. There are 16 muscles in the face. They mostly come in pairs, one on each side. The pairs work together, as when people shut their eyes; or they may work independently, as when people wink. Most facial expressions need the combined work of a group of muscles, some contracting, some relaxing. A smile, for example, requires several pairs of muscles. The muscles of the face are unusual because most of them attach to the bottom layer of skin, not to bone.

How muscles move

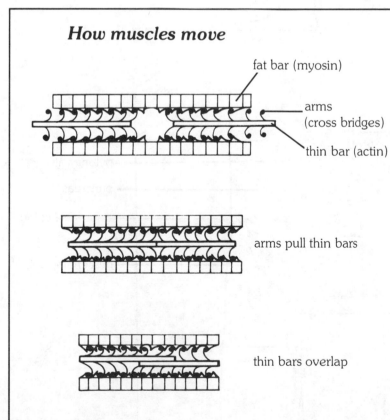

fat bar (myosin)

arms (cross bridges)

thin bar (actin)

arms pull thin bars

thin bars overlap

Each muscle fiber is made up of hundreds of thousands of tiny bars made out of protein. There are two kinds of bars. One kind is fat and doesn't move. It has lines of tiny arms. The other kind is thin and slides between the fat bars. It has little places where the arms can grab hold. When the brain sends a message to a muscle to move, the little arms on the fat bars grab hold of the thin bars and pull them along a short distance. Then the arms let go and grab hold again a little way back and pull once more. Finally the thin bars will overlap. In this way the whole muscle becomes shorter and fatter when it contracts. The arms are so tiny they are barely visible under the most powerful microscope in the world.

The digestive system

The job of the digestive system is to turn the food people eat into a form the body can use to grow and make energy. First, big pieces of food are broken up into little pieces, and then the little pieces are separated into small simple molecules. Useful molecules are taken to all parts of the body by the bloodstream, and all nonuseful material is sent on out of the body.

The digestive system is basically a long tube connected to the outside at both ends and divided into several areas that do different jobs in the process of digestion. Each area is like a chemical laboratory, adding special substances, called *enzymes,* to the food. The enzymes help the body break down the food.

Food enters the body through the mouth. Here powerful muscles of the jaw grind the food between the teeth. Three pairs of *salivary glands* release saliva, a liquid that moistens the food, making it easier to swallow.

The digestive system is a long tube with special parts and is open to the outside at each end. This group of organs breaks down food and absorbs it.

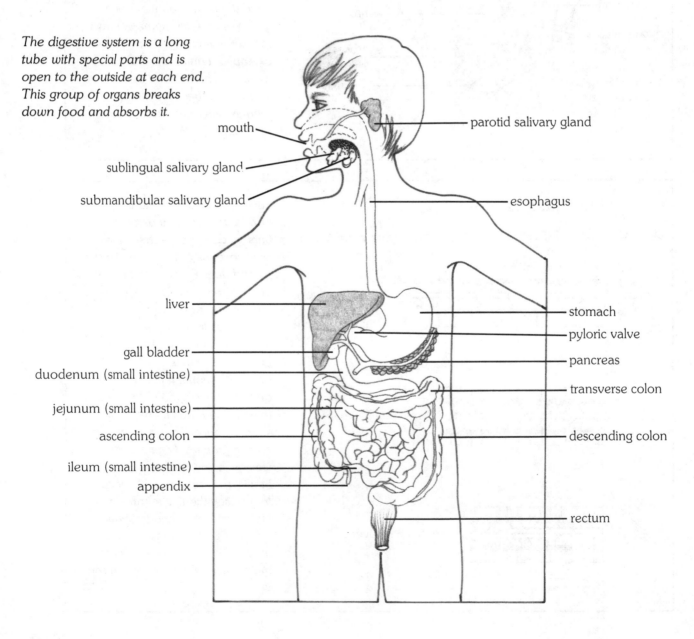

mouth

sublingual salivary gland

submandibular salivary gland

parotid salivary gland

esophagus

liver

gall bladder

duodenum (small intestine)

jejunum (small intestine)

ascending colon

ileum (small intestine)

appendix

stomach

pyloric valve

pancreas

transverse colon

descending colon

rectum

Saliva also contains enzymes that break down the carbohydrates in foods like bread and potatoes. The salivary glands are located under the tongue and below the ear.

The food is then swallowed, passing into the back of the throat and down into a tube called the *esophagus* (see page 157). Esophagus comes from the Greek word for "I carry food." Rings of muscles in the esophagus squeeze behind the food one after another, pushing it down. It's like squeezing a tube of toothpaste and sliding your finger all the way down to the cap. This motion of pushing food is called *peristalsis*, and it is the way food is moved along through the whole *gastrointestinal* (digestive) *system.*

The esophagus opens into the *stomach*, a soft muscular bag that can stretch to hold almost a quart of food. The stomach stores food so that people can eat a whole meal. Otherwise they would have to constantly eat small amounts. Cells in the stomach wall secrete *hydrochloric acid* and enzymes that dissolve protein and thicken milk so that it will stay in the stomach long enough for its protein to be digested. The hydrochloric acid kills most of the bacteria in the food. Other cells in the stomach wall secrete *mucus*, a sticky liquid that keeps the lining of the stomach from being dissolved by its own acid. The muscles of the stomach wall squeeze in a rippling motion that mixes the food with the enzymes a little at a time.

By the time the food is ready to leave the stomach it has turned into a thick, milky liquid called *chyme* (rhymes with "time"). At this point the muscular contractions of the stomach become strong enough to push the chyme through the flap called the *pyloric valve* at the bottom of the stomach.

The food then enters the

Digestion of food

Part of body	Length	Job	Time food normally spends there
Mouth	about 4"	Chews food. Breaks down carbohydrates like bread with the saliva.	Under 1 minute
Esophagus	10"	Moves food to stomach.	Under 1 minute
Stomach	about 6"	Mixes food. Stores food. Dissolves proteins like meat. Thickens or curds milk.	20 min. to 3–4 hours
Small intestine	23'	Breaks down carbohydrates, proteins, and fats, and absorbs them into the blood.	4–8 hours
Large intestine	5'	Absorbs remaining water and minerals. Stores waste products temporarily.	10–12 hours

small intestine. It is here that most of the food is broken down into molecule size and absorbed into the blood. First, the chyme is mixed with three enzymes. Cells in the wall of the small intestine itself make *intestinal juice.* The other two enzymes come from other organs. *Pancreatic juice* is made by the pancreas, a finger-shaped gland that lies behind the stomach. It is the most important of the digestive chemicals. And the liver makes *bile,* a greenish fluid that acts like a dish detergent. It breaks fats into little globules that the other enzymes can then break down. Intestinal juice and pancreatic juice break down protein from meat and dairy products, carbohydrates from bread and fruit, and fats from meat, oil, and butter.

When the food is fully digested it is absorbed into the blood through the *villi,* finger-like projections from the wall of the intestine (see pages 157–58). They bring the food in touch with the blood. What remains after this is water, leftover enzymes, mineral salts, and indigestible plant fibers.

The same peristaltic motions that have mixed the food in the small intestine move the leftover material on into the *large intestine.* The large intestine is the home of millions of bacteria. These bacteria live there normally and are helpful. They feed on the leftover plant fibers. In the process they produce many things, including vitamins B and K, which are needed by the body. In the large intestine most of the remaining water is absorbed, along with more minerals that are needed by the body.

The waste material now remaining is called *feces* (fēecēes), which comes from the Latin word for dregs or leftovers. The feces are squeezed on into the *rectum,*

In the first step in swallowing, the tongue pushes the food back. Next the soft palate rises to keep food from entering the back of the nose. And the voice box rises to keep food from going down the windpipe. Once food enters the esophagus, muscles push it down to the stomach.

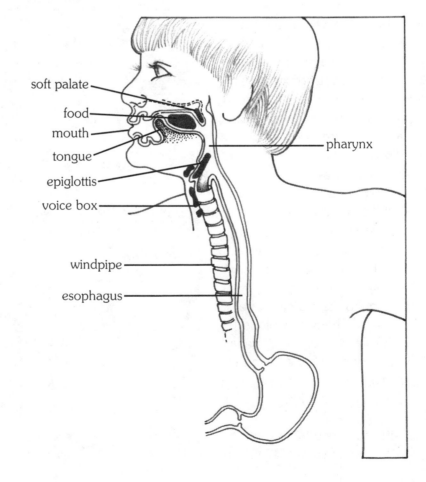

soft palate
food
mouth
tongue
epiglottis
voice box
windpipe
esophagus
pharynx

a storage area at the bottom of the large intestine. Here it is collected for a time and then expelled as a bowel movement (see page 161). The characteristic color of a bowel movement comes from left-over bile salts; the odor comes from the bacteria that live in the large intestine.

Swallowing Swallowing is the means by which food gets from the mouth to the stomach. Swallowing feels easy, but it is no simple matter because the back of the throat opens into the nose, mouth, windpipe, and esophagus, and in order to swallow properly the body has to close off all the openings except for the esophagus. Otherwise food would go into the back of the nose or down the windpipe.

First, the chewed food is pushed to the back of the throat when the tongue raises up to touch the roof of the mouth. As food touches the back of the throat, it alerts nerves there, which send messages to the swallowing center in the brain. This center automatically signals all the swallowing muscles to work together. The *soft palate,* or "roof," at the back of the mouth is pulled up and covers the opening to the nose. At the same time the vocal cords close across the windpipe and the whole voice box rises, pushing a flap called the *epiglottis* down over the windpipe (see Breathing, page 165). Thus, the mouth, nose, and windpipe are all closed off and the only opening left is the esophagus. Finally, the muscles of the *pharynx,* the back of the throat, push the food into the esophagus, where it is squeezed down into the stomach by peristalsis.

The villi Most food is absorbed into the blood through the wall of the small intestine. Only a little food can

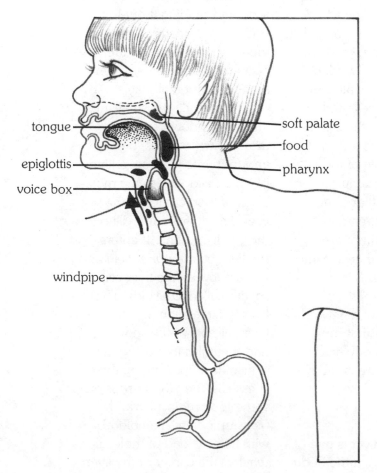

tongue

epiglottis

voice box

windpipe

soft palate

food

pharynx

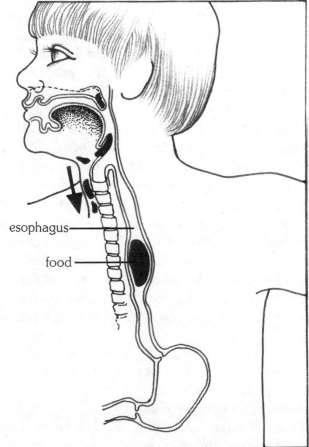

esophagus

food

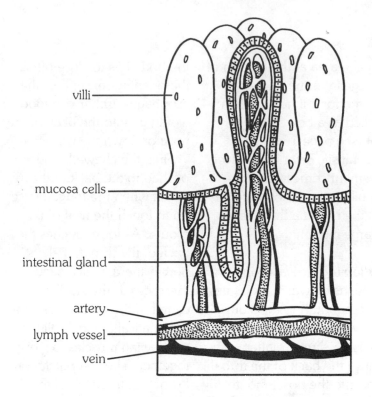

The inside of the small intestine is covered with tiny fingers called villi, which absorb food into the blood. This drawing shows how the villi look under a microscope.

villi

mucosa cells

intestinal gland

artery

lymph vessel

vein

be absorbed at any point in the wall, so the more wall space there is, the better. The small intestine is so long it loops around on itself like a pile of thick rope. In addition, the inside of the tube, instead of being smooth, is covered with big wrinkles or folds. These folds look like a shaggy carpet, with millions of little fingers called villi sticking out. Finally, the sides of the villi themselves are covered with hairlike threads (too small to be drawn on the illustration). Due to the folds, the villi, and the hairlike threads, the absorbing area of the small intestine is as big as a football field.

Sugars, minerals, and amino acids (the tiny parts into which proteins are broken down) pass through the walls of the villi into the villi's tiny blood vessels, and then go to

the liver and the rest of the body. Food does not just flow across the cells of the villi walls. It is actively pumped by chemicals that lock onto food molecules when they touch the outside of the wall, carry them across the cell, and release them into the blood vessels. Each time a carrier moves a molecule of food it uses up a little energy.

Fats, on the other hand, enter the bloodstream in a different way. Without the help of a carrier they slip into ducts called *lacteals* in the center of the villi. These lacteals are part of a network of lymph vessels that run throughout the body and enter the bloodstream above the heart.

The liver   The liver is one of the largest organs in the body.

It does a number of different jobs, including storing digested food and sending it out to the body as it is needed. This means that the cells of the body can get a steady, even amount of food all day.

After a meal, the small intestine breaks down carbohydrates, like potatoes, bread, and fruit, into glucose, a kind of sugar. Blood carrying molecules of food comes to the liver directly from the villi of the small intestine. It enters the liver by the *portal vein* and flows between the liver cells in spaces called *sinusoids*. The liver is like a sponge, with the liver cells being the sponge and the holes in it being the sinusoids. In passing by the liver cells, the blood drops off some food molecules and picks up others. The blood, with its new load of molecules, reaches the center of the liver

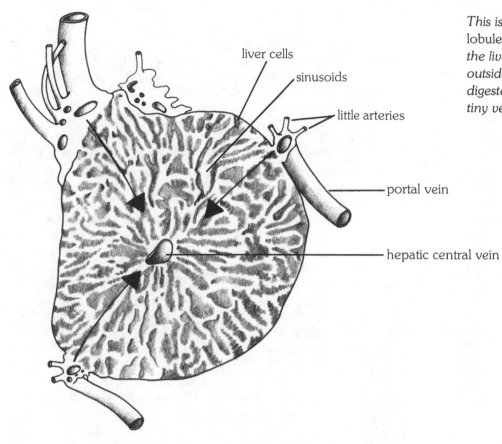

liver cells

sinusoids

little arteries

portal vein

hepatic central vein

This is a microscopic drawing of a lobule, a tiny part of the inside of the liver. Blood comes from the outside, drops off or picks up digested food, and leaves by the tiny vein in the middle.

What the liver does

Makes bile, an enzyme that digests fats

Stores sugar by making and dissolving glycogen from glucose

Breaks down and stores fat

Breaks down and stores amino acids, the building blocks of protein

Makes fat chemicals like phospholipids (for nerves) and cholesterol

Makes protein chemicals like albumin, globulin (anti-bodies), and fibrinogen (blood clotting)

Clears the blood of poisons, such as drugs, toxins, old hormones, and chemicals, and makes them harmless

Stores vitamins A, D, B_{12}

Stores extra blood

Digestion games

Swallow over and over until there's no saliva left in your mouth. Now chew a piece of bread and try to swallow it. See how important saliva is to moisten food and make it easier to swallow.

Cut off the end of an old toothpaste or shampoo tube. Fill it with a thick batter of flour and water. Now circle the tube with your thumb and second finger, and slide down the tube, squeezing out the batter. This is somewhat like how the food is moved through the digestive system by peristalsis.

Add a rennet tablet to a cup of warm milk. Rennet is the stomach enzyme *rennin,* from a cow. In a few minutes it will curd the milk. The same thing happens to milk in your stomach.

Put your hand on your Adam's apple. Now swallow. What happens to your Adam's apple? Compare what you felt with the drawings about swallowing.

Hear the sounds of digestion. Put your head against a friend's stomach, or listen to it with a stethoscope.

Thoroughly mix one-half teaspoon of cornstarch with one-quarter cup of boiling water. Let it cool. Now add one teaspoon of saliva. Every minute take a half teaspoon of the mixture and add a drop of iodine. At first the iodine will react with the starch and turn it blue. But as the saliva turns the starch to sugar, the iodine will turn the mixture less and less blue. This is how saliva begins to digest your food.

Place a very thin slice of meat in a bowl. Cover it with vinegar and leave it for several days. Vinegar is a mild acid and will soften or digest the meat. You can try this with meat tenderizer, which also contains a digestive enzyme.

Place one cup of flour, one-half cup of water, and five drops of food coloring in a plastic bag. Tie the top and knead the bag three times a minute until the mixture is all the same color. This is how the stomach churns when it is digesting food.

Ask a friend to stand on his or her head. Then have the person take a sip from a cup of water and swallow. Peristalsis will make the water go "up" to the person's stomach.

and leaves by way of the *hepatic vein,* then joins other blood going to the heart.

After a meal, so much glucose comes to the liver that it is more than the body can use at once. So a lot of the glucose is picked up by liver cells and chemically bundled into long chains of sugar. These chains, called *glycogen,* are ideal for storing. Between meals, at night, and during heavy exercise, glucose is needed by the body; at these times, the chains of glycogen

are broken down again and sent out.

The liver also stores iron, copper, proteins, fat, vitamins A, D, and B_{12}, and even blood. It stocks up these materials when the body has too much of them and later sends them out in constant, steady amounts as they are needed.

In addition to its storage functions, the liver manufactures bile and many special proteins. Bile is sent to the small intestine to aid in the digestion of fats. Using the

amino acids that come from the small intestine, the liver makes proteins necessary for blood clotting, antibodies for fighting bacteria, and many other proteins. The liver also transforms and stores the fats that are brought to it.

Finally, the liver filters out dangerous chemicals in the body and makes them less harmful. They are then attached to the bile, sent to the small intestine, and eventually eliminated from the body.

Defecation   The body's solid wastes, the feces, are stored in the middle part of the large intestine, which is called the *colon.* Wavelike motions of the colon (peristalsis) move the waste down into the rectum. The waste is held in by two muscular rings in the *anus,* a short tube that connects the rectum to the outside. These rings are called *sphincters.*

Special nerves in the walls of the rectum send a message to the bottom of the spinal cord when waste products have arrived. Nerves at the bottom of the spinal cord signal muscles in the colon and rectum to tighten and cause the inner sphincter to open. This whole part of the process is automatic and doesn't take any thought.

When the inner sphincter opens, other nerves signal the brain and one becomes aware of a need to have a bowel movement. If it is a good time to go to the bathroom, the brain will send a message back down the spinal cord to the outer sphincter telling it to relax and open. Then both sphincters are open, the muscles in the colon and rectum squeeze, and the feces come out. The whole process

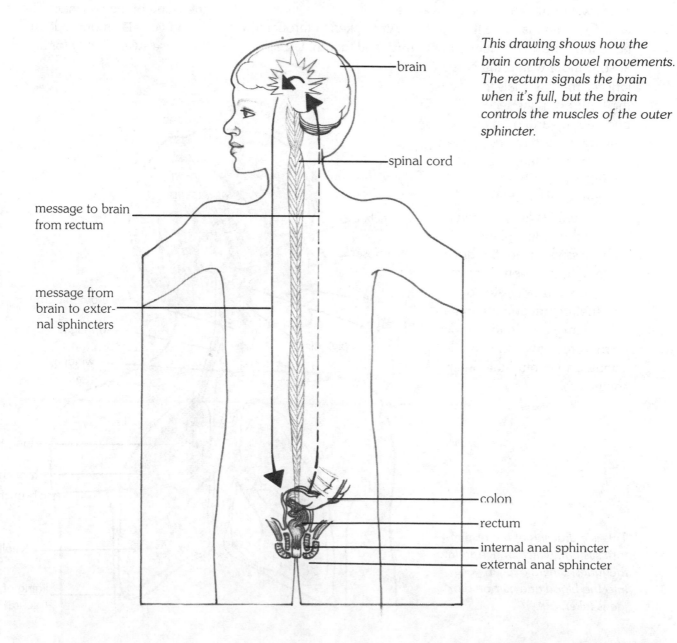

brain

spinal cord

message to brain from rectum

message from brain to external sphincters

colon

rectum

internal anal sphincter

external anal sphincter

This drawing shows how the brain controls bowel movements. The rectum signals the brain when it's full, but the brain controls the muscles of the outer sphincter.

can be helped by "pushing." This tightens the big flat muscle above the stomach (the diaphragm) and the muscles of the belly, and builds up pressure.

If it's not a good time to go to the bathroom, the brain will not send the outer sphincter a message to relax. Then the inner sphincter will automatically close, too, and the feeling of having to go to the bathroom will disappear for a while. During that time the large intestine will continue to absorb more water. If a person ignores many signals to go to the bathroom, the feces will become dry and hard and may be difficult to pass. That's why it's important to pay attention to the body's messages.

Little babies are not able to control the outer sphincter with messages from the brain. So they have a bowel movement as soon as waste comes into the rectum and the inner sphincter opens. In time they learn to recognize their bodies' signals and control the outer sphincter.

This is a drawing of the respiratory system, which brings air into the lungs, where oxygen goes into the blood and carbon dioxide is taken out.

The respiratory system

To stay alive, every cell in the body needs *oxygen,* one of the main gases that make up air. When cells use oxygen they give off another gas called *carbon dioxide,* which they have to get rid of. The *respiratory system* is the human body's remarkable way of getting oxygen and ridding itself of carbon dioxide.

Air is taken in through the nose and mouth. Usually people breathe through the nose because it warms and moistens the air and filters out dust. Inside the nose are several little mounds or folds, called *conchae,* over which air has to pass in order to reach the throat. This mazelike setup means the air moves more slowly and touches more area of the nasal walls.

The air is warmed by big blood vessels that lie under the lining of the conchae. The blood vessels on one side of the nose swell slightly for an

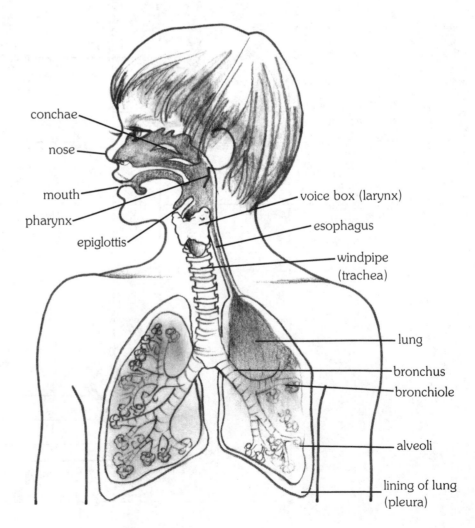

conchae
nose
mouth
pharynx
epiglottis
voice box (larynx)
esophagus
windpipe (trachea)
lung
bronchus
bronchiole
alveoli
lining of lung (pleura)

hour, slowing the air down on that side. Then the other side swells for an hour. The side that is more open does most of the breathing, while the side that is swollen does most of the warming.

The air goes from the back of the nose, down the throat. The back of the throat, called the pharynx, is divided into two tubes. One tube goes to the stomach, the other to the lungs. When people swallow, a flap called the epiglottis closes over the windpipe so food doesn't get into the lungs (see Swallowing, page 157).

When people breathe in, air goes down the *trachea* (windpipe), the front tube which is about one inch wide and is made up of many C-shaped cartilage rings covered with tough elastic tissue. At the top of the trachea is the *larynx* (voice box), which contains the *vocal cords*.

In the chest the trachea divides into two main branches, called the *bronchi*, which go to the right and left lungs. Each bronchus divides into smaller and smaller tubes like the branches of a tree. Finally, each tiny tube ends in a little sac called an *alveolus*. The lungs contain 300 million air sacs. If they were spread out flat, they would cover the floor of a classroom.

Every alveolar sac is surrounded by tiny blood vessels. The wall between the blood vessels and each air sac is so thin that the air is practically touching the blood. Red blood cells come to the lungs carrying molecules of carbon dioxide. The carbon dioxide goes from the blood into an air sac, and finally is exhaled from the lungs. Meanwhile, oxygen molecules in the air sacs cross the membrane and enter the bloodstream where they are picked up by red

blood cells and taken to all parts of the body.

The right lung has three *lobes* (parts) that are attached to three forks of the bronchus. The left lung is smaller and has only two lobes because the heart also lies in that part of the chest.

The lungs lie in two big sacs within the chest cavity, called

This drawing shows how oxygen goes into the blood from air in the lungs' air sacs (alveoli) and how carbon dioxide leaves the blood, enters the air sacs, and is exhaled when we breathe out. The alveoli can be seen under the microscope, but the oxygen and carbon dioxide molecules can't.

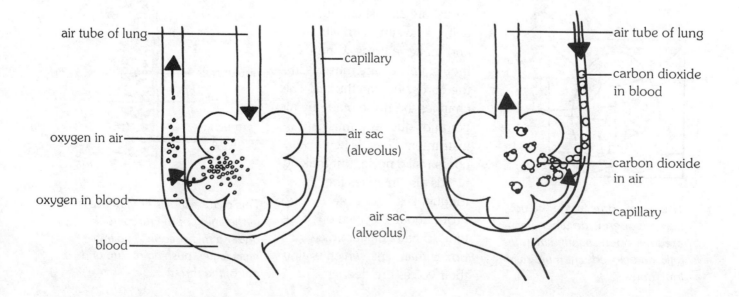

the *pleurae*. These sacs are made from a thin, clear, airtight membrane that looks a little like plastic wrap. Over this is a second membrane, which is attached to the ribs in the back and the front. A tiny bit of fluid between the two membranes allows them to slide over each other when a person breathes in and out.

The vocal cords   At the top of the windpipe is the larynx (voice box). It is a triangular box that points out in the front of the neck. The point itself is often called the "Adam's apple."

The vocal cords are lodged inside the larynx. These are two elastic bands that are open during breathing. As we have seen, the vocal cords close completely during swallowing, which helps prevent food from going down the windpipe. That is why people can't talk while they swallow. When the two bands, or cords, are almost closed, air going between them vibrates and makes a noise. When they squeeze, tiny muscles in the cords become thicker. This changes the noise made by air going by, just as a musical instrument does. (The vocal cords make noise, but making words also involves the tongue, lips, and cheeks.) From about 13 years on, boys tend to have bigger voice boxes than girls, which is why their voices are deeper.

The lining of the nose and throat   In the lining of the nose there are many *goblet* cells that make a watery fluid called mucus. When air passes over the mucus, it picks up water and becomes moist. The mucus also traps particles of dust that come in with the air. These particles are moved along by millions of little arms, called *cilia*, that stick out from the lining of the nose and throat. The cilia all move in waves, pushing bits of dust to the back of the throat where they are swallowed. This keeps most dust and dirt out of the lungs, which is important because the lungs' air sacs are so tiny they would be

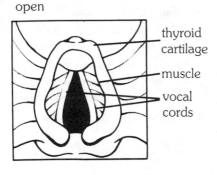

open

thyroid cartilage

muscle

vocal cords

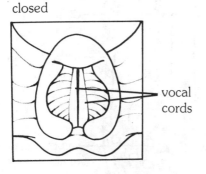

closed

vocal cords

The vocal cords inside the voice box are open wide when we breathe, open slightly when we talk, and closed when we swallow food.

goblet cells

cilia

mucous membrane cells

This picture shows how the cells in the lining of the throat look under a microscope. The tiny hairs wave, pushing dirt up and out of the throat.

Respiratory games

Hold a mirror directly under your nose. Breathe out through your nose. The mirror will fog up because the lining of your nose and throat moistens the air you breathe in and out. Notice if there is more fog from one nostril than the other. Usually one side of the nose does more breathing at any time.

Make a model of an air sac from the lung. Make five or ten pinholes in a small balloon. Attach the balloon to the end of a straw (with a rubber band if necessary). Put the balloon in a sinkful of water and gently blow on the straw. Watch the air bubbles come out in the water. This is how oxygen gets into your blood from the air sac.

Make a simple lung model. Pick a ten-inch branch that has two or three major forks, and then many little branches. This is the way the bronchi and air tubes look. Attach cotton balls onto all the little branches to represent the air sacs. Put the whole thing in a plastic bag and tie the bag tightly around the big stem. This bag represents the pleura that covers the lung. Hang the model upside down.

Mark on a paper every time you breathe in. Have a friend time you for 30 seconds. Multiply by two to get your breathing rate per minute. Now run around a field until you are tired and check your breathing rate again.

Take a normal breath. Blow into a small balloon as much as you can and then knot it. Then practice the exercise for taking a complete breath (see page 285). Now take a deep breath and blow into another little balloon and tie it. The second balloon is bigger because your lungs can hold much more air than you usually breathe in.

Get an empty plastic dish detergent or shampoo bottle with a squirt top. Cut off the bottom and cover it with a piece of rubber (use an old balloon) attached tightly with a rubber band. The bottle is like your lung, the balloon is like your diaphragm muscle. Push the balloon way up inside the bottle and feel the air come out at the top. Let go of the balloon and hear air go into the bottle as the balloon comes down. This is how air goes in and out of the lung when the diaphragm moves.

plugged by dust and then less oxygen would be able to pass into the blood.

If a lot of dirt comes into the nose and throat, the body has even faster, more powerful ways to get the dirt out. When there is dirt in the nose, it is blasted out with a sneeze. The *soft palate* at the back of the nose drops a little, blocking the mouth and forcing most of the air out through the nose. If the dirt reaches the windpipe, it is blown out with a cough. The breathing muscles automatically squeeze, building up pressure in the lungs.

At the same time, the vocal cords close, which blocks the air from getting out. Then suddenly the vocal cords open and the air rushes out of the mouth at up to 70 miles per hour, blasting out the dirt.

Breathing   Breathing brings air into and out of the lungs. The lungs themselves have no muscles, but they are elastic and can stretch. The lungs lie in a cage or compartment whose sides are the ribs. Air is moved by the muscles of the ribs and by the great thick muscle called the *diaphragm* that sits under the lungs and separates the chest from the belly. When people breathe in, the diaphragm tightens, which drops it down and makes it flat. This actually pulls down the lungs and makes the chest area longer. At the same time, the muscles *between* the ribs tighten. This raises the whole rib cage and makes the chest wider and higher. As the whole chest area becomes bigger, a vacuum forms and air is sucked in to fill the area. The diaphragm does three-quarters

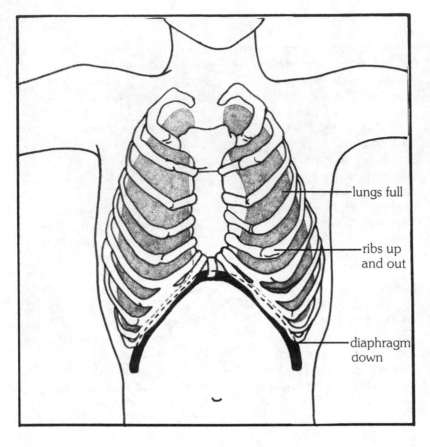

lungs full

ribs up
and out

diaphragm
down

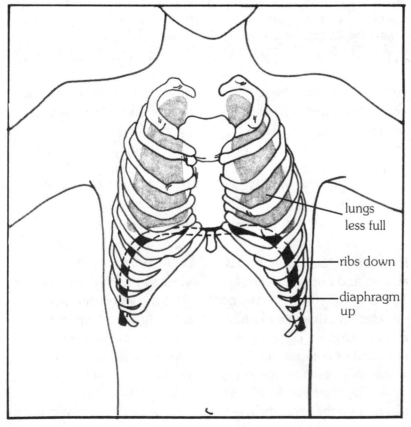

lungs
less full

ribs down

diaphragm
up

of this work, the chest muscles one-quarter.

Bringing air into the lungs is called *inhaling*. When the air goes out of the lungs it's called *exhaling*. After people breathe in, the muscles of the ribs and diaphragm relax and then the chest falls back to the way it was. Air can also be forced out of the lungs by squeezing the muscles of the ribs and belly. This makes the chest still smaller and pushes the air out.

Even though people can change their breathing on purpose, most of the time they breathe automatically. Breathing is controlled by a special respiratory center in the brain. The center sets the pace of breathing so that the amount of carbon dioxide in the blood doesn't go above a certain level. Kids usually breathe about 20 times a minute. Young kids breathe a little faster; adults breathe a little slower. When people exercise they can take in as much as 20 times the normal amount of air. The harder people exercise, the more air they need. The more often people do heavy exercise, the more air their lungs become able to take in.

These drawings show what happens when a person breathes in (1) and breathes out (2). When a person inhales, the diaphragm drops and the ribs lift, so the chest becomes bigger and air is sucked into the lungs.

The circulatory system

The circulatory system is a giant network of tubes through which blood goes to every part of the body. It is called the circulatory system because the blood travels in a circle from the heart, out to the body, and back to the heart. The bloodstream carries food and oxygen to every cell and carries away carbon dioxide and other waste products.

The *heart* is a big pump that pushes the blood through the blood vessels. Blood carrying oxygen and food leaves the heart through large vessels called *arteries*. Major arteries go to the head, the arms, the trunk, the legs, and even to the heart itself. These arteries branch into vessels so tiny they can only be seen through a microscope. They are called *capillaries*. Here oxygen and food leave the blood and go to the cells, and carbon dioxide and other wastes enter the blood. The blood is now halfway on its journey around the circle.

The blood *returns* to the heart through another set of blood vessels that run alongside the arteries. The return vessels are called the *veins*. They begin with microscopic vessels that start where the tiniest arteries leave off in the capillaries. They feed into bigger and bigger veins, and finally return to the heart.

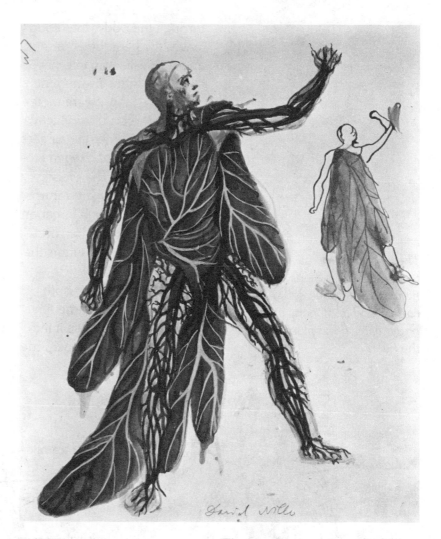

The circulatory system is a giant network of tubes.

Tchelitchew, Pavel. The Cave of Sleep: Series of 18 gouache designs for the ballet. 1941. Unproduced. Costume design, gouache. 14 × 11". Collection, The Museum of Modern Art, New York. Gift of the artist.

Actually the blood makes two loops away from the heart and back. These two loops are completely separate. Before the blood makes the circle to all parts of the body, it makes another circle to the air sacs of the lungs and back. This journey is made just to get rid of carbon dioxide and pick up new oxygen. As in its circle through the body, the blood leaves the heart by an artery, and makes its way into tiny capillaries that surround the air sacs in the lungs. Here molecules of carbon dioxide leave the blood to enter the air sacs, and molecules of oxygen cross into the blood. The blood, with its fresh oxygen, returns to the heart through larger and larger veins, which join into one large vein that enters the heart.

To pump blood to both these loops at the same time, the heart is actually split into two pumps, one on each side.

One pump sends most of the blood to the body, while the other pump sends some of the blood to the lungs. Each blood cell makes one journey and then the other. Blood leaves from the left side of the heart and goes out to the body where it drops off food and oxygen. The blood returns and goes to the *other* side of the heart, the right side. The pump on the right side pushes the blood through the lungs, where it drops off carbon dioxide and gets oxygen. The blood with fresh oxygen comes back and enters the left

These drawings show the circulatory system. It is made up of the heart and blood vessels. Arteries carry blood to all parts of the body; veins bring blood back to the heart.

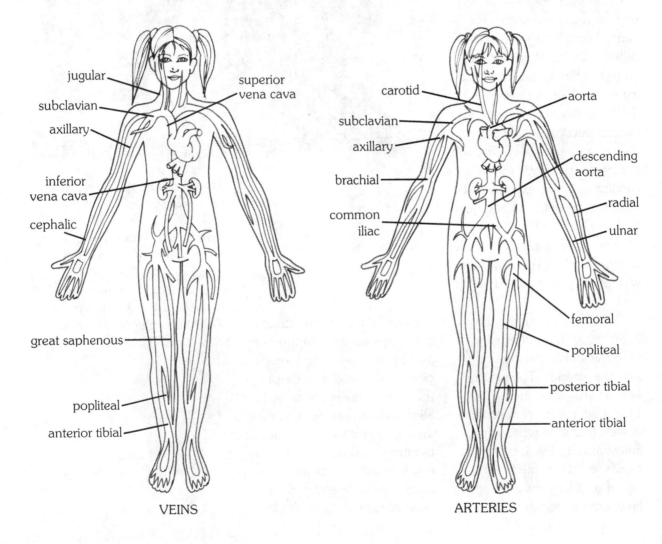

jugular

subclavian

axillary

inferior vena cava

cephalic

great saphenous

popliteal

anterior tibial

superior vena cava

VEINS

carotid

subclavian

axillary

brachial

common iliac

aorta

descending aorta

radial

ulnar

femoral

popliteal

posterior tibial

anterior tibial

ARTERIES

side of the heart and then goes back out to the body again.

The heart The heart is a hollow muscle shaped like a pine cone. It's about the size of your fist, and it's located in the center of your chest, pointing to the left. Both the pump to the lungs and the pump to the body work at the same time. Each pump has two areas or chambers: the top chambers are called the *atria;* the bottom chambers are called the *ventricles.* Each chamber is actually a pump in itself. Blood enters the two top chambers, the *left* and *right atria.* The atria are small pumps that squeeze blood into the lower chambers, the ventricles, and fill them completely. The *ventricles* are the big pumps that actually send the blood out to the lungs and body.

The heart works in *beats,* or *strokes.* That is, the chambers squeeze and send out blood, then rest and fill up again.

The heart is made up of two pumps, each of which has two parts, an atrium on top and a ventricle on the bottom. The right pump sends blood to the lungs. When it comes back, the left pump sends the blood to the body. First the blood comes into the atria which fill the ventricles, and then the ventricles pump the blood out to the lungs and body.

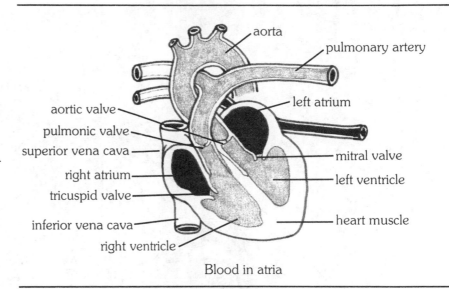

Blood in atria

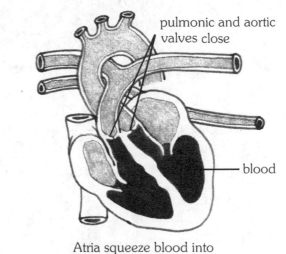

Atria squeeze blood into ventricles

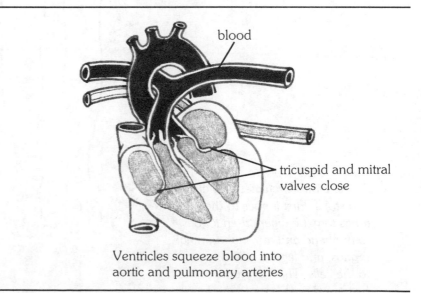

Ventricles squeeze blood into aortic and pulmonary arteries

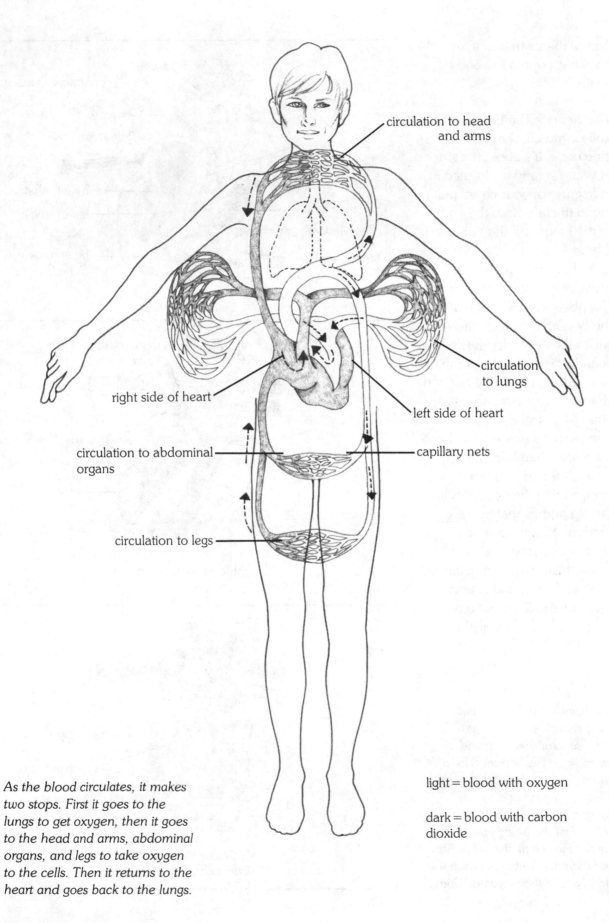

circulation to head
and arms

circulation
to lungs

right side of heart

left side of heart

circulation to abdominal
organs

capillary nets

circulation to legs

As the blood circulates, it makes
two stops. First it goes to the
lungs to get oxygen, then it goes
to the head and arms, abdominal
organs, and legs to take oxygen
to the cells. Then it returns to the
heart and goes back to the lungs.

light = blood with oxygen

dark = blood with carbon
dioxide

First, both the atria fill, then they both squeeze at the same time. This pushes blood down into both the ventricles, which are at rest. Then the ventricles squeeze. All of this happens in a fraction of a second. Then the whole heart rests for a much longer time. This pattern of squeezing and resting happens almost 100 times a minute in kids.

The chambers of the heart have *valves* to keep the blood from going backward. The valves are doorlike flaps that can only open out. When pushed hard enough from the inside, they open. If pushed from the outside, they close more tightly. When the atria squeeze, pressure builds up and the valves at the bottom open and let the blood into the ventricles. When the ventricles contract, pressure builds up in the same way, pushing open the valves that lead to the lungs and body. Meanwhile back pressure keeps the atria's valves closed so blood can't get back through them.

The heart is made of a very special kind of muscle cells. From the time they're formed these cells contract, or squeeze, automatically almost a hundred times a minute in a regular rhythm. At the top of the heart are a group of cells called the *pacemaker*. They squeeze first and then the squeezing spreads like a wave down to the cells at the bottom of the heart. This is what makes the top chambers start to squeeze a little ahead of the lower chambers. Once the pacemaker starts to contract, every cell in the heart joins in the wave and squeezes, making one big stroke, or heartbeat.

Artery, vein, and capillary net Blood leaves the heart through vessels or tubes called arteries, as we've said. It drops off its oxygen and food in tiny vessels called capillaries. And it returns to the heart through vessels called veins.

Artery walls have both elastic and muscular fibers. This makes them strong but stretchable. Every time the heart pumps, it squeezes out a spurt of blood under pressure. When this happens the arteries stretch a little. Between beats of the heart, no surge of blood comes out and the arteries shrink back a little, but they don't flatten or collapse because of the muscles in their walls.

The smallest arteries are called *arterioles*. They lead into the capillaries, a network of tiny interconnecting blood vessels. Every cell in the body needs food, so there is a capillary net almost everywhere in the body. If all the capillaries in the body were laid out flat, they would cover two acres or two square blocks in a city. The capillaries are perfect for . exchanging molecules because they have holes so small that only the tiniest things can get through.

All over the body the capillaries exchange oxygen for carbon dioxide and food for waste products. But in certain organs, the capillaries do other jobs, too. For example, in the small intestine the capillaries pick up the food the body has broken down into molecules (see page 158). In the glands, the capillaries pick up hormones that have been made (see page 206), and in the kidneys they drop off waste products (see pages 178–82).

The amount of blood that goes through any group of capillaries at a particular time depends on how tightly the arterioles squeeze. For example, during heavy exercise muscles need lots of oxygen. Both the muscle cells themselves and the nervous system send messages to the arterioles that more oxygen is needed, so the arterioles in the muscles relax and open wide, bringing in more blood.

After the blood has made its drop-offs and pick-ups in the capillaries, it feeds into larger and larger veins. By the time the blood reaches the veins, it no longer feels the pressure of the spurts of blood coming from the heart. Because the blood is under much less pressure, the walls of the veins are very thin. In fact, the pressure in the veins is so low that the blood needs help to get back to the heart. The veins have

Oxygen and food are dropped off and carbon dioxide is picked up in the tiniest blood vessels, the capillaries. The capillaries connect the arteries to the veins. This drawing shows how they look under a microscope.

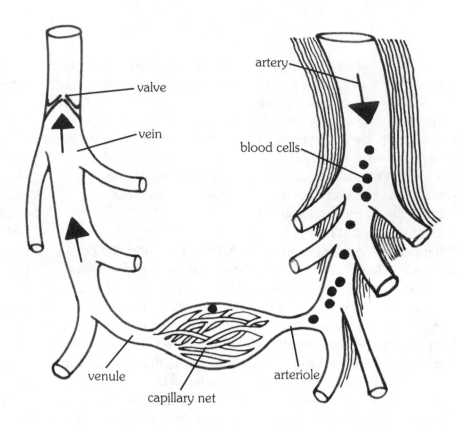

valve
vein
artery
blood cells
venule
capillary net
arteriole

Circulation games

Find your pulse. The pulse is the pressure of each surge of blood from the heart or the arteries. It can be felt in many places in the body. The easiest places to feel the pulse are under the jaw to one side of the windpipe, on the back of the wrist below the thumb, and on the line where the front of the leg meets the body. Count the beats for 15 seconds and multiply by 4 to get the number of beats per minute. Try this before and after running, and compare the number of beats.

Put your ear against the left side of a friend's chest, around the fourth rib down. Listen to the sounds of the heart beating: "lub-dub," "lub-dub." The first sound, "lub," is caused by the clos-

ing of the valves between the top and bottom chambers on each side while the lower chambers squeeze the blood out to the body. Closing of these valves keeps the blood from going backward. After the blood is squeezed out, the other valves close to keep blood from coming back into the heart. This causes the second sound, the "dub." So the "dub" sound means the heartbeat is over. Before you hear the "lub-dub" repeated, the heart rests and fills again.

Ask your butcher for a cow's heart. Notice the pine cone shape and feel how thick and rubbery the muscle is. Look at the holes where blood vessels attach to the top of the heart—a small portion of the vessels may stick out like

tubes. Carefully cut the heart in half from the top to the point at the bottom. You should be able to see a top and bottom chamber on at least one side. See if you can feel the valve between the chambers with your finger.

Make a model of the tiniest blood vessels, the capillaries. Poke a few holes in a piece of plastic tubing (or even a straw) with a safety pin. Squeeze one end of the tube closed and gently blow a mouthful of water into the other end. Water will come out of the holes. This is how the liquid part of the blood comes out of the capillaries and carries food to the cells.

Make a model of your blood. Fill a small jar with half a cup

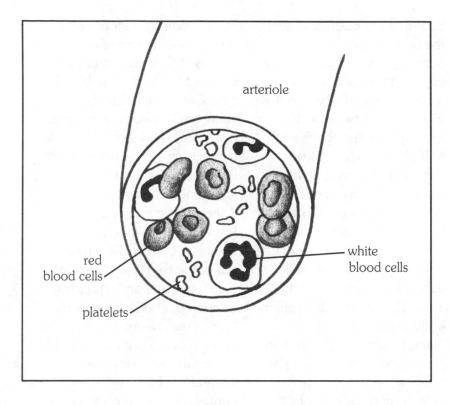

arteriole

red
blood cells

platelets

white
blood cells

There are three kinds of blood cells: red cells, white cells, and platelets. This is how they look under a microscope.

tiny valves or flaps that keep the blood from flowing backward. And when muscles around the veins squeeze and do work, they also squeeze nearby veins and help push the blood back toward the heart. It's a good setup, because this is exactly when the muscle cells need more blood. Generally half of the blood in the body is in the veins. When the muscles need more oxygen during exercise, a lot of the blood stored in the veins is squeezed back to the heart.

The blood   Blood is one of the most important substances in the body: it supplies the cells with oxygen, food, minerals, and salt; it removes waste products that are made by the cells; it helps the body defend against bacteria and viruses; and it is the means for regulating the body's temperature.

Blood is made up of about half cells, half water, and a little bit of proteins and salt. Almost all the cells in the blood are *red blood cells*. They give blood its color. A red blood cell looks like a flat Frisbee, or a doughnut that hasn't lost its hole. Actually the red blood cells are elastic

of water. Add a pinch of salt, a pinch of sugar, and a sprinkle of unflavored gelatin for protein. This mixture represents blood plasma. Meanwhile soak a half cup of Cheerios in enough grape juice to cover them. When the Cheerios look red, add this to the other mixture. These are the red blood cells that give blood its color. Take four or five round cereal pieces like puffed corn or Kix and add them. They represent the white blood cells. Finally break up a tablespoonful of cereal like cornflakes and add them. These represent the platelets, which help the blood to clot.

Make a rough model of the heart. Get a plastic detergent bottle with a push-close top and fill it with a mixture of grape juice and water. (Do this outside or in the bathroom—it's messy.) The push top acts like a valve. Push it closed, and squeeze the bottle. No "blood" comes out. This is what happens when the ventricles are filling from the auricles. Now pull up the top and squeeze the bottle. "Blood" comes out just as it does when the ventricles squeeze or pump. Each time you squeeze, it's like a heartbeat; each time you let go, it's like the heart resting. If possible, get a piece of clear plastic tubing. Pull off the snap top and stick the tubing over the hole. Now squeeze the bottle and watch the "blood" go through the tube, which is like the aorta, the artery that leads away from the heart.

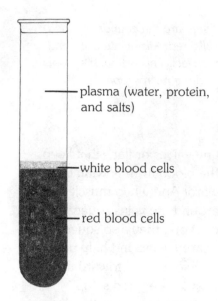

plasma (water, protein, and salts)

white blood cells

red blood cells

Blood is made up of about half red blood cells, a little white blood cells, and the rest water with some salts and proteins.

What's in blood?

Cells (red, white, platelets)

Water

Minerals (calcium, copper, iron, magnesium, sodium, zinc, and so on.)

Food and vitamins (amino acids, sugar, vitamins A, B, C, fats)

Waste products (acetone, ammonia, urea)

Hormones

Antibodies

Clotting proteins

Dissolved gases, oxygen, carbon dioxide

bags that are pushed around the body at high speed, bumping into things and twisting into funny shapes. They spend their whole lives in the blood vessels because they are too big to fit through the tiny holes in the capillary walls. The job of the red blood cells is simply to carry oxygen from the lungs to the capillaries and bring carbon dioxide back. They can do this because they have a special protein called *hemoglobin,* which contains iron. It is the iron which chemically grabs hold of the oxygen, while the globin part picks up carbon dioxide. Each red blood cell can carry millions of molecules of oxygen or carbon dioxide.

The body makes red blood cells constantly because they only last about four months. They are manufactured in a special place in the center of the bones called the *marrow.* When the body needs more red blood cells because it is growing or bleeding, a chemical is sent out by the kidney that tells the marrow to produce more. So the body always has just the right number of red blood cells to see that it gets the oxygen it needs. And that number is enormous—every drop of blood has half a million red blood cells!

The other cells in the blood are called *white blood cells.* They aren't red because they don't contain any hemoglobin. Their job is to protect the body against infections caused by germs—either bacteria or viruses. There are a number of different kinds of white blood cells. Some kill germs by eating them (see Phagocytosis, page 238), and some kill germs by making antibodies to fight the germs (see The lymph nodes, page 177). Although they are much bigger than red blood cells, the white blood cells can get out of the capillaries by changing their shape and squeezing through the holes in the walls. Once they are out of the capillaries, they go back to their old shape and ooze along by themselves, hunting for germs. Some white blood cells stay in the blood, and some wander around between the cells. Others go to live permanently in the liver, the lungs, and the lymph nodes. The ones in the liver kill bacteria that have gotten in with digested food; the ones in the lungs fight bacteria that have been inhaled; and the ones in the lymph nodes fight bacteria that have spread through the body or gotten in through cuts.

Like the red blood cells, the white blood cells are made in the bone marrow, but they last a much shorter time and there are fewer of them. In fact, there are only 150 white blood cells per drop of blood. Any time cells are injured or attacked by germs, chemicals are given off that signal the bone marrow to make more white blood cells. The more the body needs, the more white blood cells are made. Within six hours, the marrow can make four times the total number it normally has.

Platelets are the third kind of cell found in the blood. They are very tiny bumpy pieces that have broken off from special big cells in the marrow. Their job is to help stop bleeding. They are very sticky and they clump together whenever there is a break in a blood vessel, making a plug like a cork (*see* Blood clotting, page 232).

The rest of the blood is made up of water and all the substances that are going to and coming from the cells. These substances include dissolved food, salts and minerals, proteins, wastes, and hormones. But mostly it is water. This fluid mixture, called *plasma,* is light yellow in color.

The lymph system

Every cell in the body is surrounded by a fluid that is a lot like sea water. This fluid carries molecules of food and oxygen from the tiniest blood vessels to all the cells. And it carries all wastes back. The fluid moves in little circles, out of the blood vessels, in and around the cells, and back to the blood vessels. Most of the fluid is absorbed back into the blood vessels, but a little isn't.

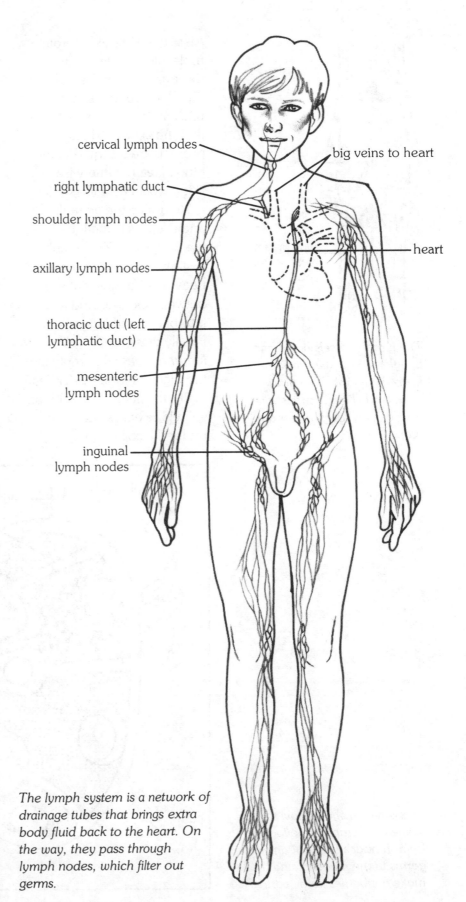

The lymph system is a network of drainage tubes that brings extra body fluid back to the heart. On the way, they pass through lymph nodes, which filter out germs.

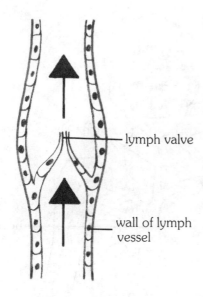

— lymph valve

— wall of lymph vessel

The lymph vessels have many tiny flaps, or valves, inside that keep the lymph from flowing backward. This picture shows how a valve looks under a microscope.

Also, there are extra protein molecules that leak out through holes in the walls of the blood vessels and can't get back in. It's very important that the extra fluid and proteins are returned to the bloodstream. Otherwise the body would actually swell up.

Returning the extra fluid and proteins is the job of the *lymph system.* The lymph system is like a giant one-way network of drains that start between the cells and lead into bigger and bigger tubes. Finally these tubes, called *lymphatic vessels,* empty into the biggest blood vessels leading to the heart. These blood vessels lie below the neck under the collarbone.

The mixture of fluid and proteins is called *lymph.* It is pushed into the tiniest lymph vessels when too much builds up around the cells. There is no big pump, like the heart, that moves the lymph along. It moves because the tiny lymph vessels themselves tighten and push it along. Like the veins, the lymph vessels have little valves or flaps inside that keep the lymph from flowing backward. When the space between two valves gets full, the lymph vessels automatically tighten and squeeze the fluid past the next valve. Exercise also helps return the fluid. There are lymph vessels all through the muscles of the body. When these muscles

This drawing shows how the inside of a lymph node looks. Lymph nodes filter out and eat germs in the medulla, and they make antibodies in the cortex.

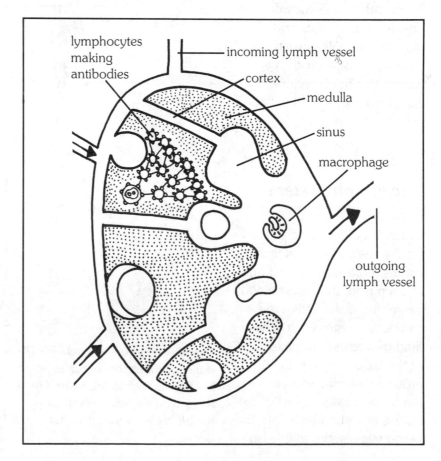

lymphocytes making antibodies

incoming lymph vessel

cortex

medulla

sinus

macrophage

outgoing lymph vessel

work and tighten they squeeze the lymph vessels, too.

On their way to the heart, the lymph vessels pass through tiny oval organs called *lymph nodes*. The nodes filter out bacteria, viruses, and poisons. The nodes range from the size of a pea to the size of a grape, and they are arranged in chains. Each chain filters all the lymph from one area of the body.

The lymph nodes The lymph nodes help to protect the body against dangerous germs and poisons. They do this in two ways: one part of the node captures and breaks down dangerous substances; another part of the node makes special proteins called antibodies, which can trap and kill germs anywhere in the body.

Lymph comes into the nodes from the lymphatic vessels and flows inside through tubes called *sinuses*. The sinuses are filled with a fine net of fibers that lets the lymph fluid pass, but filters out bacteria, viruses, and clumps of poison. In the net of fibers are many special white blood cells called *macrophages*. Their name comes from the Greek words for "big eater." They actually eat and digest dangerous substances (see Phagocytosis, page 239). After eating a dangerous substance, the macrophage spits out proteins that were part of the substance. These proteins are

Lymph games

Make a rough model of a lymph vessel. Make a number of little holes in a plastic straw. Flatten both ends of the straw and tape them closed. Now submerge the straw into a pan of salty water. This represents the fluid between the cells. Hold it down for a minute, then lift it out. Water will have drained into the straw just as extra fluid from between the cells drains into the smallest lymph vessels. Hold up one end of the straw and untape it. Pinch your fingers around the other end and slide them up the straw, pushing the water up and out of the straw. This is how the big muscles around the lymph vessels squeeze the lymph fluid toward the heart.

Push a coffee-filter paper into a funnel. Pour a glass of water with a pinch of sugar and salt dissolved in it through the filter paper. This is how pure lymph fluid, passes through a lymph node. Now add rice to the water and pour it through the filter paper again. This is how a lymph node traps bacteria, viruses, and dead cells.

picked up by another kind of white blood cell, called a *lymphocyte*. When a lymphocyte picks up one of these proteins, it moves it from the sinus to the other part of the node, the *cortex*. Here the lymphocyte makes an *antibody* that fits only this protein. Then the lymphocyte divides over and over into many lymphocytes. Each of the new lymphocytes knows how to make antibodies against the particular protein. These lymphocytes enter the bloodstream by the thousands and go all over the body hunting for any substances that have the dangerous protein.

When a person gets sick, the lymph nodes become very active, filtering out the dangerous substance and manufacturing antibodies against it. When the lymph nodes are active, they get bigger temporarily. For example, when a person has a sore throat from a virus cold, the lymph nodes in the neck go to work to kill the virus and keep it from spreading to other areas of the body. The nodes become so big they can be felt as little lumps at the back of the jaw and down the sides of the neck. These little lumps mean your body is working to fight an infection. (For more information on how antibodies protect the body, see the sections on Antibodies and Phagocytosis, pages 238–42.)

The urinary system

Every cell in the body contains fluid and is surrounded by fluid. Like sea water, this fluid contains water, salt, and a number of other minerals. For the body's cells to remain alive the amount of salt and minerals has to be just right. This fluid also contains chemicals that are left over after the body has used up food. If these chemicals were allowed to build up high levels, they would be poisonous, or toxic. Since the cells are using up food all the time, the body has to get rid of the wastes all the time.

The salts and minerals, as well as the toxic waste materials, all enter the bloodstream sooner or later. Most of this material enters the blood directly, but some enters through the lymph system (see page 175). At one point on its travels around the body, the blood passes through the *kidneys*. In fact, one quart of blood passes through the kidneys each minute. It is here that the toxic wastes are drawn out of the blood. Salts and minerals are drawn out *only* if there is too much of them.

The kidneys are two bean-shaped organs, about four and a half inches long, that lie behind the belly button near the spinal column. The right kidney is a little lower than the left in order to make space for the liver, which is quite big. Each kidney contains a million *nephrons,* groups of cells that make *urine,* which contains the toxic wastes, salt and minerals, and mostly water.

All the nephrons join into bigger and bigger tubes until they reach a central area called the *renal pelvis.* Here they join ten-inch tubes that lead to the bladder. These tubes, called *ureters,* have strong muscles in their walls. The muscles squeeze drops of urine down into the bladder.

The *bladder* is a muscular bag that lies directly behind the pubic bone, where the insides of the legs join the trunk. The bladder has many folds inside that can stretch out to hold as much as two cups in an adult. Urine is made continuously in the kidneys, squeezed down the ureters, and stored in the bladder.

At the bottom of the bladder is a ring-shaped muscle called a *sphincter.* The sphincter is tightly closed except when a person is going to the bathroom. The bladder is connected to the outside through a tube called the *urethra.* The urethra is different in boys and girls. In boys the urethra is long and passes through a gland called the *prostate* (see page 211) and then down through the *penis,* ending at its tip. In girls, the urethra is short and comes out above the vagina (see pages 213–15).

The nephrons—the working units of the kidneys
The nephrons are the part of the kidneys that filter out poisonous or toxic wastes from the blood and make urine. Each nephron has two parts: the *glomerulus* and the *tubule.* The glomerulus is a tiny, microscopic filter through which the blood passes. Inside is a mesh of blood vessels whose walls contain very tiny holes. Blood cells and proteins are too big to fit through these holes, but water, minerals, salts, and toxic wastes go through the holes easily and pass into the tubules. The blood in the glomerulus is under high pressure, which helps to push the water and salts through the holes in the walls.

The tubule is a microscopic tube that goes down from the glomerulus, makes a sharp loop, goes back up, and empties into a *collecting tube.* Wrapped around each tubule is a tiny blood vessel, which

What's in urine?

Water

Minerals (chlorine, sodium, potassium, sulfur, phosphorus, calcium, magnesium)

Waste products (ammonia, urea)

A very small amount of amino acids and hormones

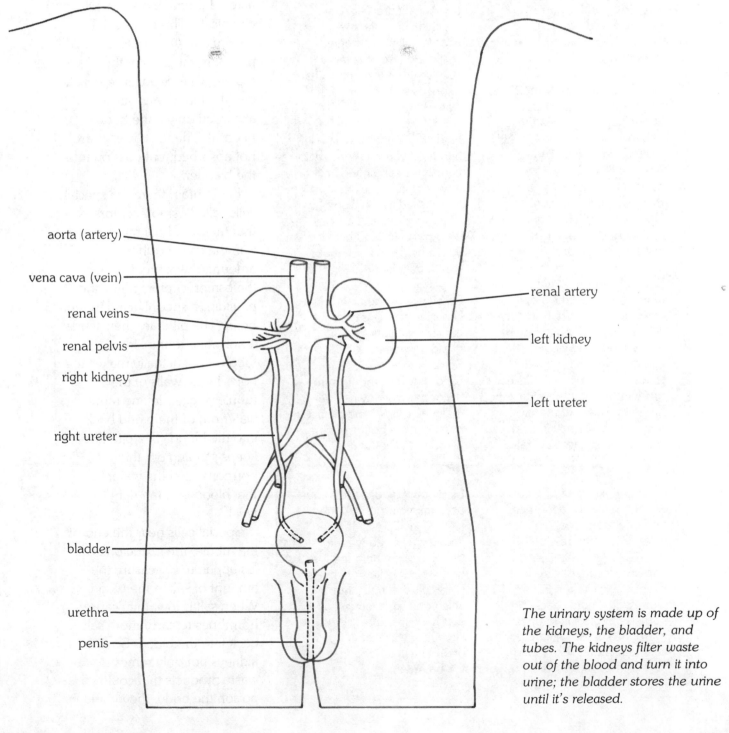

aorta (artery)

vena cava (vein)

renal veins

renal pelvis

right kidney

right ureter

bladder

urethra

penis

renal artery

left kidney

left ureter

The urinary system is made up of the kidneys, the bladder, and tubes. The kidneys filter waste out of the blood and turn it into urine; the bladder stores the urine until it's released.

Urinary tract games

For one whole day, collect all your urine in a bottle. Count the number of times you go, how much urine there is each time, and the total for the day. Most kids release about one quart of urine per day. (Remember, urine has no bacteria, so there is no harm in using kitchen measuring cups.)

Collect a small amount of urine in a clean jar. Use litmus paper to check the pH. The numbers on the pH scale go from 0 to 14 and tell how acidic or basic a chemical is. The more acid something is, the lower its pH. Urine is usually between five and eight on the pH scale—just about neutral.

Let a cup of urine evaporate in the sun or on the stove over low heat. When all the liquid is gone a white powder will remain. This powder contains salt and urea. In small amounts, these waste products are not the slightest bit poisonous, but they will make the body sick if it can't get rid of them for several days.

Make a mixture of one cup water, one tablespoon rice, and one tablespoon salt. Stir it well. Pour the mixture through a piece of filter paper or a coffee filter. The filter paper, like the kidney's *glomerulus*, holds back big particles but lets little ones through. The rice, like blood cells and proteins, is too big to pass. But the salt and water pass through easily. Taste the water to prove to yourself that the salt has come through.

Now try the experiment again, substituting a couple of drops of yellow food coloring for the salt. The food coloring, like toxic wastes, will pass through easily. Pour several more cups of water through. What happens to the color of the water?

Find your kidneys. Rest your hands on your hipbones with your thumbs pointing back toward your spine. Your thumbs will rest in a soft space in your back above your hipbones and below your ribs. This is just about where your kidneys lie.

Fill a large balloon with one cup of water. This is about the size and shape of the bladder when it's full. Squeeze the neck of the balloon tightly and turn the balloon upsidedown. Your fingers are like the sphincter muscle at the bottom of the bladder. Relax them slightly and the water will come out.

Find your bladder. Rest your hand on your pubic bone (see page 213). Slide your fingers up just above the bone. This is where the top of the bladder lies when it is partly filled. If you press a little you may even feel as if you have to urinate. Pressure like this is what signals your brain that you need to go to the bathroom.

comes from the glomerulus and leads out of the kidney. As liquid goes down the tubule, anything that the body needs leaves the tubule and goes back into this blood vessel. At the top of the tubule sugar and vitamins are carried across into the blood vessel by chemicals. This takes a little energy and works like a pump. In the loop of the tubule, water is absorbed back into the blood, and salt is absorbed *only* if the body needs it. The toxic wastes are not absorbed, but pass on into the bladder.

In the brain there are special cells called *osmoreceptors* that measure how much water is in the blood. When the amount of water gets too low, the osmoreceptors notify the *pituitary*, a special gland in the brain. The pituitary then sends a hormone to the kidney tubules that actually makes the holes in the walls of the tubules bigger, letting more water out of them and back into the blood. The pituitary keeps sending out this hormone until the water in the blood is at the right level.

Special cells near the end of the tubule, the *juxtaglomerulus apparatus,* measure the amount of salt in the blood. When salt is low, they cause hormones to carry more salt back into the blood. So the kidneys not only remove waste products that could poison the body, they manage

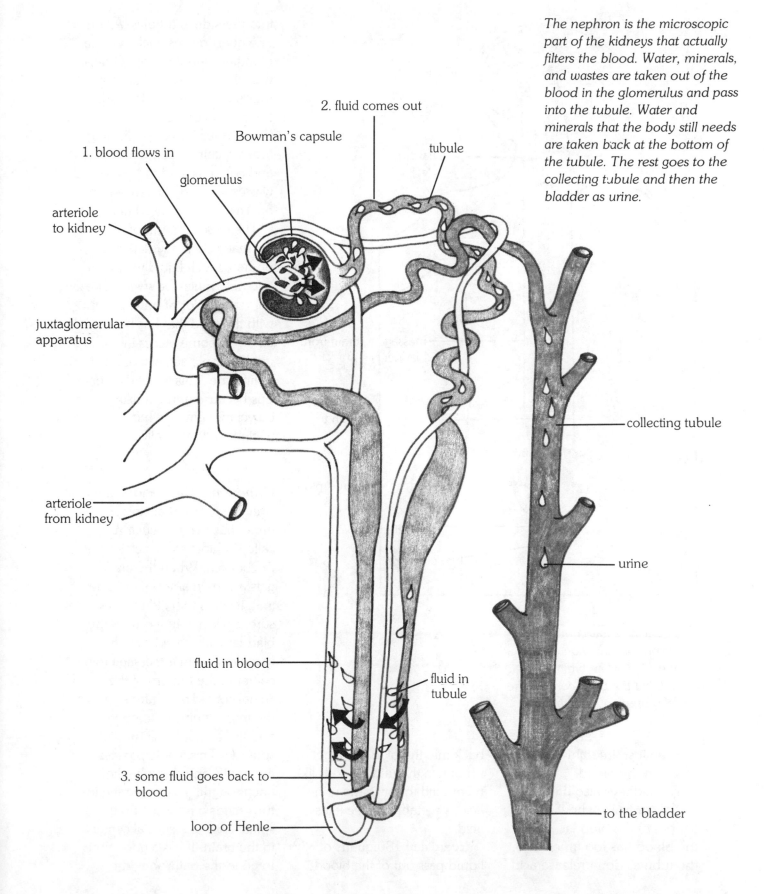

1. blood flows in

Bowman's capsule

2. fluid comes out

tubule

glomerulus

arteriole to kidney

juxtaglomerular apparatus

arteriole from kidney

The nephron is the microscopic part of the kidneys that actually filters the blood. Water, minerals, and wastes are taken out of the blood in the glomerulus and pass into the tubule. Water and minerals that the body still needs are taken back at the bottom of the tubule. The rest goes to the collecting tubule and then the bladder as urine.

collecting tubule

urine

fluid in blood

fluid in tubule

3. some fluid goes back to blood

loop of Henle

to the bladder

Anatomy and physiology **181**

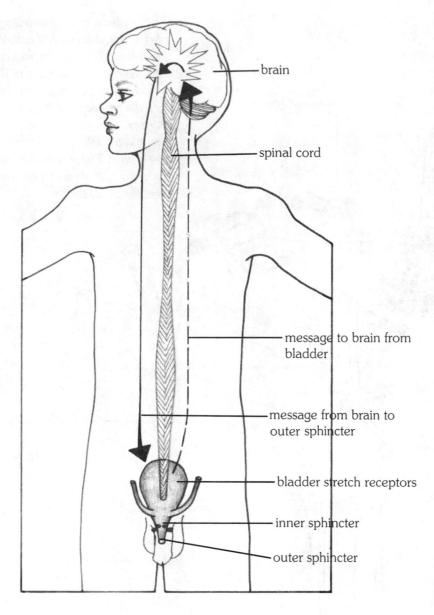

into the kidney tubules. All but one quart passes back into the blood around the loop. Otherwise the body would become totally dried out within a few hours. The one quart that slowly drips into the collecting tube contains water, extra salts and minerals, and the poison wastes the body has to get rid of. This liquid is called *urine.*

The exact amount of urine we make each day depends on how much liquid we drink and how much we sweat. The color and odor of urine varies with the food that has been eaten. In some places in the world people actually drink their urine. This is not dangerous because urine, unlike bowel movements, has no bacteria in it normally.

brain

spinal cord

message to brain from bladder

message from brain to outer sphincter

bladder stretch receptors

inner sphincter

outer sphincter

This drawing shows how the brain controls urination. The bladder signals the brain when it's full, but the brain controls the muscles of the outer sphincter.

Urination   The bladder, the stretchable bag that stores urine, has two muscular rings called sphincters that close it at the bottom. When the bladder gets a certain amount of urine in it, it starts to build up pressure. Special nerve cells in the bladder wall, called *stretch receptors,* send a message to a center in the bottom of the spinal cord. The center signals the *inner sphincter* to open and the bladder wall to squeeze. This whole process is automatic and doesn't take any thought. The squeezing in turn sends a message up the spinal cord to a special center in the brain. If it is a good time to go to the bathroom, the

to keep just the right amount of salt in the blood.

The kidneys also have the job of controlling how acidic (or basic) the blood is. When the blood has too much acid, the tubules don't release acid

back into the blood, but get rid of it in the urine. Foods like meat tend to make the urine acid; vegetables make it less acid.

Every day 180 quarts of liquid pass out of the blood

brain will send a message back down the spinal cord to the *outer sphincter* telling it to relax and open. Then both sphincters will be open, the bladder will squeeze, and urine will come out. If the brain doesn't send a "relax" message to the outer sphincter, it stays closed and the inner one closes again. No urine comes out and the feeling of having to go disappears for a while. Babies who have not yet learned to consciously control the outer sphincter just urinate as soon as their inner sphincter opens. For this reason they go to the bathroom more frequently than older children.

The nervous system

The nervous system is a very complicated network that carries messages back and forth all over the body. Since the body is so big, cells in one area don't know what cells in another area are doing. For the whole body to work together smoothly, all the different parts have to be told what to do by cells that know what's happening. For example, if a hungry lion is about to attack you, your leg muscles don't know about the danger, so they have to be told to run. Seeing the lion, understanding the danger, and sending messages to the muscles are all jobs of different parts of the nervous system.

Twelve billion nerve cells make up the nervous system. Basically, the nerve cells act very much like telephone wires, sending messages in the form of little bursts of electricity. There are three kinds of nerve cells: "feelers," "thinkers," and "doers."

Sensory nerve cells are designed to "feel" what's going on around them. They send messages about things happening both inside and outside the body. Outside sensory cells pick up touch, sound, skin temperature, smell, taste, and sight. Inside receptors respond to tilting,

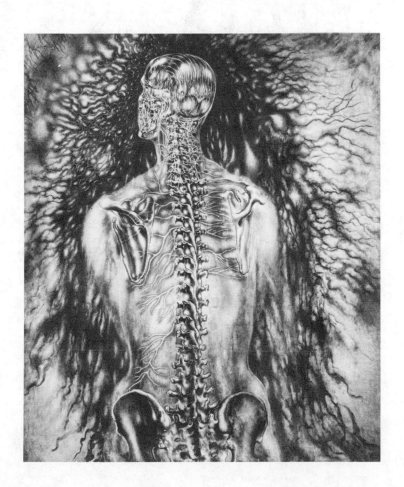

The nervous system is a communication network that connects the inside of the body with the outer world.

Tchelitchew, Pavel. Anatomical Painting. *c. 1945. Oil on canvas. 56 × 46″. Collection, Whitney Museum of American Art, New York. Gift of Lincoln Kirstein. Photograph by Geoffrey Clements.*

The nervous system is a network of nerves that carries messages back and forth between the brain and all parts of the body. "Feeler" nerves report messages from the eyes, ears, nose, and skin to the spinal cord and brain. There "thinker" nerves figure out what to do, and send messages to muscle cells along "doer" nerves.

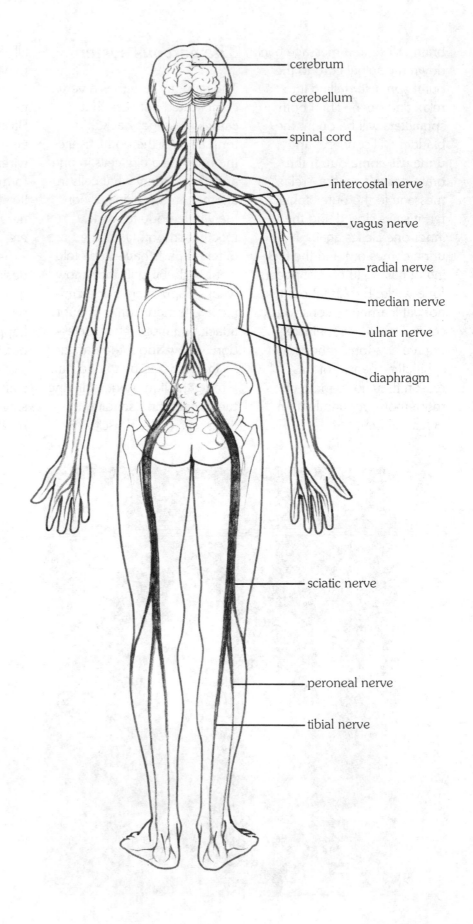

cerebrum

cerebellum

spinal cord

intercostal nerve

vagus nerve

radial nerve

median nerve

ulnar nerve

diaphragm

sciatic nerve

peroneal nerve

tibial nerve

pressure inside the blood vessels, amount of oxygen in the blood, and body temperature. They also send messages about how all the body organs are working and tell if any area is hurt and in pain.

Integrative nerve cells take the messages coming in from the sensory cells, "think" about them, and then figure out what to do. The more complicated groups of integrative nerve cells may even compare the incoming messages with old memories, decide if the messages are good or bad, and then make a decision about what should happen.

The decision about what to do is sent to the final group of cells, the *motor nerve cells*. These are the "doers." They make things happen. They make big muscles move, they make smooth muscles in organs squeeze, and they make certain glands send out chemical messengers. For example, they make the body run, digest its food, and speed up the heartbeat.

These feelers, thinkers, and doers are found in different parts of the body. The integrative cells (the thinkers) are in the spinal cord and brain. They make up the *central nervous system*. The sensory and motor cells (the feelers and the doers) are all over the body. The feelers and the doers make up the *peripheral*, or outer, *nervous system*.

The peripheral system is

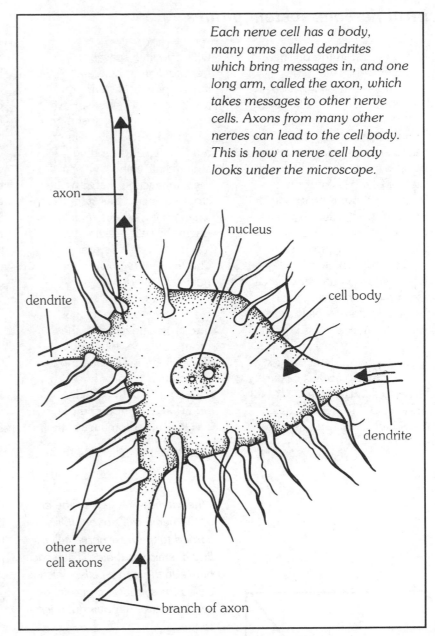

Each nerve cell has a body, many arms called dendrites which bring messages in, and one long arm, called the axon, which takes messages to other nerve cells. Axons from many other nerves can lead to the cell body. This is how a nerve cell body looks under the microscope.

axon

nucleus

dendrite

cell body

dendrite

other nerve cell axons

branch of axon

made of *nerves*. Nerves consist of many nerve cells bundled up inside of a tough connective tissue covering, or sheath. Both sensory and motor cells are often side by side in the nerve sheath, but are separated by special fatty cells that don't let messages for one type pass to the other.

These fat cells are like the rubber insulation that is wrapped around telephone and electrical wires. Without insulation, the messages of the nerves would get totally mixed up.

All the motor and sensory nerves eventually lead to the spinal cord and brain, where

Central nervous system games

Call a friend on the phone. Tell him or her what the room you're in is like. You are like a "feeler" cell in the eye sending messages to the brain. Your friend is like a "thinker" cell who can figure out the messages and form a picture of what the room is like even though he or she is not in it. If your friend were to tell you to do something like shut a door, he or she would be a "thinker" cell who's figured out what needs to happen, and you would be like a "doer" cell that makes a muscle move.

You can get an idea of how a nerve impulse travels down a nerve cell and excites another cell that it touches. Stand ten dominoes in a line with only little spaces between them. Leave a larger space and stand up another ten dominoes. Push the first domino against the second. This is like exciting a nerve cell and sending sodium into the cell. It starts a chain reaction that can't be stopped once it has started. The impulse moves rapidly down the cell, hesitates as it jumps the gap (the synapse), and then starts down the next cell (see drawing).

Have a friend sit in a chair and cross one leg over the other so it's not touching the floor. Find the soft area right below your friend's kneecap. Tap it firmly with the edge of your hand. Your friend's leg will kick up automatically (if it doesn't, try tapping a little higher or lower). This is the knee-jerk reflex. It's caused by exciting feeler nerves in the end of the muscle.

Cut open a piece of old electric wire (not plugged in!) or, better yet, a piece of extra telephone wire. Inside the big wire you will find two or more metal wires covered with rubber or plastic insulation. This is like the nerve cells inside a nerve bundle, which are covered with a fatty kind of insulation. This insulation keeps nerve messages from getting mixed up.

Ask your butcher for an uncut beef or lamb brain. Notice the two sides (hemi-

When a message gets to the end of the nerve cell's axon, it is carried to the next nerve cell by tiny chemical bubbles. The space between the nerve cells, which is called the synapse, can only be seen under very powerful microscopes.

axon of first nerve

mitochondria

synaptic knob

chemical transmitter sacs

synaptic space

cell body of second nerve

they connect with the integrative nerve cells. The integrative cells in the spinal cord and the brain are arranged in groups based on what they do.

How nerves send messages Nerve cells are some of the largest and most complicated cells in the body. But each nerve cell has three basic parts: a body and two types of arms. The *body* contains the nucleus and is the control center for the cell. Although the body is very tiny, the nerve cell cannot live with-

spheres), the thin membrane or layer that covers the brain, and the blood vessels coming to it. Look at the folds and see if the lower brain, the cerebellum, is still there. Carefully cut the brain in half —you may be able to see gray areas of nerve cell bodies and white areas of nerve fibers that connect the brain to all parts of the body.

Have a friend sneak up behind you and make a loud noise. If you are really surprised you'll feel your heart start to pound faster and your hair stand up. You may also feel your stomach tighten and your breath stick in your throat. These feelings are caused by the autonomic nervous system.

out it. The first type of arm is called a *dendrite*. Each nerve cell has many dendrites. They bring messages to the body of the cell from many different places. The other type of arm is called an *axon*. There is only one axon for each cell and it can be very long, up to three or four feet. The axon takes the message away from the body of the cell.

Nerve messages are simple signals. In fact all the nerves send only one kind of signal, and it travels only in one direction. That signal is a very tiny burst or impulse of electricity that shows that the nerve has been excited. This burst of electricity only lasts for the tiniest part of a second. It starts at the far end of one dendrite, travels across the body, and out the axon. The electrical impulse is started by a chemical called sodium flowing into the nerve cell. The cell then pumps out the extra sodium all the way down the axon. This carries the burst of electricity from one end of the cell to the other. It's like setting a match to a trail of gunpowder. The fire starts at one end and burns rapidly down the line, using up the gunpowder as it goes.

The arms, both the axons and the dendrites, never actually touch another nerve cell. They come very, very close, but they always leave a little space. The name of this space is the *synapse,* which is Greek for union, or joining. When the burst of electricity gets to the synapse something special happens. The far end of the axon has a bulb, or bump, which is almost touching the next nerve cell. When the electricity reaches the bulb it causes little sacs of a chemical to cross the synapse and excite the other nerve cell. These little sacs are like ferry-boats crossing a river. When they touch the next nerve cell, sodium flows into it. If enough sodium flows in, a burst of electricity flows down that cell. Sometimes many messages from many nerve cells are needed to start the next nerve cell firing.

Synapses carry messages in just one direction. That's because only the bulb-shaped end of the axon can make the sacs that take sodium across the synapse. This means that all nerves are like one-way streets—the burst of electricity can only go in one direction. Messages on sensory nerves travel inward to the spinal cord and the brain; messages on motor nerves travel out to muscles.

Reflexes The whole nervous system works by combining the jobs of the three different kinds of nerve cells—the feelers, the thinkers, and the doers. The feeler picks up what's happening and sends a message to the thinker in the spinal cord or brain. The thinker figures out what to do and sends a message to the doer. The doer sends a message to its muscle causing it to move. These three steps form an arc, or circuit, along which a message comes in and goes back out.

The simplest circuits are called *reflexes*. They don't require a person to think or do something on purpose; they just happen. The thinker cells decide what to do automatically. In fact, much of the body works like this. Reflexes control breathing, heartbeat, balance, even pulling away from something painful.

One of the simplest reflexes

The body has many muscle reactions, called reflexes, that take place automatically when certain "feeler" nerves are excited. When stretch receptors in the knee are excited by a tap, the foot swings forward without the brain even thinking about it.

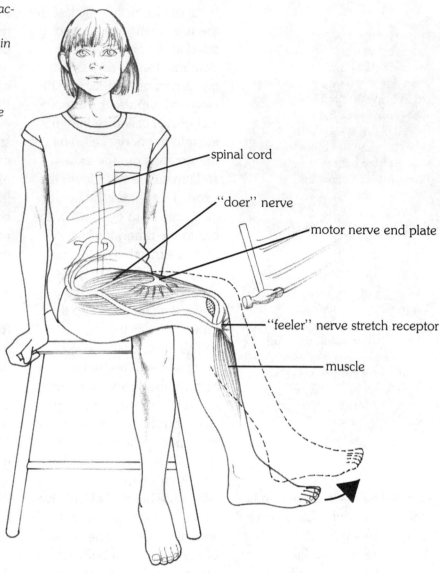

spinal cord

"doer" nerve

motor nerve end plate

"feeler" nerve stretch receptor

muscle

is the knee-jerk. When a person is tapped just below the kneecap, his or her leg will automatically kick. This happens because the tap hits hundreds of little sensory nerve endings at the tip of the muscle. These feeler nerves, which constantly measure how tight the muscle is, send a message to the spinal cord saying that the muscle has been stretched. A message is then sent back along the motor nerve telling the big muscle on the top of the thigh to tighten. This tightening is what causes the lower leg to swing out. Simple reflexes like this help to make all muscle movements smoother. Most reflexes are even more complicated than this and involve thinker nerve cells in the brain and combine the movement of several muscles.

The central nervous system The brain and spinal cord are filled with groups of thinker cells working together to do a particular job. The spinal cord is the simplest part. It is here that feeler cells bring in messages and motor cells leave with messages. The spinal cord also has groups of nerves that connect feeler and doer nerves with thinker nerves in the brain. These groups of nerves are called *tracts*. There are matching groups on either side of the spinal cord for the two sides of the body. Separate tracts carry up pain messages, touch messages, temperature messages, and so on. There are also motor tracts that carry messages from the brain down to the muscles. So the spinal cord is like a big cable that contains many bundles of wires. And each bundle carries just one kind of nerve. As sensory nerves enter the spinal cord they join with similar sensory nerves in the right bundle or tract.

Most of the thinker cells are in the brain. The brain is divided into different areas, each with a particular job. The jobs get more complicated and less automatic as they get higher in the brain. The *medulla* and the *pons* at the bottom of the brain have control of many of the functions that keep us alive— breathing, heartbeat, blood pressure, swallowing, and digestion. The *cerebellum* has control of balance and coordination of groups of muscles. It makes sure that movements are smooth, not jerky, and that all the muscles are working together.

The biggest part of the brain is the *cerebrum*. It is so big that it has to be folded up so it

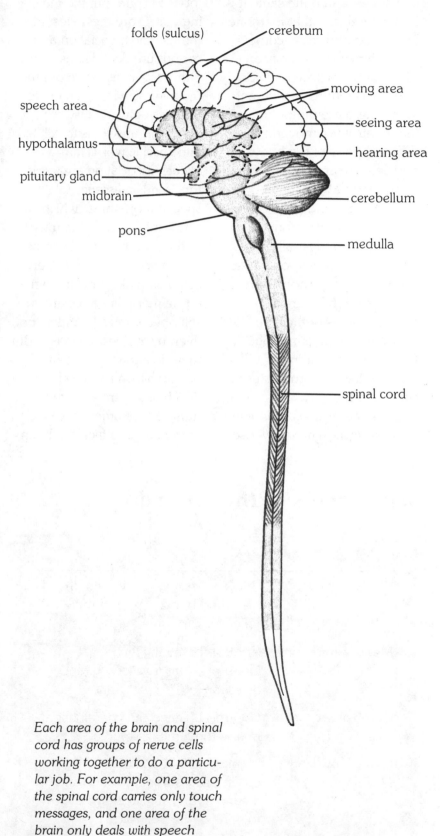

Each area of the brain and spinal cord has groups of nerve cells working together to do a particular job. For example, one area of the spinal cord carries only touch messages, and one area of the brain only deals with speech messages.

can squeeze into the skull. It is in the cerebrum that memories are stored and really complicated thinking takes place. The cerebrum itself is divided into areas that have different jobs: There are motor areas that control the movements of different parts of the body, and sensory areas that receive information about touch, temperature, and pain. The sensory areas are grouped by parts of the body—all nerves from the face are in one area, from the legs in another area, and so on. There are also separate areas of the cerebrum that receive messages from the eyes and nose. Other areas of the cerebrum cause a person to feel pleasure, anger, and other emotions. There are also *association areas*, whose job is to figure out the meaning of sensory messages. In the hearing association area, sounds are decoded as words. Other big areas figure out the meaning of whole sentences and decide what answer to give. This answer is translated into specific words in the speech association area. It in turn sends messages to a speech motor area, which sends messages to the muscles of the mouth and voice box.

Just how the firing of nerve cells can make a person write a poem or paint a picture is still not completely understood even by the best scientists. But they do know that the brain has 10 billion nerve cells, all of which are interconnected with hundreds of other nerve cells in the brain. In fact, the brain has many more interconnections and circuits than the largest computer on earth.

The autonomic nervous system The *autonomic nervous system* takes care of unconscious, or automatic, things like breathing, heartbeat, and digestion. It keeps different organs in the body running at the right speed. When organs are working too hard, it slows them down; when organs are working too slowly, it speeds them up.

The autonomic nervous system is controlled by the bottom of the brain, especially by an area called the *hypothalamus*. The hypothalamus also regulates the endocrine glands, which are the body's *chemical* way of controlling digestion, heartbeat, and breathing.

The autonomic nervous system has two different parts: the sympathetic nerves and the parasympathetic nerves. Basically, they do opposite things. The job of the *sympathetic nervous system* is to prepare the body for action, especially in times of emergency. This is called the *fight-or-flight* response. The job of the *parasympathetic nervous system* is to help the body rest, store food, and heal.

The sympathetic nervous system is made up of nerves that start in the spinal cord and lead out to various organs

What areas of the brain do

Area	Job
Spinal cord	Brings messages to and from the brain and body; controls simple reflex actions
Medulla and pons	Controls breathing, heartbeat, blood pressure, swallowing, and digestion
Cerebellum	Controls balance and coordination; makes movements smooth
Cerebrum	Thinks and solves problems; figures out messages from the body and the world and sends out messages to parts of the body to act

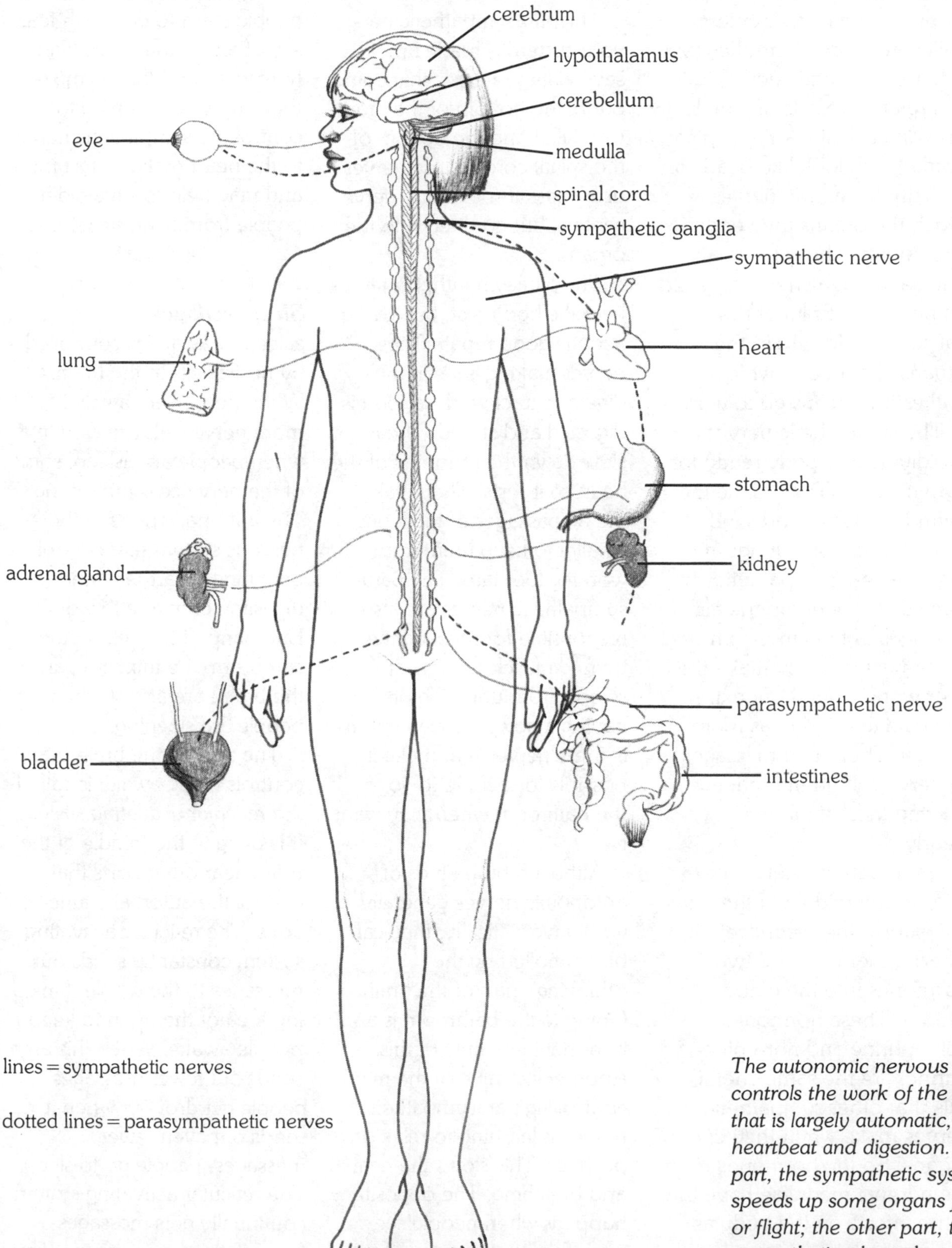

cerebrum

hypothalamus

cerebellum

medulla

spinal cord

sympathetic ganglia

sympathetic nerve

eye

heart

lung

stomach

kidney

adrenal gland

parasympathetic nerve

bladder

intestines

lines = sympathetic nerves

dotted lines = parasympathetic nerves

The autonomic nervous system controls the work of the organs that is largely automatic, such as heartbeat and digestion. One part, the sympathetic system, speeds up some organs for fight or flight; the other part, the parasympathetic, slows down organs to rest and digest food.

Anatomy and physiology **191**

in the body. Just outside the spinal cord, these nerves pass through little nerve centers, called *ganglia,* where they join other sympathetic nerves. There are two sets of ganglia, one on each side of the spinal cord, which look like beads on a chain. When the nerves reach the organs they end in special tips. These tips make and send out a chemical called *epinephrine.* Epinephrine causes muscle cells in the organs to squeeze, which makes the organs go to work.

The sympathetic nerves rapidly get the body ready for fight or flight. They make the heart beat faster and send more blood to the lungs and big muscles. Sympathetic nerves also open up the air passages of the lungs so more air can get in. They make the liver work to send out extra sugar so the body has more energy. They send messages to nerve cells in the brain, making them think more clearly.

A sympathetic nerve also goes to the middle of the *adrenal glands,* the *medullae,* causing them to send two hormones into the bloodstream. These hormones, epinephrine and nor-epinephrine, are the same chemicals that other sympathetic nerves make when they end in organs. So the hormones from the adrenal medullae have the same effects on the body as the sympathetic nerves them-

selves and boost all their actions.

The parasympathetic nervous system is made up of several large nerves that come out of the bottom of the brain (medulla) and the bottom of the spinal cord. These nerves *don't* pass through any nerve centers, but go directly to the organs.

The parasympathetic nerves help the body rest, build, and keep in good repair. These nerves make glands in the digestive tract work so food is digested and stored. They slow down the pumping of the heart so it rests. They make the air passages of the lungs smaller to keep them from working too hard. The parasympathetic nerves are also responsible for relaxing the trained muscles that keep people from urinating or having a bowel movement. It is these nerves that make it possible for people to go to the bathroom when they want to.

Although both kinds of autonomic nerves generally work automatically, they can be controlled by the "thinking" part of the brain. Going to the bathroom is an important example of this. Another example of the mind controlling parasympathetic nerves is learning to relax on purpose. This slows the heart and breathing. The opposite happens when people see something frightening. Then

their sympathetic nerves speed up the heart and breathing. If people learn to deal with fear, say of a test, then they learn how to control their sympathetic nerves. Learning to control the sympathetic nerve to the heart makes it rest more and may help to save older people from heart attacks.

Sleep feedback   Being asleep or awake is controlled by nerve cells in the brain. When people are awake, more nerve cells are working; when people are asleep, some of the nerve cells are resting. The automatic parts of the nervous system that control breathing, heartbeat, and digestion continue to work. But many of the cells in the cerebrum, the thinking part of the brain, are at rest when people are sleeping.

The area of the brain that controls being awake is called the *reticular activating system.* It is deep in the middle of the brain near other parts that control the automatic functions. The reticular activating system constantly sends out messages to the whole thinking area of the brain to keep people awake. When this area sends out fewer messages, people get drowsy; when it sends out even fewer messages, people go to sleep. The reticular activating system continually gets messages from all the sense organs. This

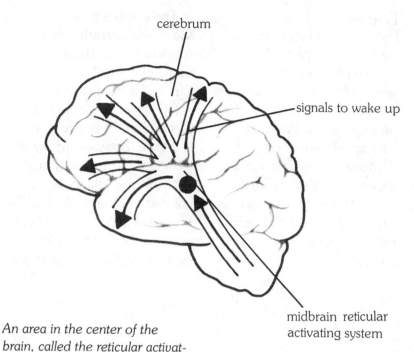

cerebrum

signals to wake up

midbrain reticular activating system

An area in the center of the brain, called the reticular activating system, sends many messages to the rest of the brain to keep people awake.

they happened. In other words, this side of the brain does a lot of the schoolwork—math and reading.

The *right side* of the brain keeps track of where all parts of the body are in space. This means it's important in dance, sports, and making things. The right brain gets its ideas in flashes—this is where hunches and intuitive feelings come from. It has to do with art, creativity, and seeing things all at once. At school, the right side has to do with art and sports. Also, when a number of facts come together clearly or when we get a new idea about how to solve a problem —it happens in the right brain.

means that people can be awakened by being shaken, by a loud noise, or by a light suddenly going on. The reticular activating system also gets messages from the thinking brain. This means that people can keep themselves awake by sending messages to the reticular area.

Another part of this system helps decide what people will concentrate on out of all the images, sounds, and feelings that are coming into the brain. It helps people to focus on one thing by filtering out all the other incoming messages.

Right and left brain The thinking brain, the cerebrum, is divided into two halves that are connected by a big group of nerve fibers. The whole thing looks like two sides of a shelled walnut. Although both sides of the cerebrum are involved in memory and thinking, each side controls different functions.

The *left side* of the brain thinks about words and numbers. It's good at figuring out how things work in a step-by-step way. It deals with facts, putting things in groups, and putting things in order as

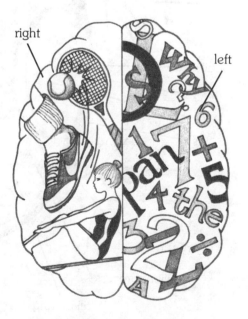

right

left

The left side of the brain deals more with words and numbers; the right side deals more with body position and ideas.

The eye

The eye is a special organ of the nervous system. Cells in the back of the eye are feeler cells whose job is to feel or pick up light and send the messages to the brain. These sensing cells are directly connected to the brain by a large nerve called the *optic nerve*. The eye's sensing cells actually grow outward from the brain when a baby is first developing.

The eye is a hollow ball, or sac, made of thick, white, rubbery fibers. This white area of the eye is called the *sclera*. The ball is filled with a clear, Jell-O-like liquid called *vitreous humor*. This gives the eye its shape. Because the liquid is clear, light can pass through it. In the front of the eye is a colored ring called the *iris*. The iris varies in color in different people—blue, brown, green, or gray. The amount and color

The eye is the sense organ that picks up light messages and sends them to the brain. The back of the eye is lined with two kinds of "feeler" cells: the rods see in the dark, the cones see color and sharp images. The insert shows how they look under the microscope.

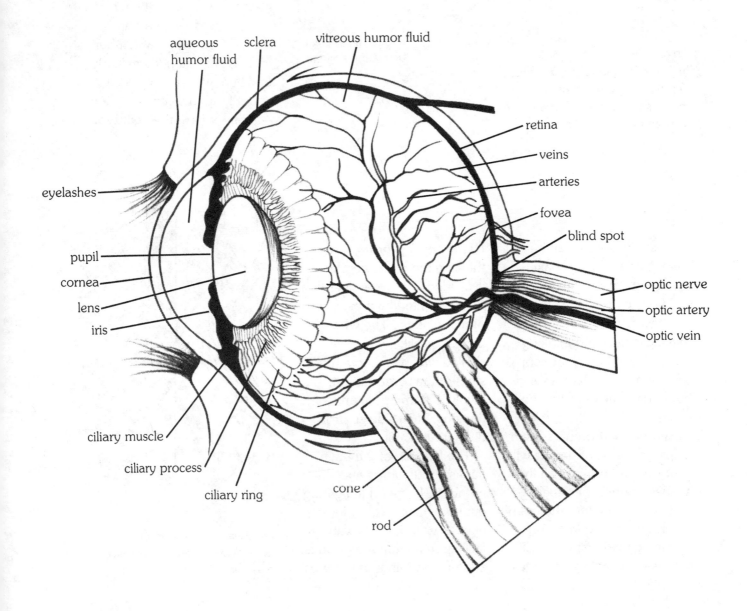

of pigment in people's irises are inherited from their parents. The job of the iris is to control how much light gets into the eye. The iris is a muscular ring that automatically opens wide in low light and closes down in bright light.

In the center of the iris is a black hole called the *pupil*. This is where light actually enters the eye. It is dark because the lining of the eye is dark colored so that light won't bounce around inside. This dark lining is called the *retina*. It contains the special light-sensing cells that send messages to the brain.

Directly behind the iris is a clear, rubbery disk called the *lens*. This is what focuses the light on the cells of the retina and makes it sharp. Around the lens is a muscle called the *ciliary muscle*. It pulls the lens to change its shape and adjust the focus of the eye. The very front part of the sclera, over the pupil, is clear rather than white in order to let light pass through it. This part of the sclera is called the *cornea*. It focuses light on the lens, but it can't be adjusted. Between the cornea and the lens is a small bulge filled with clear fluid that is called the *aqueous humor*. It brings food to the cornea.

Light is focused, or bent, as it goes through the cornea. Then it passes through the aqueous humor and the open-ing of the pupil. Next it goes through the lens and it is bent again at the back of the lens. Then the light passes through the vitreous humor and hits the cells in the retina that line the back of the eye. The eye is actually like a soft camera that captures the light and focuses it on special sensing cells.

The retina lining the eye contains two different types of nerve cells. These sensing cells are called *rods* and *cones*. Most of the cells in the retina are rods, which pick up very low amounts of light. They are responsible for seeing at night and in other dark situations. They create a general picture of light and dark and are especially important in picking up what people see out of the corners of their eyes. The cones need bright light to work. They make a sharp, detailed picture. Most of the cones are located in one area in the middle of the retina that is called the *fovea*. This is why people look straight at things they want to see sharply.

Cones are also responsible for color vision. There are three types of cone cells—red, blue, and green—and each one picks up only one color. Colors that are mixtures, like purple or orange, are picked up by two types of cone cells. About one boy in fifty lacks one kind of cone cell. When this happens, a boy sees colors but has trouble telling the difference, usually between red and green. This special condition is called *color blindness*. Boys inherit it from their parents; girls rarely do.

There is one spot on the retina where there are no rod or cone cells. This spot is where the "arms" of all the rod and cone cells join to make up the optic nerve. It is called the *blind spot* because it can't pick up light (see "Eye games," page 198).

Basically, rod and cone cells work the same way. They join Vitamin A to a protein to make a special chemical that fires the nerve cell when a ray of light hits it. Once the chemical is hit by light it is used up.

The nerve message, or impulse, is passed from one nerve cell to another until it gets to the back of the brain. Each cell works to decode the message and give it a more exact meaning: First the message is simply registered as light or dark; then the brain decides just how far away the light source is and what color it is; then the brain figures out the shape of the light coming in; finally, the brain decides exactly what object the light is coming from.

The eye muscles The eye moves easily in all directions. This enables it to follow moving objects. It also helps it to focus the sharpest area of light-sensing cells on an object

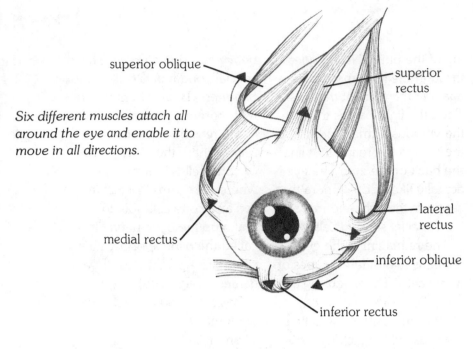

superior oblique

superior rectus

Six different muscles attach all around the eye and enable it to move in all directions.

medial rectus

lateral rectus

inferior oblique

inferior rectus

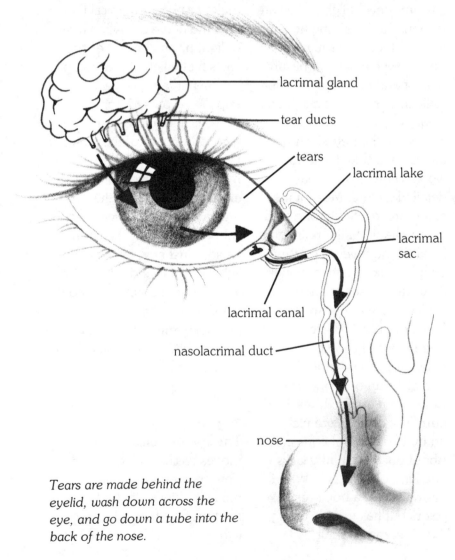

lacrimal gland

tear ducts

tears

lacrimal lake

lacrimal sac

lacrimal canal

nasolacrimal duct

nose

Tears are made behind the eyelid, wash down across the eye, and go down a tube into the back of the nose.

without requiring people to turn their heads.

The eye is moved by six muscles that attach to the white covering of the eye behind the lids. The top and bottom muscles pull the eye up or down. The side muscles pull the eye to the left or right. The last two muscles help the eye to roll around.

Generally, both eyes move together. This is not because the muscles of the two eyes are attached, but because a special area of the lower brain automatically sends out the same "moving" message to each eye.

The tear ducts The eye is kept wet with tears all the time. Tears are a clear fluid made up of salt, a little mucus, and a chemical that kills bacteria. They are made constantly by the *lacrimal gland*, which is located above the eye, toward the side of the head.

When people blink, tears are pushed down across the eye and then flow into the inner corner next to the nose. Here they collect in the *lacrimal lake* and finally flow down two little tubes into the back of the nose.

When something irritates the eye, many more tears are made than usual. Often this is enough to wash a tiny speck of dirt down the back of the nose. When people are very sad or even very happy, they also make many more tears than usual. This is called *crying*. No one really knows why this happens.

How the eyes focus   The job of the lens is to turn a big scene outside the eye into an extremely tiny scene inside the eye. The lens actually shrinks the outside picture so it can fit on the back of the retina.

Light rays bend whenever they pass through anything thicker than air. When light rays pass through a curve that bulges out, they are bent closer together on the other side. This is how the lens of the eye bends a scene to make it smaller.

The lens has to bend a scene just the right amount to make it land sharply on the retina. The light from objects that are far away and from objects that are close has to be bent differently. The closer an object is, the more the light from it has to be bent; the farther away an object is, the less the light from it has to be bent. To bend light in different amounts, the lens has to change its shape. This is done automatically by the brain. The brain controls the ciliary muscle, which can flatten out the lens, making it bend light less.

Light from the top of a scene is bent down and comes out the bottom of the lens on the other side. Light from the lower part of a scene does just the opposite—it comes out the top of the lens. Thus the whole picture that lands on the retina is not only smaller, it is also upside down! In the brain the picture is flipped again, so people believe they are seeing right side up.

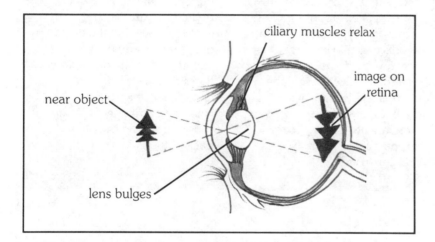

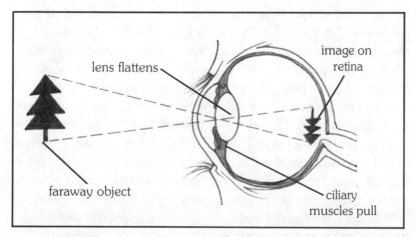

The lens of the eye sharply focuses an image of an object on the back of the eye as muscles automatically change its shape. The image is upside down, but the brain knows to flip it over.

Eye games

Look at a camera and compare it with the illustration of the eye. Both have a lens that focuses the light. If you can, switch the camera's F-stops to see the diaphragm open and close. This is what the iris of the eye does. Open the back of the camera and look where the film goes. This is like the retina; the image or picture is focused here.

Look at a magnifying glass. It's a lens like the eye—it's curved out on both sides. Hold the magnifying glass up to a bright light or the sun. Move a piece of paper back and forth about two or three inches under the magnifying glass. At one position all the light rays will be bent in to the same point and will focus a point of light on the paper. This is how the lens of the eye focuses a big scene on the small retina at the back of the eye.

Look at a friend's eye from the side to see the cornea, the clear area over the lens. In a darkened room notice how big the pupil, the black area of the eye, looks. Then shine a small flashlight into your friend's eye for a few seconds. Watch how the pupil quickly and automatically closes and gets small in the light. Also have your friend look up, down, diagonally, to each side. Watch how smoothly and beautifully the muscles move the eye.

On a piece of paper draw a cross, and about two or three inches to the right, draw a dot. Cover your left eye and stare at the cross with your right. Slowly move the paper in closer to your eye. When the paper gets about six inches from your eye, the dot will disappear. This is because the dot is right in front of the place where the big optic nerve attaches to the back of your eye, and there are no "seeing" cells in this part of the retina (see drawing, page 194).

Have a friend hold a pencil out in front of his or her eyes and focus on it. Then have your friend slowly bring the pencil in toward his or her nose, keeping it in focus all the time. Watch to see how your friend's eyes turn inward to keep the pencil in focus. Try it yourself and feel your eye muscles at work.

Stare at something straight ahead. Without moving your eyes, notice what's to either side. Now actually look to the left and right and notice how much sharper and clearer the things are when you look directly at them. That's because the cones, the cells that see sharply in bright light, are mostly in one spot (the fovea) in the center of the retina. Try the same experiment in the dark. Now the side objects will be very clear. That's because the cells that see in the dark, the rods, are spread over the back of the eye.

***How eyeglasses
work*** Sometimes the lens of the eye can't bend the right amount to make light rays from a scene land sharply on the light-sensing cells of the retina. This is when people need glasses. Glasses are just another pair of lenses that help the lenses of the eyes.

If the lens of the eye can't flatten out enough, or if the eye is too narrow, an object will be in focus *behind* the retina. Right at the retina, the picture will be fuzzy. This is called being *farsighted*. People who are farsighted can see objects far away easily, but objects that are very close (like a book) are blurry. Glasses that bulge (convex lenses) help to focus the light right on the retina and make it sharp for farsighted people.

When the lens of the eye flattens too much or the eye is too long, an object will be in focus in *front* of the retina. Right at the retina, the picture will be blurry. This is called being *nearsighted*. People who are nearsighted see close objects well, but have trouble seeing things far away. Glasses that are bent inward (concave lenses) help to focus distant light right on the retina and make it sharp for nearsighted people.

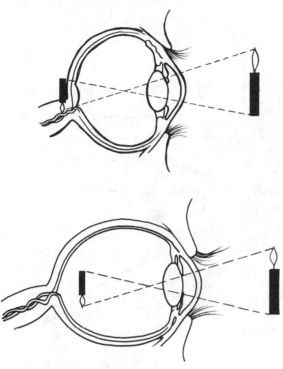

Farsightedness:
image focused behind retina

Nearsightedness:
image focused in front of retina

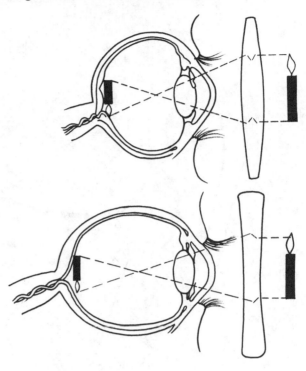

Farsightedness corrected:
image focused on retina convex lens

Nearsightedness corrected:
image focused on retina concave lens

The ear

The ear is a very complicated organ whose job it is to pick up sounds and turn them into nerve impulses that are sent to the brain. The brain learns to make meaning out of these messages.

Sounds are actually waves that travel through the air. You can't see them, but you can feel them against your body if they are very loud. Your ears are much more sensitive—they can "feel" even very soft sounds. To make a sound, something has to move back and forth, or vibrate. You can feel this if you put your hand on the front of your neck as you talk. The vibrations of your voice box jiggle the molecules in the air close to them. These molecules in turn jiggle the molecules next to them, and so on. The sound waves or vibrations spread out equally in all directions. That is why everyone in a room hears the same sound. As sound waves move away from the object that made them, they become less and less loud. The waves use up their energy as they jiggle more and more molecules. Eventually the vibrations stop and the sound "ends." How far a sound travels depends on how much energy it starts

Sometimes the lens of the eye focuses an image in front of or behind the retina at the back of the eye. Glasses can adjust this image so it falls right on the retina.

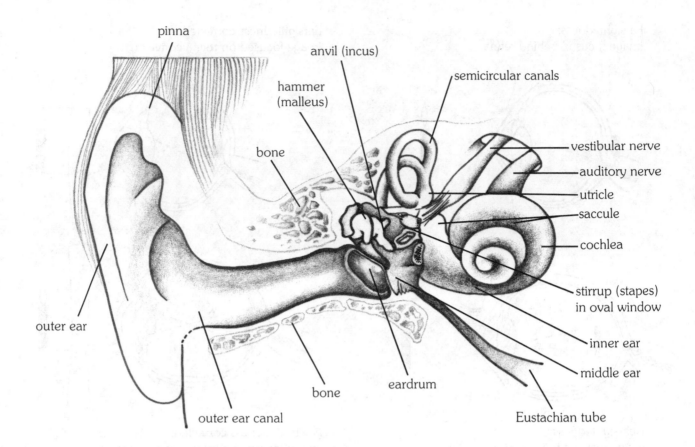

pinna

anvil (incus)

hammer
(malleus)

semicircular canals

bone

vestibular nerve

auditory nerve

utricle

saccule

cochlea

stirrup (stapes)
in oval window

inner ear

middle ear

outer ear

outer ear canal

bone

eardrum

Eustachian tube

*The ear has three parts. The
outer part catches sounds, and
the middle part strengthens and
carries the sound to the inner ear,
which excites nerve endings in
the cochlea and carries the
message to the brain. The rest of
the inner ear has special nerve
endings that help a person keep
in balance.*

with. Different noises make
different patterns in the air. To
make a high sound, something
has to vibrate very quickly,
many times per second. Low
sounds are made when
objects vibrate more slowly.

The ear is divided into three
parts. The part we see is called
the *outer ear*. It consists of a
wrinkly funnel on the outside
and a tube leading inside. The
funnel, called the *pinna*, helps
to gather in sound waves. It is
made of rubbery cartilage
covered with skin. The tube,
called the *external canal*, goes
through the bones of the skull.
The end of the canal is
covered with a tightly
stretched, elastic piece of skin
called the *eardrum*. The

eardrum can bounce or
vibrate just like the head of a
drum. Whenever sound waves
reach the eardrum, it vibrates
in and out.

Beyond the eardrum lies the
middle ear. It is a walled-off
area with no outside opening.
It's like a cave. The middle ear
is surrounded by bone except
for a tiny tube that connects
the middle ear to the back of
the throat. This tube, called the
Eustachian tube, keeps the
pressure the same on both
sides of the eardrum (see "Ear
games," page 201) so it can
vibrate freely.

Inside the middle ear are
three tiny bones—the smallest
bones in the body. The first
bone, the *hammer*, is actually

Ear games

Put your fingers below your Adam's apple. Say a few words and feel the vibrations from your voice box. Make a loud noise; make a soft noise. Try singing a high note, a low note. Feel the difference in the vibrations.

Put several big rubber bands around an old tissue box that has a wide hole in the top. Pluck the rubber bands. Listen to the sound they make and watch how they vibrate. Pull one rubber band tighter and pluck it again. The sound will be higher. Try playing a guitar or a drum and watch how the strings and drumhead vibrate.

Put your hand directly over a stereo, radio, or TV speaker when the volume is fairly high. You will feel vibrations, especially if the speaker is only covered with cloth. You may even be able to feel sound waves moving the air in front of the speaker.

To see how sound travels through the air, you can make a model with marbles. Set five or ten marbles close together in a straight line. Tap the first marble toward the second. Each marble will push the next. This is how sound is transferred from one air molecule to the next.

Listen to a watch ticking with your bare ear. Now hold a kitchen funnel to your ear and listen again. The sound will be much louder because the funnel directs the vibrations into your ear. This is how the outer ear helps to gather sound waves. To see how much the outer ear helps, listen to a radio playing softly in front of your ear and then behind it.

Make a model of the middle ear using a small cardboard box with an open top. Cut a round, two-inch hole in one side of the box. Stretch a cut piece of balloon tightly over the hole and attach it with thumbtacks. Through the top of the box, stick a piece of

clay onto the inside of the balloon. Stick a toothpick into the clay. The balloon represents the eardrum and the toothpick represents the tiny bones in the middle ear. Tap gently on the outside of the balloon and see how it wiggles the toothpick. This is how sounds move the eardrum and the bones of the inner ear.

Make a model of the inner ear to see how the tiny hairs move. Take a piece of brown, hairy rope or string and unravel one end until all the little hairs stick out. Cut off the rope about an inch above and attach the unraveled end to the inside of the bottom of a small glass jar with a piece of clay. Fill the jar with water. Stretch a cut balloon over the top and hold it in place tightly with a rubber band so it won't leak. Turn the jar on its side (in the sink). Tap on the balloon and watch how the hairs on the rope shake. This is how the fluid moves in the inner ear and shakes the hairs on the nerve endings.

attached to the eardrum. The second bone, the *anvil*, is attached to the hammer on one side and to the *stirrup*, the third bone, on the other side. The stirrup touches the *oval window*, the opening to the inner ear.

The *inner ear* consists of two hollow parts in the bones of the skull. One part, the

vestibular apparatus, has a central area and three loops. It helps people keep their balance (see page 200). The second part, the *cochlea*, looks almost exactly like a snail shell. It helps to conduct sounds to the brain. The spiral tube of the cochlea is filled with fluid. It has a thin lining inside that has many hairs that

stick out into the fluid. Each of these hairs has many special nerve cells with *very* tiny hairs on them.

When a sound reaches the eardrum, it vibrates the drum, which pushes the three little bones back and forth. The last bone jiggles the fluid in the cochlea and starts waves going through it. These waves shake

When a sound wave hits the inner ear, it jiggles a big hair, which in turn rubs little hairs against a wall on top called the tectorial membrane. This drawing shows how the sound receptor, the organ of Corti, looks under a microscope.

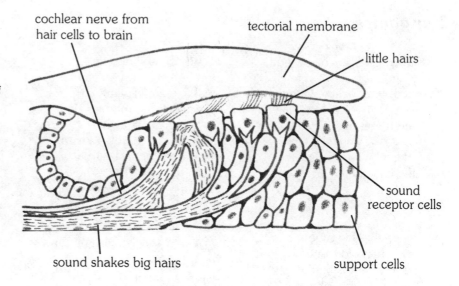

cochlear nerve from hair cells to brain

tectorial membrane

little hairs

sound receptor cells

sound shakes big hairs

support cells

the big hairs, which makes the smaller nerve hairs shake. When the hairs of the nerve cells are shaken, they start a nerve signal that passes from cell to cell until it reaches the brain.

In a series of steps, the brain figures out what the nerve signals mean. First the brain decides whether the message came from the right or left side. Then it figures out whether the notes are high or low, and what rhythm, or pattern, they have. Then the brain figures out if the ears are hearing music, noise, or speech. Finally, it figures out what the music or sentences mean.

The inner ear and balance Inside the inner ear is a special organ whose job is to figure out whether the head is upright, tilted, or upside down. This organ, called the vestibular apparatus, also signals the brain when the head moves suddenly. Being aware of tilting and moving is necessary in order for people to keep their balance; without this awareness people would fall down when they ran or played sports.

The vestibular apparatus has two parts—the *semicircular canals,* and the *saccule and utricle.* Inside the saccule and utricle are special nerve cells covered with hairs. These hairs are stuck in a Jell-O-like

A special part of the inner ear, called the macula, *signals the brain when the head is tilted. Inside, little grains shift, moving a layer of gel underneath, which rubs against tiny sensing hairs. This is how these cells look under a microscope.*

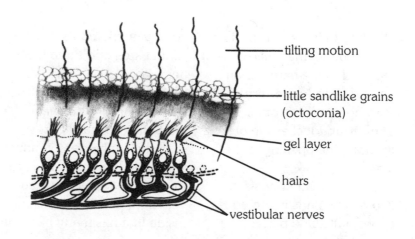

tilting motion

little sandlike grains (octoconia)

gel layer

hairs

vestibular nerves

Balance games

substance that is covered with little sandlike grains. When a person's head moves, the grains move and bend the nerve hairs, and these nerve cells send a message to the brain that the head is out of balance. The brain answers by sending messages to the muscles that will keep the person from falling.

There are three semicircular canals; each measures or senses when the head moves in a different direction. One canal is sideways; one is straight up and facing front to back; and one is straight up, facing side to side. The canals are filled with fluid. At the bottom of each canal are tiny nerve cells with hairs on them. These nerve hairs are also stuck in a Jell-O-like

substance. When people turn their heads quickly, fluid rubs against the Jell-O-covered hairs. Then whichever nerve cells are rubbed send a message to the brain. The brain figures out which way the head is moving and sets muscles to work to keep the person from falling.

The taste buds

Taste buds are nerve cells in the mouth that enable people to tell whether foods are salty, sweet, bitter, or sour. There are 10,000 taste buds. Most are located in mounds on the top and sides of the tongue. Each taste bud is made up of special long skin cells that have tiny hairs that stick out

through little holes in the mound. Packed between the skin cells are nerve endings. The skin cells react to certain chemicals in the mouth and make the nerve cells send messages to the brain.

Each skin cell, or *taste cell*, basically picks up one of the four "flavors." Most taste cells of the same kind are located in the same area of the tongue. The bitter ones are in the back; the sour ones are on the sides, toward the back; and the sweet and salty ones are toward the front. Most foods are a combination of the four flavors. Different foods have different combinations that the brain learns to recognize.

Thousands of years ago the different taste cells were probably very important to help

The tongue is covered with taste buds that pick up sweet, sour, bitter, and salty tastes.

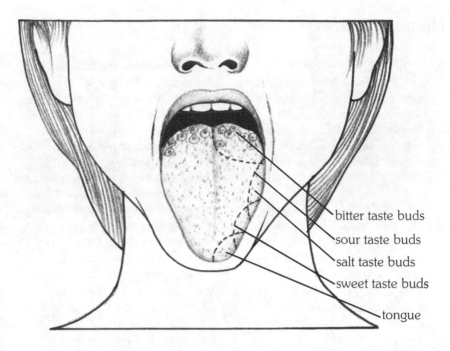

bitter taste buds
sour taste buds
salt taste buds
sweet taste buds
tongue

Taste games

Try a taste test with a friend. Blindfold your friend and then put a drop of salty water, white vinegar, sugar water, and finally an unflavored vitamin C tablet on his or her tongue. Let your friend try and guess what each taste is—sweet, sour, bitter, or salty. Be sure your friend rinses his or her mouth in between tastes.

Sprinkle a few grains of salt, then a drop of salty water on your tongue. Which do you taste fastest? Try putting a drop of salt water on different areas of your tongue. Use a chopstick or a plastic drink mixer to apply the salt solution so it doesn't run all over your tongue. Which parts of the tongue taste salt the best?

Make a simple model of a taste bud. Make a tongue out of pink clay (or Play-Doh). Poke many tiny holes in the top of the tongue and fill the holes with red clay. If you want to, use slightly different colors for taste buds that pick up sweet, sour, bitter, and salty tastes (see illustration). Place three or four bristles from an old toothbrush into each taste bud, so they stick out. These represent the hairlike endings of the taste buds (see drawing).

Get a beef tongue from the butcher. They are so large that you can actually see taste buds on the back and the fuzzy hair endings all over the top. Cut into the tongue to see the muscle fibers and the fat.

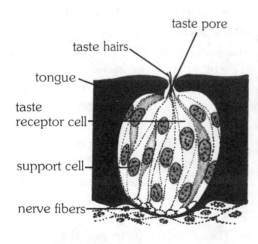

taste pore
taste hairs
tongue
taste receptor cell
support cell
nerve fibers

This drawing shows how a taste bud looks under the microscope.

early peoples survive in the woods. Bitter taste cells help to identify poisonous foods, which are often bitter. Salt taste cells help to identify foods with salt, which the body needs to stay alive. Sour taste cells help to identify acid foods, which may be rotten. Sweet taste cells help to identify sweet things like ripe fruits, which have lots of food energy and vitamins.

The nose

The sense of smell makes it possible for us to be aware of molecules in the air. People smell the odor of food, flowers, smoke, and even dangerous chemicals. In other animals, smelling is the major way they find food, recognize other animals who are friends or enemies, and figure out where they are.

In humans the sense of smell is not so sharp, but it's still very helpful in recognizing dangerous situations like fire, and pleasurable things like food. The sense of smell is probably more important to people than they realize. Even though people may not be aware of it, smells affect the way they act. For example, people often become hungry when they smell food they like. Newborn babies can

Way up inside the nose there are nerve cells with tiny hairs that react to odors. This drawing shows where the hairs are; the insert shows how they look under the microscope.

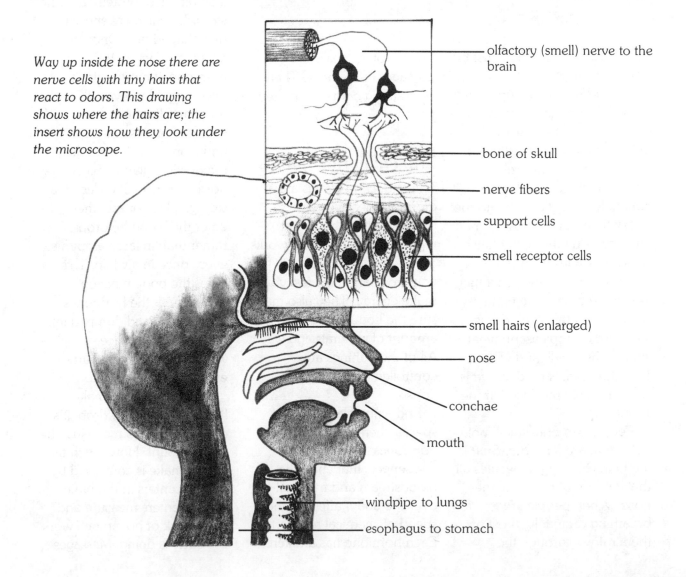

olfactory (smell) nerve to the brain

bone of skull

nerve fibers

support cells

smell receptor cells

smell hairs (enlarged)

nose

conchae

mouth

windpipe to lungs

esophagus to stomach

Smell games

recognize their mothers just by their special scent!

The cells that pick up odors or smells are located in the top of the nose. There are 100 million of these special nerve cells in an area the size of a square inch. The cells have tiny hairs that stick out into the moist lining of the nose. When molecules hit them, the hairs send messages from one nerve cell to another until they reach the brain. The brain decides whether the odor is pleasant or unpleasant, what makes the smell, and what it is. If the smell is food, saliva is automatically produced in the mouth.

People can only smell molecules that are airborne. *Sniffing* helps to bring molecules all the way up to the top of the nose. When people are breathing ordinarily, most of the air flows through the bottom of the mazelike passages of the nose. Then only strong odors are picked up.

The endocrine glands

The *endocrine glands* are a group of special organs throughout the body that regulates how the body works. These organs control how fast you grow, and how fast you make energy. They also make sure the body has just the right amount of minerals and water. All of these things are controlled by chemical reactions.

Endocrine glands make special chemicals called *hormones.* Hormones are messengers that enter the bloodstream and travel all over the body, affecting the speed of chemical reactions. Each hormone has a different function. Some hormones affect every cell in the body, some affect only the cells in one organ. (When a hormone affects just one organ, it is called a *target organ.*) The hormones are so powerful that it only takes a few drops for them to do their job. For this reason, most of the endocrine glands are very small.

Each endocrine gland contains cells that make a particular hormone. There are two basic kinds of hormones: the *polypeptides,* which are little pieces of protein, and the *steroids,* which are special ring-shaped fats. Once the cells manufacture the hormone, it moves directly into a tiny blood vessel, not a tube, and then into the bloodstream. For this reason the endocrine glands are called the ductless glands. Since the hormones do not collect in a storage place or sac, they enter the blood by drops, rather than in large amounts every once in a while. This helps the body function smoothly. If the hormones were stored and dumped into the blood all at once, people would have a great spurt of energy and then none.

Since the glands make hormones drop by drop, it's easy for them to make just the right amount. How much the glands make is controlled by special centers in the brain. These centers measure and keep track of how much work the body is doing. Messages are continually sent to the glands telling them to make more or less of a hormone, depending upon how much is needed. Making tiny adjustments based on how well things are working is called *feedback*. It is a basic way the body maintains itself and keeps healthy.

The hormones themselves don't know where in the body to go. But the cells that use the hormones have special sites on their walls that lock onto the hormone. Some hormones actually enter the cell after they lock onto it and then trigger the work that goes on. But most hormones don't enter a cell directly. They trigger other chemicals that work inside the cell.

The most important endocrine gland is the *pituitary*. It is called the *master gland*

The endocrine system is a group of glands that makes chemicals called hormones, which affect cells all over the body. Some hormones control growth, some control energy production, some keep the body's minerals in balance.

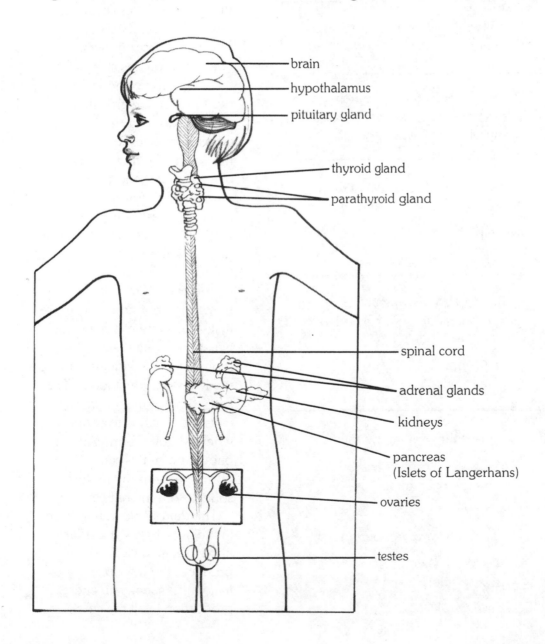

brain
hypothalamus
pituitary gland

thyroid gland
parathyroid gland

spinal cord

adrenal glands

kidneys

pancreas
(Islets of Langerhans)

ovaries

testes

What each gland does

Gland	Job
Pituitary	Tells other glands what to do—the "master gland"
	Tells the body to grow
	Controls the kidney; tells it how much water to save
	Tells the uterus to contract when a baby is born and the breasts to make milk after a baby is born
Thyroid	Tells all the body's cells to make energy
Parathyroids	Raises calcium level in the blood to the right amount for nerves and muscles to work well
Pancreas islets	Keeps sugar in the blood at the right level to maintain energy
	Helps sugar get into all the body's cells
Adrenals	Keeps the right amount of sodium and potassium in the blood to keep all the cells alive
	Helps the body react to an emergency or fight
Ovaries	Causes the growth spurt in girls
	Makes girls' breasts and bodies grow to adult shape
Testes	Causes the growth spurt in boys
	Makes boys' penises and bodies grow to adult shape

because it makes hormones that tell the other glands how much of their hormones to make. The pituitary is the size of a lima bean and lies in a cavity in the middle of the brain, directly under the *hypothalamus.* The hypothalamus controls the pituitary, and has special cells that measure how all the hormones are working.

The pituitary is divided into two parts. The front part of the pituitary produces six important hormones. *Growth hormone* causes growth. Even after a person has stopped growing, this hormone continues to cause the growth of new cells to replace old ones. Other hormones tell the adrenal cortex, the thyroid, the ovaries, and the testes how much of their hormones to make. The last hormone controls the production of milk after a woman has had a baby.

The back of the pituitary makes two hormones. The first, ADH, controls how much water the kidneys save. The more water the kidneys save, the less salty the blood is. The second hormone (oxytocin) causes the uterus to contract when a baby is born. After the baby is born, this same hormone helps the mother to squeeze out the baby's milk.

The *thyroid gland* is located in the neck below the Adam's apple (see page 207). It produces the hormone *thyroxine,* which speeds up energy production in all the cells.

Endocrine games

Cells make energy through a chemical process in which a special sugar and oxygen are turned into water and carbon dioxide. Thyroxine tells the cells to make more enzymes, which speeds up the whole process. Thyroxine also affects how fast children grow.

Sitting on the thyroid gland are four tiny round glands called the *parathyroids*. They send out a hormone that regulates how much calcium is in the blood at any given time. Nerves and muscles need just the right amount of calcium to work. Parathyroid hormone raises calcium in the blood in three ways: It keeps the kidney from sending out calcium in the urine; it makes the small intestines take more calcium out of food; and it causes special bone cells to dissolve bone and release calcium into the bloodstream.

The *islets of Langerhans* make two hormones that regulate how the body uses glucose, the sugar that comes out of digested foods. The islets are scattered throughout the *pancreas,* a long gland that lies under the stomach. (The rest of the pancreas makes digestive enzymes that are dumped into the small intestine.) The islets make insulin, a hormone that makes it possible for glucose to pass from the blood into the body's cells. Without insulin, sugar can't be used to make energy —it just builds up in the blood. Insulin is released whenever the level of blood sugar rises; it stops being released when the level of blood sugar drops. The islets also make *glucagon,* a hormone that does the opposite of insulin. It raises the amount of sugar in the blood by making the liver send out stored glucose when the body needs more energy.

The *adrenals* are a pair of endocrine glands that sit one on top of each kidney. The outer part of the gland is named the *cortex.* It produces a number of hormones called *steroids.* The steroids do two basic things. One group constantly regulates the amounts of sodium and potassium in all the fluids of the body. This group makes the kidney save sodium and get rid of potassium. A second group of steroids helps the body react to stressful or frightening situations. It makes the liver cells release sugar, fat cells release fat, and other cells release protein. The sugar, fat, and protein are all sent into the bloodstream, ready to aid the body in running and fighting. While an emergency occurs, this group of steroids also keeps the body from swelling and making antibodies. This probably allows people to continue running or fighting even though they're hurt. For a brief time the body continues to act as if it were well.

The inside of the adrenal glands is called the *medulla.* The medulla is actually made up of special nerve cells that make two hormones called *epinephrine* and *nor-epine-phrine* (see pages 190–92). These hormones help regulate all the work the body does automatically: heartbeat, breathing, blood flow, and so on. They do the actual work of making a body run or fight in an emergency. They make the lungs open and the heart pump harder. They also take blood away from kidneys and digestive track and send it to the big muscles and the brain. Like the adrenal cortex, the medulla makes cells send sugar into the blood. Like the thyroid, the medulla speeds up energy production. All together the hormones of the medulla help people to act quickly, intelligently, and with greater than normal strength. Epinephrine and nor-epine-phrine help kids when they run a race, take a test, or get scared.

The male and female sex organs are also part of the endocrine system (see pages 211–15). The female glands, the *ovaries,* make two hormones, *estrogen* and *progesterone,* which cause girls' adolescent growth spurt. The male sexual glands, *testes,* produce *testosterone,* the hormone that causes the teen-age growth spurt in boys.

The reproductive system

A baby grows from one special cell that divides over and over again. The information that tells the cell how to grow into a baby is in the nucleus in the center of the cell. The information is stored on long rods called *chromosomes.* Every human cell has 46 chromosomes. Half the chromosomes in the nucleus come from the mother, half from the father. This means a baby is not an exact copy of the mother or the father, but is a special mixture of both. Both men and women make cells that contain half the amount of chromosomes (23) that cells usually have. In men these

Reproductive games

Kids get their features from their parents, but kids are a special mixture, not a copy. Look at your hair color, eye color, skin color, the shape of your nose, dimples (or lack of them), and the shape of your ears. Which things are like your mother? Your father? Your grandparents?

Make a model of the male reproductive system. Make an oval ball about one inch high out of clay to represent a testicle. Take a ten-inch piece of string and make a couple of loops on top of the testicle. This represents the epididymus. About four inches down the string, wrap a little piece of clay around the string. This represents the seminal vesicle. Below the vesicle, put a large round ball of clay around the string to represent the prostate gland (see drawing).

Make a model of the female reproductive system. Make two little balls of clay about one inch in diameter. These represent the ovaries. Take two little pieces of string and unravel one end of each. Put the fuzzy ends of the string on top but not quite touching the ovaries. These represent the fallopian tubes and the *fimbria* that catch the eggs as they pop out of the ovaries. Curve the strings down and attach them to the top of another ball of clay shaped like a three-inch upside down pear. This represents the uterus (see drawing).

To see how an egg comes out of an ovary, put a marble in a small plastic bag. Squeeze the plastic bag until the marble pops out. This is what happens when an egg bursts out of the follicle (see drawing).

special cells are called *sperm;* in women they are called *eggs.* When one sperm and one egg join, they make one new cell with 46 chromosomes. This is a new combination of chromosomes that has never existed before. From this cell, a new baby, unlike any other, will develop.

The male reproductive system

The male reproductive system is what makes it possible for a man to be a father. The parts of the system work together to make sperm, and to enable the sperm to join an egg from the mother.

Sperm are made in the *testes,* two oval balls the size of tiny plums. Sperm start to be made when a boy is between 10 and 16 and his sexual organs start to grow up rapidly. From then on, the testes constantly make millions of sperm. The testes also make testosterone, the male hormone that makes teen-age

The male reproductive system makes it possible for a man to become a father. The insert shows the inside of a testis, where the male reproductive cells called sperm are made.

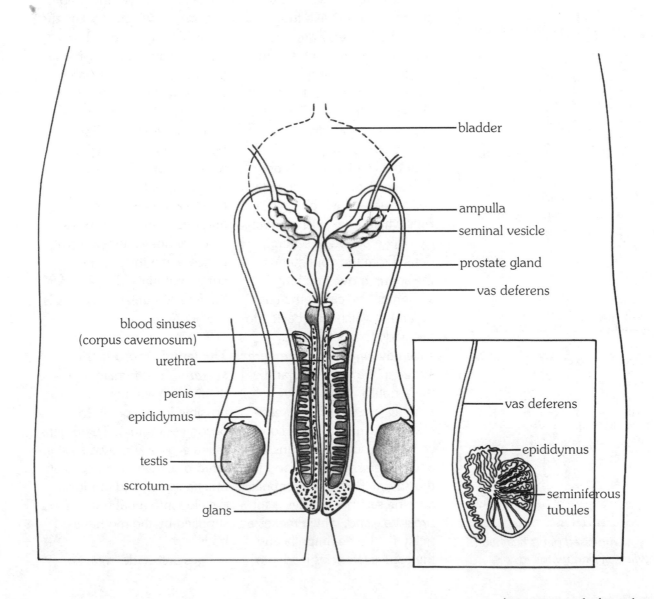

blood sinuses (corpus cavernosum)
urethra
penis
epididymus
testis
scrotum
glans

bladder
ampulla
seminal vesicle
prostate gland
vas deferens

vas deferens
epididymus
seminiferous tubules

boys' bodies grow and mature. The testes rest in a pouch of skin called the *scrotum,* which hangs outside the body behind the penis. Being outside the body keeps the testes several degrees cooler than inside. Sperm have to stay at this temperature to grow. The perfect temperature can be kept because the muscles in the wall of the scrotum pull the testes up when it is cold and relax, letting them down, when it is warm.

Inside the testes are tiny coiled tubes. In each tube special cells divide and produce sperm. Each sperm cell looks something like a tadpole, with an oval head and a long thin tail. The tail waves back and forth and makes the sperm move along at about eight inches an hour. The sperm move into a wide, coiled tube called the *epididymus* where they finish growing up over a period of several days. From the epididymus the sperm move into long straight tubes, called the *vas deferens,* which lead back into the body to a wider area called the *ampulla.* Sperm are stored in the wide tube and the ampulla. Next to the ampulla are the *seminal vesicles.* They make a thick liquid containing sugar, vitamins, and proteins, which is food for the sperm. Below the ampulla and the seminal vesicles is the *prostate gland,* which makes a milky fluid. The ampulla and the seminal vesicles lead into

the prostate gland and join the *urethra,* the tube that runs from the bladder to the tip of the penis. The fluids from the seminal vesicles and the prostate mix with the sperm and make a fluid called *semen.* It contains almost half a billion sperm and enough food to keep them alive until they reach an egg.

Circumcision   All baby boys are born with a small fold of skin, called the *foreskin,* that comes down over the tip of their penis, which is called the *glans.* For centuries it has been a custom among many people to cut off this skin in the first few days after birth. Cutting off the foreskin is called *circumcision.* Some people do this for religious reasons, some because they believe it makes it easier for a boy to keep his penis clean and free of infection. Boys who are not circumcised will notice that a thick, white, curdy material collects under the foreskin unless this area is washed.

The female reproductive system   The female reproductive organs make it possible for a woman to become a mother. The organs make eggs and provide a sheltered place where an egg can meet a sperm and gradually develop into a baby with food supplied by the mother's body.

Eggs are made in a

Uncircumsized

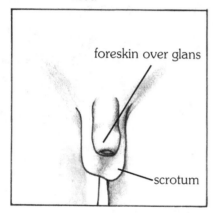

foreskin over glans

scrotum

The end of the uncircumcised penis is covered by a flap of skin that a boy is born with.

Circumsized

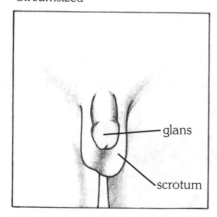

glans

scrotum

The circumcised penis has had the flap of skin removed.

woman's *ovaries.* The two ovaries are almond-shaped bodies located within the circle of the hips. All of a woman's eggs are actually made before she is even born! Girls have hundreds of thousands of eggs, but only a few hundred ever come out of their ovaries.

Like men's sperm, these eggs have only 23 chromosomes—half the information needed for a baby to grow. The eggs don't start to change or grow until a girl reaches 10 to 16 years of age and her sexual organs start to mature rapidly. At this time a girl's pituitary gland starts sending out FSH, a hormone that makes a few of the eggs in her ovaries start to develop. A tiny fluid-filled sac grows around these eggs, which are then called *follicles.* One of the follicles grows fastest and moves to the edge of the ovary. This egg develops into the biggest cell in the body. Pressure builds up as the egg grows and it finally bursts out of the follicle and through the wall of the ovary. This is called *ovulation.* It takes place in one ovary or the other about every 28 days. Once one egg has been released, all the other follicles stop growing and die.

The female reproductive system makes it possible for a woman to become a mother. The ovaries make the female reproductive cell called the egg. If an egg is fertilized by a sperm from the father, a baby will grow.

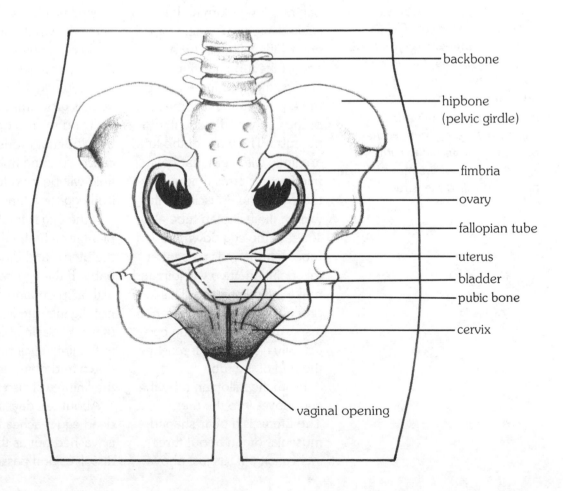

backbone

hipbone (pelvic girdle)

fimbria

ovary

fallopian tube

uterus

bladder

pubic bone

cervix

vaginal opening

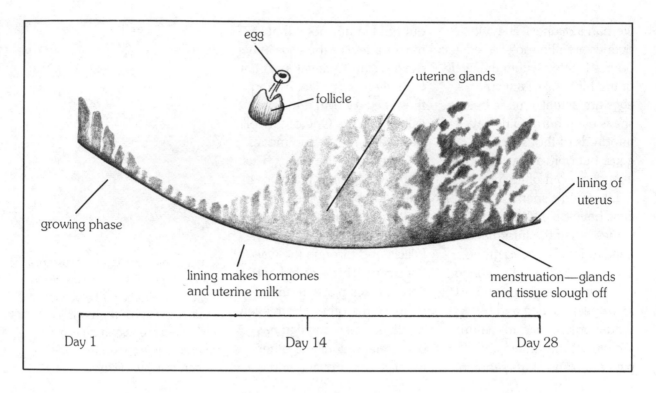

egg

follicle

uterine glands

lining of
uterus

growing phase

lining makes hormones
and uterine milk

menstruation—glands
and tissue slough off

Day 1   Day 14   Day 28

This drawing shows how the inside lining of a woman's uterus changes each month. The lining thickens in preparation for a baby to grow. If an egg is fertilized by a sperm, it then burrows into the lining around the twenty-first day.

If the egg is not fertilized, the lining breaks away and washes out of the uterus along with the egg at the end of the month. This process is called menstruation.

The newly freed egg then begins a long journey. It is sucked into the funnel-shaped end of the *fallopian tube.* This end of the tube has tiny fingers, the *fimbria,* that catch the egg wherever it comes out of the ovary and guide it into the tube. The walls of the tube are lined with cells that have microscopic arms that push the egg along. Muscles in the wall of the fallopian tube also squeeze the egg down the tube. If a sperm is present at this point, the two will join and make a *fertilized egg.* This process is called *fertilization.* If a sperm is not there, the egg actually dies before it reaches the end of the tube.

From the fallopian tube the egg moves into the *uterus.* The uterus is a pear-shaped, muscular organ about three inches long. It sits just above

and behind the bladder. For several weeks before the egg comes down the tube, the lining of the uterus grows thicker, and gets ready for a fertilized egg. Many new blood vessels grow in the uterine wall and microscopic glands develop that produce a fluid called "uterine milk." This fluid will be food for the fertilized egg for a time.

If the egg is fertilized, it will plant itself in the thick lining of the uterus and develop into a baby. If the egg has not joined with a sperm and dies, it will not dig into the lining of the uterus. The tiny blood vessels in the lining will start to close down and many of the cells in the lining will also die.

About ten days after the dead egg reaches the uterus, it is washed out as the lining dissolves and passes out of the narrow opening at the bottom of the uterus. This opening is called the *cervix*. The cervix opens into a 3-inch muscular tube, or canal, called the *vagina,* which opens to the outside of the body.

The washing out of the lining and the dead egg is called *menstruation*. It takes place once a month and goes on for about four or five days. The fluid that comes out is bright red because of the blood that was in the lining. But it is not like blood from a cut. It also contains clear fluid from the dissolved lining cells and the dead cells themselves. Once menstruation is over, the whole cycle starts again. Another group of eggs begins to grow rapidly and the lining of the uterus begins to thicken once more.

The whole female cycle is controlled by hormones. Two hormones from the pituitary gland start the process by making eggs grow and pop out of the ovary. They also cause the cells in the ovaries to produce another hormone called *estrogen,* which makes the walls of the uterus start to thicken. Then the follicle that surrounds the egg makes a hormone called *progesterone,* which makes the glands in the uterus wall produce "uterine milk." If the egg has not been fertilized, progesterone and estrogen stop being produced. Then the lining of the uterus dissolves, causing a menstrual period, and the cycle begins again.

Female genitalia   The vagina is the tube that connects the uterus to the outside of the body. The opening of the vagina lies between the legs, in front of the anus. In young girls the vagina is partly covered by a circular flap of skin called the *hymen.* Just above the vagina is the opening for the urethra, which connects the bladder with the outside and through which urine passes (*see* page 178). Above the opening of the urethra is a hooded round body called the *clitoris.* It contains many nerve endings (like the penis), and it swells and becomes hard when it is rubbed. Surrounding the clitoris, urethra, and vagina are two folds of skin called the *labia,* which cover and protect the opening. The inner labia are small and thin: the outer labia are larger and thicker.

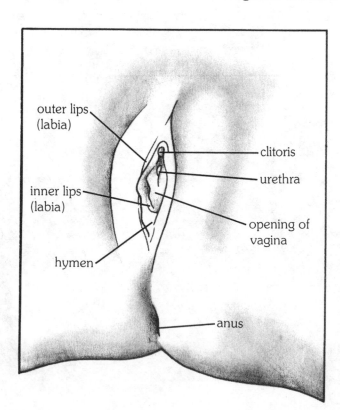

outer lips (labia)

clitoris

urethra

inner lips (labia)

opening of vagina

hymen

anus

This drawing of a girl shows the opening of the vagina, the tube that leads to the uterus, and the urethra, the tube that leads to the bladder.

Puberty

Men's and women's reproductive organs, which make it possible for them to create a baby, are formed before they are even born. But unlike the rest of the organs in the body, they don't begin to work or grow in size for about ten years. During this period, the reproductive organs are inactive; it's almost as if they were asleep. This is no accident. A young girl is not physically big enough to have a healthy baby. Girls' bodies need time and energy to grow—which would take energy away from a growing baby. Just as important, girls and boys need time for their minds and feelings to grow. They would not be able to care for and raise babies by themselves. In fact, all animals have a period of time when they are growing up and can't make babies. But in the case of humans, it's a much longer time than for most other animals.

The human body begins to start preparing to have babies at about ten years of age. Changes begin to take place both inside and outside the body. The exact age at which all this starts varies from one child to another. Changes generally start earlier in girls than boys.

These changes begin in both boys and girls when the area of the brain called the hypothalamus sends a signal to the master gland, the pitui-

During puberty boys develop body hair, wider shoulders, bigger muscles, and the penis and testes grow larger.

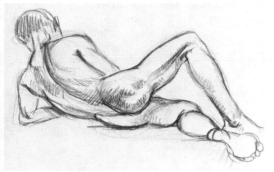

Matisse, Henri. Man Reclining. 19th–20th cent. Pencil on paper. 9¼ × 12⅛". The Metropolitan Museum of Art, New York. The Alfred Stieglitz Collection, 1949.

Karfiol, Bernard. Boy Bathers. 1916. Oil on canvas. 28 × 36". Collection, Whitney Museum of American Art, New York. Purchase (and exchange). Photograph by Geoffrey Clements.

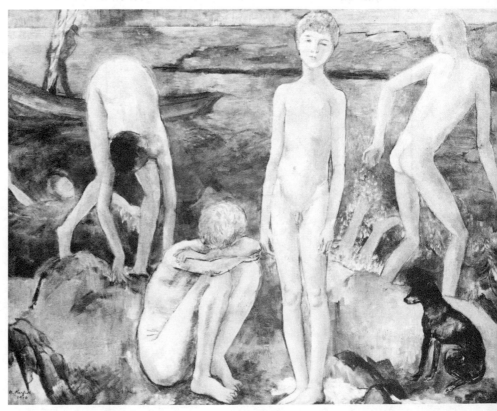

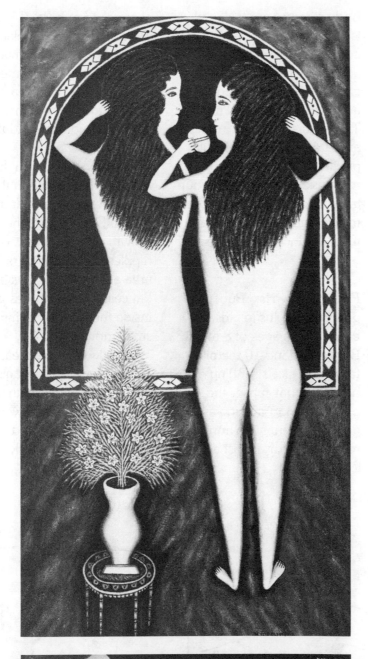

During puberty girls develop breasts, body hair, and wider hips.

Hirshfield, Morris. Girl in a Mirror. 1940. Oil on canvas. 40⅛ × 22¼". Collection, The Museum of Modern Art, New York. Purchase.

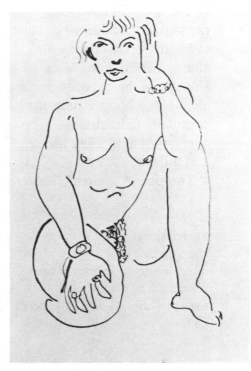

Matisse, Henri. Nude. 19th–20th cent. Pen and ink on paper. 12⁹⁄₁₆ × 8¹³⁄₁₆". The Metropolitan Museum of Art, New York. The Alfred Stieglitz Collection, 1949.

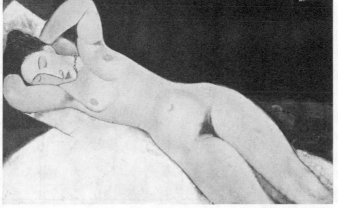

Modigliani, Amedeo. Nude. 1917. Oil on canvas. 28¾ × 45¾". Collection, The Solomon R. Guggenheim Museum, New York.

Anatomy and physiology **217**

tary. This happens by itself, and no one knows exactly what causes it. In response to this signal, the pituitary begins to make large amounts of special hormones. These hormones cause girls' ovaries to make estrogen, and boys' testes to make testosterone.

Over the next few years, these hormones create enormous changes in the body. First, they cause a tremendous growth spurt that affects the whole body. Second, they cause the reproductive organs inside the body to grow and change. Third, they cause changes in the outside appearance of the body. Finally they contribute to immense changes in kids' inner feelings and the way they act.

The period when all these body changes are taking place is called *puberty*. Puberty comes from the Latin word for adult. All over the world, the change from childhood to adulthood is a special time. Teen-agers find new interests and are given certain adult privileges, as well as new responsibilities. In many countries there are important ceremonies marking the passage from childhood to adulthood.

Puberty in girls   Puberty generally begins in girls between the ages of 8 and 13. Between 7 and 10 the pituitary gland starts sending out a hormone that causes the ovaries to start making estrogen. Estrogen is the hormone responsible for almost all the changes of puberty in a girl. These changes take place gradually over several years, in more or less the same order. But some girls are just starting to enter puberty while others already have adult-looking bodies.

Estrogen speeds up the making of new cells in the reproductive organs and in the bones. First, it starts the growth of the breasts. The nipples lift and the darkened area around them gets bigger. Fat cells and tiny tubes grow inside the breasts, forming small mounds.

Shortly after the breasts start to develop, most girls go through a rapid growth spurt. This spurt occurs between 9½ and 14½, slowing and stopping much more quickly than

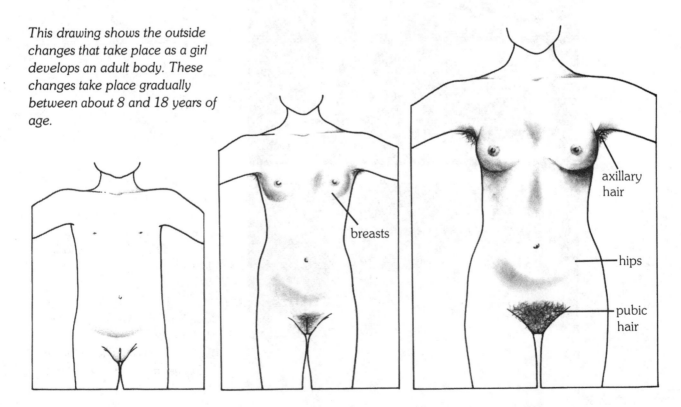

This drawing shows the outside changes that take place as a girl develops an adult body. These changes take place gradually between about 8 and 18 years of age.

breasts

axillary hair

hips

pubic hair

the burst of growth in boys. As girls grow taller, their hips grow wider. This makes for a larger opening in the pelvis, through which a baby can pass. Not only do the hipbones grow wider, but the amount of fat around the hips and thighs increases. In fact, girls begin to have more fat than boys over most of their body.

Between 11 and 14, girls start to develop special body hair. Coarse dark hair begins to grow under their arms, and around their vagina. This hair growth is caused by *androgen,* a hormone made by the adrenal glands.

At about the same time, the estrogen from the ovaries causes tremendous growth and change in the uterus,

vagina, and fallopian tubes. Both the uterus itself and the muscles in its walls become much bigger. Also the glands that make "uterine milk" develop (see page 222). The fallopian tubes develop many more cells with cilia, and the vagina grows a new, stronger lining. Also the labia around the opening of the vagina grow bigger.

Shortly after the fastest part of the growth spurt, girls' bodies begin to make estrogen only for a part of each month, and they have their first menstrual period. This can happen anywhere between 10 and 16, but most often happens between 12 and 13.

Puberty in boys   Puberty generally begins in boys

between the ages of 9 and 13. This means that some boys are just starting to enter puberty while other boys their age already have rather adult-looking bodies. Between 7 and 12 the pituitary gland in boys starts sending out testosterone. It is testosterone that is responsible for almost all the changes of puberty that take place in boys. Testosterone is the hormone that speeds up the making of new cells in the reproductive organs and in the bones. The changes of puberty take place gradually in more or less the same order in all boys.

The first thing that happens is that the testes and the scrotum start to grow. As the testes grow, they begin to make sperm for the first time (see

This drawing shows the outside changes that take place as a boy develops an adult body. These changes take place gradually between about 9 and 21 years of age.

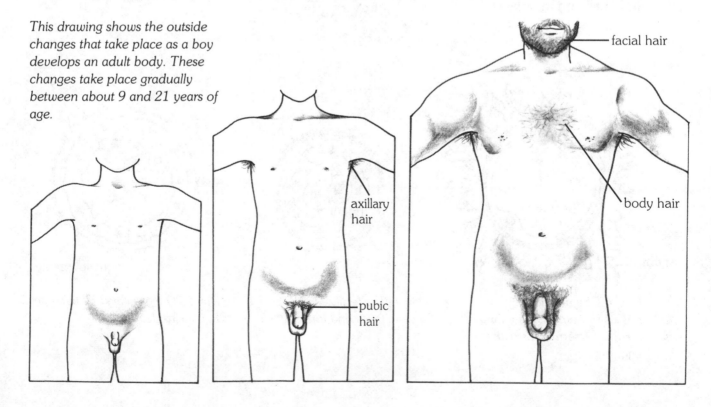

facial hair

axillary hair

body hair

pubic hair

page 212). This starts between 9½ and 13. About a year later the penis begins to grow in length, then width.

Somewhere between 11 and 16, boys enter a period of tremendous growth in height. This growth spurt occurs somewhat later in boys than in girls, but it tends to last much longer. Boys undergo much more muscle growth than girls, and their bones become thicker. Even their skin becomes thicker. Their voice box, or larynx, also becomes larger, causing boys' voices to crackle and squeak unpredictably and eventually to deepen.

Finally, between the ages of 12 and 20, boys begin to grow special body hair. Coarse hair develops around their penis and scrotum, on their chest, and finally on their face.

Puberty games

Here's a model to show the steps in puberty; that is, how kids' bodies start to take on grown-up form. Set up two jars, the first half-full with clear water, the second half-full with water that contains 5 to 10 drops of yellow food coloring. Also have a bottle of blue food coloring on hand. Set a timer for 30 minutes and go about your business. These minutes represent 7 to 10 years—the time from birth until the hypothalamus begins making the hormone that triggers the pituitary to start puberty. When the timer goes off, slowly drip 5 to 10 drops of blue food coloring into the first jar. This represents the pituitary sending its special hormones into the blood. These hormones cause the ovaries in girls and the testes in boys to start making their own hormones. To show this, slowly pour the first jar into the second. The change of color to green represents the body gradually taking on grown-up form.

To see what changes take place in the body and to see at what different ages kids' bodies start to change, just look at kids from third grade to eighth grade. In girls you notice breast growth, then the growth spurt and widening of the hips. These changes are accompanied by the growth of special body hair, the release of eggs, and getting a period (menstruation). In boys you notice the growth spurt, widening of the shoulders, and eventually a voice drop. These changes are accompanied by growth of the testicles and the penis, and growth of special body hair and the making of sperm.

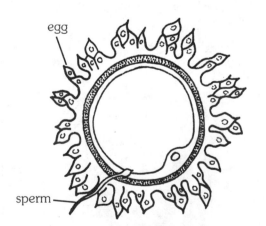

Day 1. The developing baby passes through many changes. First, the sperm joins with the egg.

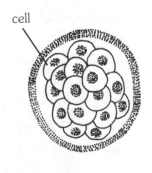

Day 4. The fertilized egg divides several times and forms a ball.

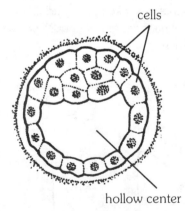

Day 5. The growing ball becomes hollow inside.

Growth of a baby

A baby grows from the joining of two cells—an egg from the mother and a sperm from the father (see pages 210–15). A woman sends out a single egg from one of her ovaries once a month. A man sends approximately 400 million sperm out at a time. But only one sperm can join the egg. The joining usually takes place in the top of a woman's fallopian tube, the tube that leads from the ovary to the uterus. The sperm reach the fallopian tube from the vagina by making swimming motions with their tails. They are also squeezed along by the muscles of the uterus and fallopian tubes. This journey takes between five minutes and an hour.

When a sperm reaches the egg, a remarkable series of things happens. Special chem-

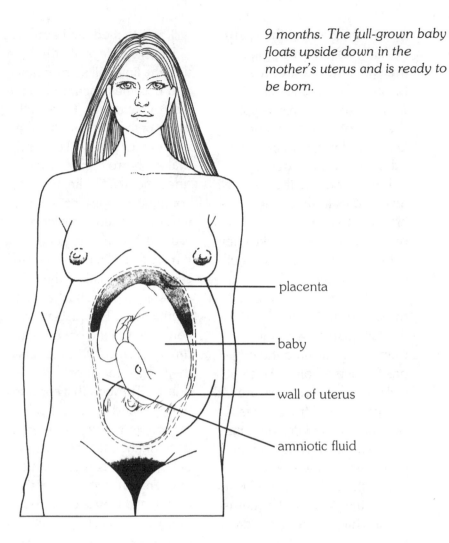

9 months. The full-grown baby floats upside down in the mother's uterus and is ready to be born.

placenta

baby

wall of uterus

amniotic fluid

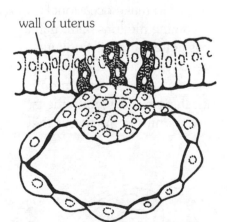

wall of uterus

Day 7. The fertilized egg burrows into the wall of the uterus.

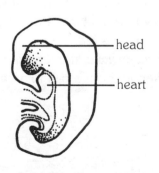

head

heart

Day 14. The fertilized egg forms a beginning head and heart.

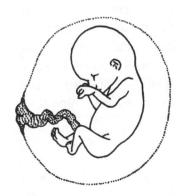

Day 49. The baby is basically formed and is fed by an umbilical cord.

icals in the head of the sperm actually dissolve the wall of the egg, and the sperm enters the egg. This is called *fertilization*. As soon as this happens the wall of the egg becomes like a tight net, preventing any other sperm from getting in.

For over a day the new cell just readies itself for the changes to come. Then it divides in half and makes new cells every 15 hours (see cell division, pages 128).

It takes the fertilized egg three days to be pushed down the fallopian tube to the uterus. By this time the egg has formed a ball of 16 to 32 cells. The dividing cells are fed by special fluid from the fallopian tubes and later by "uterine milk" from special glands in the wall of the uterus.

For the next 4 or 5 days the egg floats freely in the uterus. Meanwhile, it continues dividing and forms a hollow ball. By this time the cells have already become different and started to do special jobs. This process is called *differentiation*. Some cells start to form parts of the baby, some start to form a special lining that

will help to feed the baby.

By 7 or 8 days after fertilization the tiny ball stops floating and becomes anchored to the wall of the uterus. Cells in the lining of the egg dissolve the wall of the uterus a little and make a burrow. For almost three months the lining cells continue to digest cells in the wall of the uterus, making food for the growing baby. Finally these lining cells form a special organ, called the *placenta*, which attaches to the uterine wall. The placenta is connected to the baby by the *umbilical cord*, which enters the baby's *navel*, or *belly button*. Through this cord, the baby's blood continually passes out to the placenta and back. In the placenta the baby's blood gets food and oxygen from the mother's blood, and leaves off carbon dioxide and wastes. All this happens across the thinnest wall, or membrane—so the baby's blood and the mother's do not touch. For the last six months until birth, this is how the baby is fed.

Meanwhile, the fertilized egg changes from a ball to a pear-

shaped body with a head, tail, and heart. These parts are very, very simple at first, and become more and more complicated as the baby grows and develops inside the uterus. By the end of eight weeks the growing baby looks like a human being. All of its organs and parts are basically formed, but the baby is only one inch long and weighs almost nothing!

By the end of the third month the baby has fingernails and toenails and is starting to move on its own. By the fourth month the baby has begun to swallow small amounts of the *amniotic fluid* that surrounds it. By the fifth month the baby makes its first sucking movements and can grip things with its hands. But the baby is still incredibly small —only three inches long and weighing about one ounce.

By the sixth month the baby begins to make occasional breathing motions, although it has gotten and will continue to get oxygen from the mother's blood. By the seventh month it can perceive light. In the last two months in the uterus the

During birth, the baby makes a complicated series of movements as it emerges from the mother's uterus. These movements allow the baby to fit the narrowest part of itself through the tight space as it comes out.

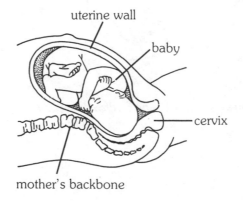
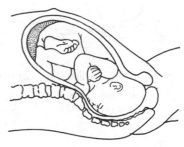

uterine wall

baby

cervix

mother's backbone

Baby games

Make a model of how a baby begins to grow. Draw a large round circle on a piece of paper. In the center, put 23 little pieces of colored yarn. This represents the chromosomes in the egg from the mother. Now take 23 pieces of yarn of another color. These represent the chromosomes from the father. Mix these pieces of yarn with the ones in the circle. This is what happens when the sperm joins with the egg.

Make a model of a baby floating in the uterus. Tape a string to the belly button of a small plastic or rubber doll. This represents the umbilical cord. Put the doll head-down in a clear plastic bag, attaching the free end of the cord to the inside wall of the bag with a large round piece of tape. The tape represents the placenta, which attaches to the wall of the uterus and brings the baby food and oxygen. Fill the bag with water and tightly close the end with a rubber band. This is how the baby grows for almost nine months (see drawing, page 221).

Make a model of the first steps in the growth of a fertilized egg: for several days the egg doesn't grow much in size, it just divides into more and more cells. Cut a small round ball of clay (or a red potato) in half. Put it back together. This is roughly how a two-cell egg looks. Now cut each half in half and put it back together. This represents a four-cell egg. Keep cutting each piece in half until you can no longer get all the pieces back together (see drawing, page 220).

To get some idea of what it's like to be born, get into a sleeping bag feet first and have someone hold or tie the end closed (about the width of your shoulders). Have the person try to squeeze you out from the bottom, while you try to slowly wiggle out, keeping your hands at your sides!

To get some idea of how tightly a baby's head is squeezed during birth, pull a tight turtleneck shirt over your head.

baby grows rapidly in length and weight. And all of the baby's organs become grown up enough so that the baby is ready to exist outside the uterus.

For almost 40 weeks, or 9 months, the baby grows inside the uterus. For most of this time the baby floats comfortably in the amniotic fluid, but by the last weeks the baby has become so large that it lies in a curled-up position with its arms and legs folded against its chest. At this point most babies are upside down with their head at the bottom of the uterus. This is also the position in which most babies are born.

Birth Birth begins when the mother's uterus starts squeezing in a steady rhythmic pattern. These squeezes, or *contractions,* begin at the top of the uterus and move down in a wave that pushes the baby downward. The contractions are a long time apart at the beginning, but they eventually get closer and closer until they are coming one after another. They also tend to last longer and longer. The

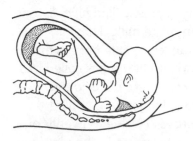 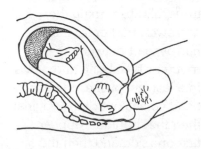 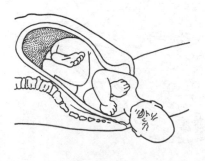

contractions happen by themselves, but they are very hard work for the mother. It is like climbing a steep mountain. It is such hard work, in fact, that it is called *labor*. It can take anywhere from a few hours to a day. The better shape the mother is in, and the more relaxed and happy she is, the easier labor generally is. The hardest part of labor usually comes right before the baby is born. But this is also the most exciting time because the mother knows that in a few minutes she will see her baby for the first time.

All the contractions and the baby's pushing cause the narrow tube at the bottom of the uterus, the cervix, to shorten and stretch open. This allows the baby's head to squeeze through into the vagina. At this point the baby's head is actually held between the muscles of the mother's backbone and pelvis, and it can't go back. Now the mother feels an overwhelming need to push down or squeeze as hard as she can. With each contraction and each push the baby moves further down. To make it through the tight space the baby naturally makes a series of twists and turns, always turning the narrowest part of itself to the narrow part between the mother's backbone and pelvis. In a last few pushes the baby's head comes out of the vagina; then the shoulders appear, first one side and then the

other; and finally the rest of the baby emerges.

The baby takes its first breath of air within a few seconds or minutes. This means it is no longer relying on the mother's blood, but is using its own lungs to get oxygen. Just as miraculous, the baby will immediately begin to suck at the mother's breast for milk, instead of getting food through the placenta. The doctor cuts through the umbilical cord to the placenta and clamps it. Within a few days the little piece remaining dries up and falls off. So in just a matter of minutes, the baby has undergone great changes and begun a whole new part of its life.

How the female breast makes milk   The breasts are special organs that only women develop. Their job is to produce milk after a baby is born. All female animals that are mammals have breasts— this is the way they feed their young. The breasts in young girls are undeveloped. They don't begin to grow until the brain signals the ovaries to start making estrogen.

Inside the breasts are lots of tiny glands, called *alveoli,* that can make milk. They are arranged in little groups that lead into tiny tubes called *milk ducts.* These ducts join to make bigger tubes called *sinuses.* Twelve to twenty of these open up in the *nipple,* a

Milk is made in the tiny glands inside the mother's breast after a baby is born.

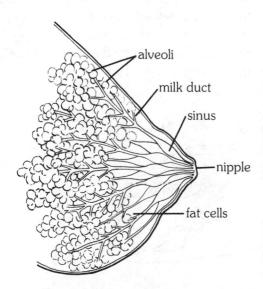

- alveoli
- milk duct
- sinus
- nipple
- fat cells

Breast games

Make a model of the breast. Take five or six short pieces of string and attach three or four little balls of clay at one end. Lay these on a piece of cardboard or a dish. Around the pieces of clay put balls of cotton. Bring the loose ends of the strings together and put them into an old baby-bottle nipple. The clay balls represent the milk glands, the strings are the milk ducts that lead to the nipple, and the cotton balls are areas of fat (see drawing).

Baby formulas are made to be as much like breast milk as possible. Here is an old recipe for baby formula. Mix 10 ounces of evaporated milk with 20 ounces of water, and 2 tablespoons of corn syrup or regular sugar. Another recipe calls for 10 ounces of cow's milk, 8 ounces of water, and 2 tablespoons of sugar. Taste the formula and notice how much sweeter it is than plain milk. All formulas lack a mother's protective antibodies and differ in the amount of vitamins, minerals, fats, and proteins they contain.

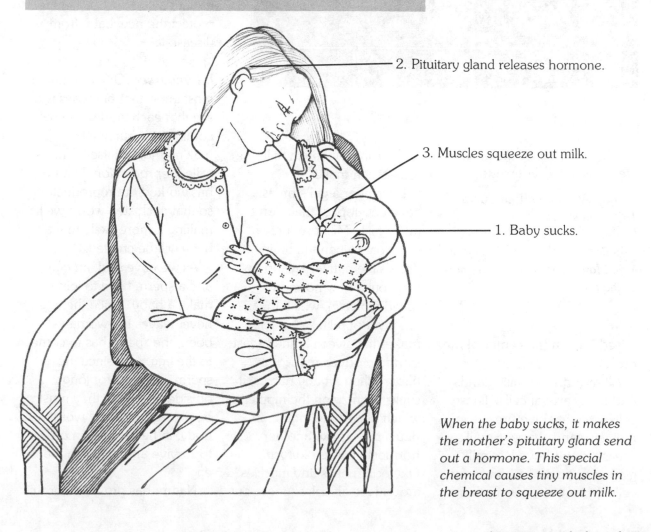

2. Pituitary gland releases hormone.

3. Muscles squeeze out milk.

1. Baby sucks.

When the baby sucks, it makes the mother's pituitary gland send out a hormone. This special chemical causes tiny muscles in the breast to squeeze out milk.

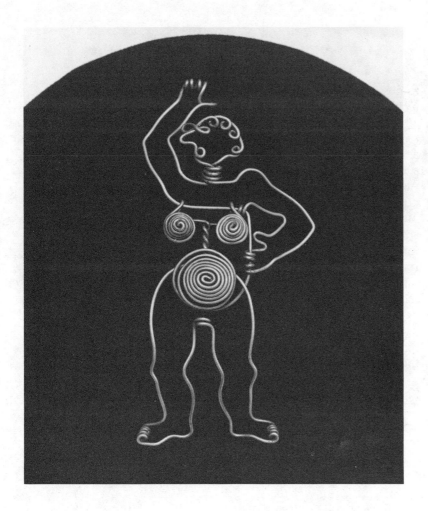

A baby is fed first by the mother's uterus, then by her breasts.

Calder, Alexander. Belt Buckle. 1935. Brass. 8 × 5 × ½". Collection, Whitney Museum of American Art, New York. Gift of Mrs. Marcel Duchamp in memory of the artist.

raised area in the center of the breast.

All around the milk glands and ducts are fat cells. These cells are what give breasts their size and shape. Small breasts don't have less milk glands or ducts, just fewer fat cells. In fact, size has nothing to do with how much milk the breasts can make.

Even after a girl's breasts have developed, they don't make milk. Milk production starts only when the brain signals the pituitary gland to send out a new hormone called *prolactin,* which means "in favor of milk." Prolactin makes the alveoli in the breast start to produce milk for a baby. When a baby nurses, it sucks strongly on the nipple, which signals the mother's pituitary to make another hormone, called *oxytocin.* Oxytocin makes tiny muscles around the alveoli squeeze out the milk. This is why milk comes out only when the baby sucks.

At first, the mother's breasts produce only a little milk. But as the baby nurses more and grows bigger, the breasts produce more and more milk. By the time the baby is three months old, the mother is making six cups of milk a day.

Human milk contains fat, sugar, protein, minerals, and water. Like all other milk, it is mostly water. But it contains much more sugar and less protein than cow's milk. Human milk also contains special antibodies from the mother's body. They help to protect the new baby from disease.

Intercourse One of nature's most important purposes is to see that each kind of animal continues to survive by making more of itself. This is called *reproduction.* Nature has worked out reproduction so that each step works well, making it more likely that a baby will be created.

As we have said, an egg and a sperm have to join to make a baby. Since the egg never leaves the woman's body, the sperm has to come to the egg. And since the sperm can't live for long outside the body, they must be placed inside the woman's body, in her vagina, in order to survive and join with the egg.

Nature has provided for this

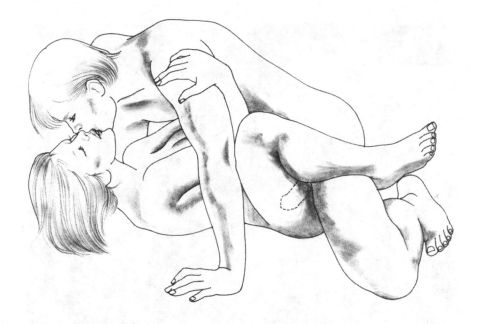

Intercourse is nature's age-old way of getting the male sperm to meet the female egg in the protected environment of the mother's body. Mating is a basic event in the animal world and a celebration of life.

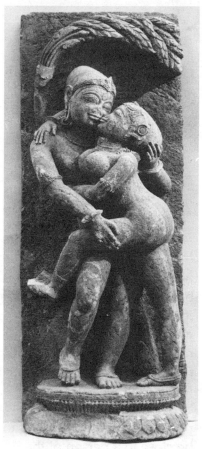

Indian. Mithuna Couple. 12th–13th cent. Stone. Height: 6'. The Metropolitan Museum of Art, New York. Florance Waterbury Fund, 1970.

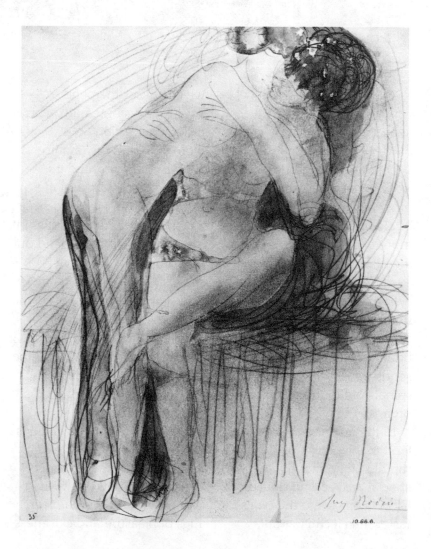

Rodin, Auguste. The Embrace. 19th–20th cent. Lead pencil, watercolor, and gouache. $12^{13}/_{16} \times 9^{7}/_{8}$". The Metropolitan Museum of Art, New York. Kennedy Fund, 1910.

Anatomy and physiology **227**

When people share strong feelings of love they want to join their minds and bodies together.

Chagall, Marc. Birthday. 1923. Oil on canvas. $31\frac{7}{8} \times 39\frac{1}{2}''$. Collection, The Solomon R. Guggenheim Museum, New York.

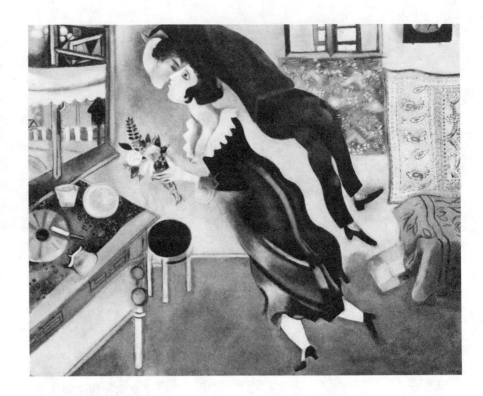

by giving men and women both the body parts and the feelings that will lead them to make babies. As people's reproductive organs grow up, their feelings about reproduction also grow up. People begin to have thoughts and physical feelings of wanting to be close to a person of the opposite sex. They want to be with someone, share experiences with him or her, and be close and touch him or her.

When a man and a woman are feeling this close, this loving, things naturally start to happen inside their bodies. They start to feel warm and tingly. Their bodies become very sensitive, and every touch and stroke starts to feel wonderful and special. Both the man and the woman begin

to enjoy themselves and feel very pleasant. And they want to share those feelings with the other person. These feelings become so strong that people want to become one with each other and join their minds and bodies together. So they touch more and more. As they do, they begin to feel a sense of excitement as well as pleasure. Nerves all over the body send signals of excitement and pleasure to the brain. When the brain gets these signals, it sends messages down the spinal cord to the reproductive organs.

In the man the arteries that lead to the penis open up and rapidly pump blood into special areas called sinuses. Blood comes into the penis faster than it can get out,

which causes the penis to swell and become hard. This is called an *erection*. In a woman, blood rushes into sinuses in and around the vagina, the clitoris, and the nipples, causing them to swell also. At the same time, cells in the wall of the vagina send out tiny drops of a fluid that makes the whole vagina moist and slippery. Glands inside the penis also make a small amount of a slippery fluid. Once the penis is hard and the vagina is wet, the penis can slip easily into the vagina. As the man and woman move back and forth, nerve endings are excited more and more in the end of the man's penis, the glans, and in the woman's clitoris and vagina. The feelings of pleasure and closeness and oneness become stronger and stronger. And all the muscles in the walls of the reproductive organs begin to squeeze in rhythmic waves. In the man these rhythmic contractions squeeze sperm from the tubes and fluid from the seminal vesicles and the prostate gland. This fluid mixture, semen, comes out of the penis in strong spurts called an *ejaculation.* It puts millions of sperm high in the woman's vagina, next to the opening of the uterus. Rhythmic contractions in the woman's vagina, uterus, and fallopian tubes squeeze the sperm up to the top of the fallopian tube where an egg may be. All this makes it likely that the egg and the sperm will meet and join.

The strong muscle contractions that propel the sperm out of the man's penis and up to the woman's fallopian tube are called an *orgasm,* or *climax.* They give both the man and the woman tremendous feelings of pleasure and completeness. And they leave both partners feeling relaxed, tired, and peaceful. It's wonderful that the act of creating a baby can bring so much pleasure to both the mother and father. And it is not an accident that this is so. This pleasure is one of the reasons that people want to have babies.

Chapter 6

Healing

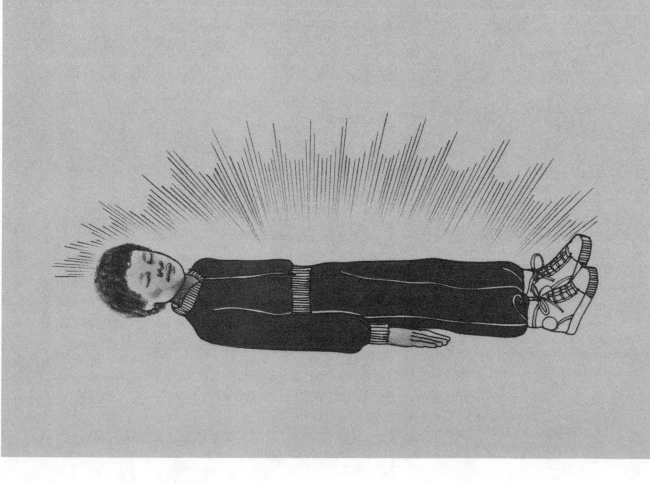

Blood clotting

The body is filled with millions of tiny blood vessels, many of them right under the skin. So whenever a person gets a scratch, a cut, or even a hard bump, blood vessels break and bleed. Not surprisingly, the body has a miraculous process to stop bleeding. The process is called *hemostasis,* which comes from the Greek words for stopping blood.

As soon as a blood vessel is broken, tiny muscles in the wall tighten and squeeze the vessel closed. This squeezing slows the bleeding but doesn't stop it completely. The squeezing effect can last as long as a half hour.

Where the wall of the blood vessel is broken, tiny collagen fibers stick out like threads from a piece of fabric that has been torn. Meanwhile, platelets (see page 175), the tiniest white blood cells, begin to stick to the fibers. Normally the platelets just flow along in the blood, but when they bump into collagen fibers they suddenly undergo a change. They swell and become extremely sticky. They also send out a chemical that makes other passing platelets become sticky, even though they have not actually touched the fibers. Since there are about 20,000 platelets in a drop of blood, the break in the blood vessel becomes plugged with sticky platelets within a few seconds. This plug is enough to stop the bleeding from a small blood vessel. Without platelets people would have hundreds of tiny bleeding areas all over their body from every bump.

In bigger cuts the blood itself has to *clot.* The watery

As soon as a blood vessel is cut, its walls begin to squeeze closed.

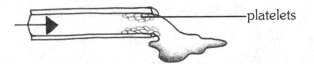

Blood platelets get sticky and begin to block the hole.

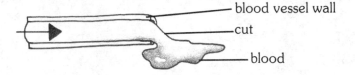

A special blood chemical makes fibrin threads, which block the cut further.

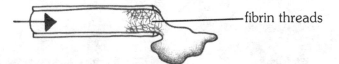

Blood cells stick to the fibrin net and make a plug.

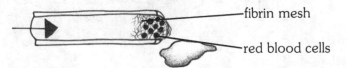

In a few minutes the clot shrinks and stops the bleeding.

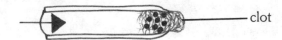

part of blood contains millions of molecules of a protein called *fibrinogen*. Whenever a blood vessel is broken, the walls of the vessel, the platelets, and the blood all release special chemicals that affect fibrinogen. These chemicals somehow make the little pieces of fibrinogen join together into long threads called *fibrin*. These threads then form a net, or mesh, that sticks to the walls of the blood vessel and covers the break. The mesh catches blood cells and platelets. Together, they all form the *clot*.

Clotting begins as quickly as 15 seconds after an injury, and stops bleeding in as little as 3 to 6 minutes. After 20 minutes the platelets actually shrink back and the fibrin fibers squeeze, closing the hole even more tightly. Press-ing on a cut stops bleeding by squeezing the blood vessel closed from outside. This also makes it easier for the body to form a clot because the clot isn't washed away by the bleeding. But outside pressure doesn't speed the clotting time. Clotting time depends on how quickly the chemicals in the blood work.

Clotting games

Next time you get a small cut, look at it closely and see how long it takes to become sticky and form a clot. To get an idea of how your body stops bleeding, peel a carrot over the drain in the kitchen sink. Along with the carrot peels, sprinkle in cereal flakes. The peelings represent the body's fibrin threads and the flakes represent the sticky platelets in the blood. Turn on a gentle stream of water. The water won't drain well through the "clot" that you've formed.

Skin healing

A cut breaks apart the cells in the skin. If it's deep enough, the cut also breaks through the tiny blood vessels called capillaries. The body begins to heal the cut immediately. The broken ends of blood vessels plug and the blood clots within minutes. This stops the bleeding (see page 232). Meanwhile the broken cells in the area release a special chemical called *histamine*. Histamine makes nearby blood vessels widen, which brings more blood to the area. Histamine also widens the tiny holes in the capillaries, so much more blood plasma leaks out into the spaces between the cells. Plasma is the watery part of the blood that has no blood cells (see page 175); but it does contain the protein that makes the fibrin threads in a clot. Within minutes, all the plasma that has leaked out clots. This clotted plasma is what makes the *scab*. The reddish color of the scab comes from blood that has

Skin-healing games

Next time you get a small cut, don't cover it with a Band-Aid. Examine it several times a day until it heals. Notice the blood clotting, any swelling or redness, the scab, and the new pink skin that forms around and under the scab. Watch what happens to the scar in the next few days.

leaked out. The strength comes from the fibrin threads. A scab is nature's own bandage. It protects the cut from dirt and bacteria while it is healing.

The plasma that has leaked out between the cells and clotted is what causes the swelling around a cut. The swelling protects the body by blocking the spread of germs from the area. This means that if the cut was caused by something covered with bacteria, those bacteria would be kept near the wound and wouldn't be able to get to other parts of the body.

Meanwhile chemicals released by the injured cells cause many white blood cells to come to the area around the cut. This process starts almost immediately and goes on for hours. The white blood cells start eating damaged cells and any bacteria or viruses in the area. Eventually, the white blood cells even begin to eat the clotted plasma and the scab.

Within minutes after someone gets a cut, a clot begins to form.

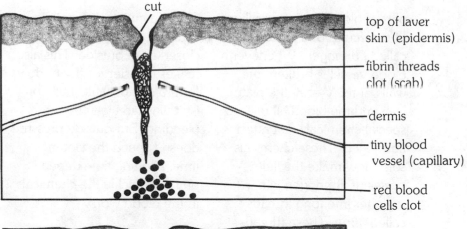

cut

top of layer skin (epidermis)

fibrin threads clot (scab)

dermis

tiny blood vessel (capillary)

red blood cells clot

Within hours, white blood cells come in to clean up, new blood vessels start to grow, and the top layer of skin begins to grow down into the cut.

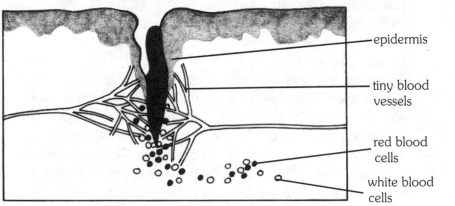

epidermis

tiny blood vessels

red blood cells

white blood cells

Within several days the blood vessels and skin from each side meet.

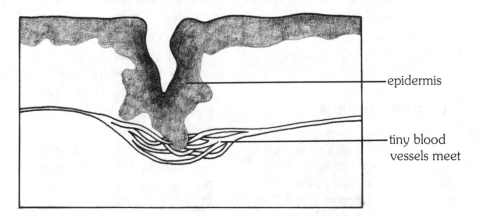

epidermis

tiny blood vessels meet

Within a week or two the cut is completely healed.

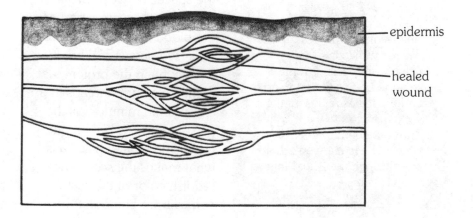

epidermis

healed wound

Cells in the lining of the ends of the cut blood vessels start splitting into more and more cells, making many new little blood vessels. They grow right into the clot along the fibrin threads, and join other new blood vessels from the opposite side of the cut, allowing blood to flow through.

Within a day or two, cells in the top layer of skin start forming new cells at 20 times their usual rate! These cells actually roll over one another down into the cut. Burrowing under the scab, they go down from each side of the cut. When they meet at the bottom, they stop dividing.

Beneath the skin, many of a new kind of cell called a *fibroblast,* move in. They start to make collagen fibers, which hold the two sides of the wound together, and keep the cut from being reopened. After they are formed, the collagen fibers actually shrink, closing the wound more tightly. All of this takes from days to weeks, depending on how big the cut is. That is why the doctor doesn't take stitches out of a big cut for a long time.

Because a cut heals from side to side, it doesn't take any longer to heal if it's one inch long or three inches long. It's how deep a cut is and where it is that determines how long it takes to heal.

Three substances help to make a wound heal: vitamin C, zinc, and protein, which is needed to make collagen fibers and new cells. So it's important to eat a good diet when healing is going on.

If a wound is filled with a lot of dirt, bacteria, or even injured cells, many white blood cells have to come in to fight the bacteria and clear away the dirt and cells. Many white blood cells die while doing the work. All the dead cells, dirt, and dead bacteria make up a creamy white fluid that is called *pus.* The pus either comes out of the top of the wound or it has to be broken down and cleared away by the body's lymph system (see page 175).

A large cut often leaves a scar. A scar is different than regular skin. It has no hair or sweat glands. Scars have more collagen fibers, which is what makes them raised and rubbery. Big scars may look wrinkly because the collagen fibers shrink as the wound is healing. Scars also have fewer blood vessels, which is why they are lighter in color than the skin around them.

Bone healing

A broken bone is a big event for the body and requires much time and energy to heal. The cast the doctor puts on doesn't heal the bone, it just holds the broken ends straight and still. The body itself repairs the damage step by step.

When a bone breaks, many blood vessels are broken, just as with a cut. Even if the skin isn't broken there is bleeding all around in the bone and in the muscles. Within minutes the blood clots and the bleeding stops. Injured cells let out histamine, the chemical that causes the blood vessels to widen and leak out plasma between the cells. The plasma forms clots between cells, and causes the hard swelling around the break. Meanwhile, white blood cells are attracted by chemicals released by the injured cells. Large numbers of white blood cells come in and begin to eat up the dead cells and the clotted plasma.

A day or two after the break, the cells in the lining of the blood vessels begin to grow and form networks of tiny new blood vessels in the injured area. Connective tissue cells around the bone start dividing rapidly and cover the whole area inside and outside the break. Some of these cells turn into *osteoblasts,* which make new bone cells; some turn into *chondroblasts,* which make cartilage; and some turn into *fibroblasts,* which make fibers for connective tissue. So the big mass of connective tissue cells begins to turn into special cells with different jobs.

The cells in the center of the break make a rough bridge of bone from one side of the break to the other. The osteoblasts make proteins that twist into the long threads

Within hours, a clot forms and white blood cells begin to clean up the area.

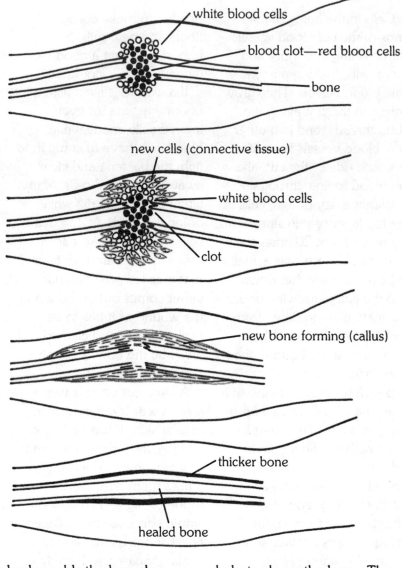

white blood cells

blood clot—red blood cells

bone

Within a day or two, new cells start to grow around the break.

new cells (connective tissue)

white blood cells

clot

Within a week, the new cells start to form bone and cartilage.

new bone forming (callus)

For many weeks the bone remains thicker around the break.

thicker bone

healed bone

called collagen fibers. Calcium crystals are then laid down all along these fibers, making them hard. Around the bone bridge, other cells make the tough tissue called cartilage. This whole mass of cells forms what is called the *callus*, a temporary bulge around the break. The callus acts like a splint, keeping the broken ends of the bone from moving. It also acts like a framework to guide the final shape of the bone. Over a period of many weeks, the body molds the bone by laying down hard bone where it is needed and by dissolving bone in the callus that is not needed. The cells called *osteoclasts* make enzymes that digest the calcium crystals and collagen fibers in the hard bone.

Even after the cast is removed the broken bone continues to change and grow stronger. Moving the bone pushes and pulls it. These forces are called mechanical stresses, and they continue to help to shape the bone. The parts of the bone where the forces are great become stronger. Where the forces are not great, the bone is dissolved further. These processes go on all the time in all bones, but happen more after a break. By six months after the break, the bone has completely healed and the callus around the break has disappeared. Eventually it becomes very difficult to tell that the bone has ever been broken.

Bone-healing games

Make a model of a broken bone that's healing. Break a small stick in half. Fit the pieces back together. Lay little pieces of string you have dipped in white glue across the break. Build up a bump over the break without moving the stick. Sprinkle fine sawdust or bread crumbs onto the sticky strings. The string represents the collagen fibers that are being laid down. The glue stands for the calcium that makes bone hard, and the sawdust represents new bone cells. The whole bump represents the callus that forms around a break. Once the glue has hardened, you can pick up the stick, but if you pick it up before that, it will break.

With your parents' help, put a cast on your arm. Wear old clothes because making a cast is messy. First cut the toe off an old sock and pull it over your forearm. Roll a strip of fabric or cotton tape *very loosely* around the sock. If the strip of fabric is too tight it can stop blood from going to your hand! Then dip strips of gauze in a thick mixture of water and quick-drying plaster of Paris. Wrap these strips *loosely* around the arm and let them dry. This is the same way a cast is made. To get the "cast" off, squirt it with a garden hose or stick it in a bucket of water. Don't leave the cast on for more than a half hour.

Nerve healing

Nerves consist of bundles of tiny nerve fibers covered by a tough sheath of connective tissue. Nerve cells are the most complicated cells in the body. They can't divide and make copies of themselves, but the long fibers can regrow when cut, as long as the cell body is unhurt (see page 185).

When the nerve is cut, tiny blood vessels nearby are also cut and they bleed. Within minutes the blood clots. Later, fibrous tissue threads grow across the cut nerve and hold the sheath or covering of the nerve together. The fibers within the sheath, cut off from the cell body, die and are removed by white cells. Gradually some of the live fibers on

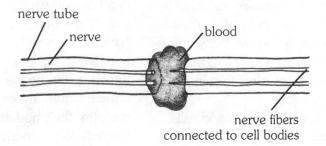

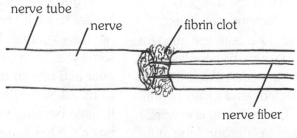

When a nerve is cut, a clot forms.

The end of the nerve that is not attached to the cell body dies and is removed.

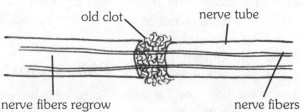

The end of the nerve connected to the cell body grows across the cut and back down the nerve tube.

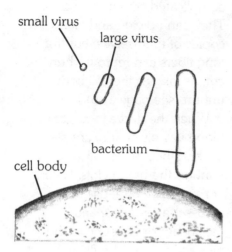

small virus

large virus

bacterium

cell body

The average body cell is much bigger than any virus or bacterium.

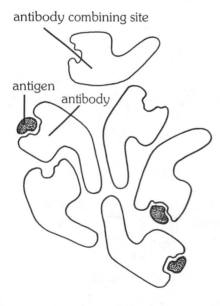

antibody combining site

antigen

antibody

The white blood cells make proteins called antibodies, which "lock" onto bacteria and viruses and make them harmless. Each kind of antibody fits only one kind of germ.

the near side grow across the cut and down the sheath to reconnect to the muscle or feeling receptor they were attached to.

Nerves do not heal as well as skin or bone. Because of this, a person may lose some feeling or movement after a nerve is cut. When a big nerve is cut, the doctor will suture or sew the two nerve ends together. This allows the fibers to regrow down the right tube. Nerve fibers grow at a rate of 2.5 millimeters per day.

Antibodies

The body has a special way of recognizing and dealing with dangerous substances. All bacteria and viruses, and the poisons that they release, have chemicals on the surface. These chemicals, called *antigens,* are unlike any others in the body. So the body immediately recognizes them as foreign invaders that may be dangerous.

Special white blood cells make big proteins that are attracted to the antigens. These proteins, called *antibodies,* lock onto the antigens and make them harmless. There is a particular antibody for each different kind of antigen. The antibody is specially shaped to fit around the antigen as if they were pieces of a puzzle. When an antibody finds the right antigen, they stick together. When the body sees a new antigen for the first time, it slowly begins to make

special antibodies that will fit that particular antigen. The next time the body sees that antigen, it will already have a number of white blood cells that will know how to produce the antibody with the right shape. In a short time these white blood cells will be able to turn out huge numbers of antibodies.

Vaccinations use the antibody reaction to do their work. Kids are given very small amounts of different antigens. In this way the body is "introduced" to the antigen, so that if it ever sees it again, the body rapidly and easily can make antibodies against it. For example, children are given small shots of special measles viruses. These viruses have been treated so they can't actually make children get the measles, but they still have their special antigens on their surfaces, so a matching antibody can be made. Later, if the children are exposed to measles, their bodies will immediately recognize the virus and make many antibodies to kill it and they will not develop measles. For the same reason, if children have ever had certain diseases such as measles, they can never get it again because their body has already learned to recognize that particular virus.

Phagocytosis

Some cells have a special way of dealing with things that

might be dangerous to them: they simply eat the harmful substances! In fact, many of the body's white blood cells spend all their time eating bacteria, viruses, cancer cells, and dead or broken-down cells. The way cells eat bacteria is called *phagocytosis*. The name comes from the Greek words for a cell eating.

White blood cells recognize

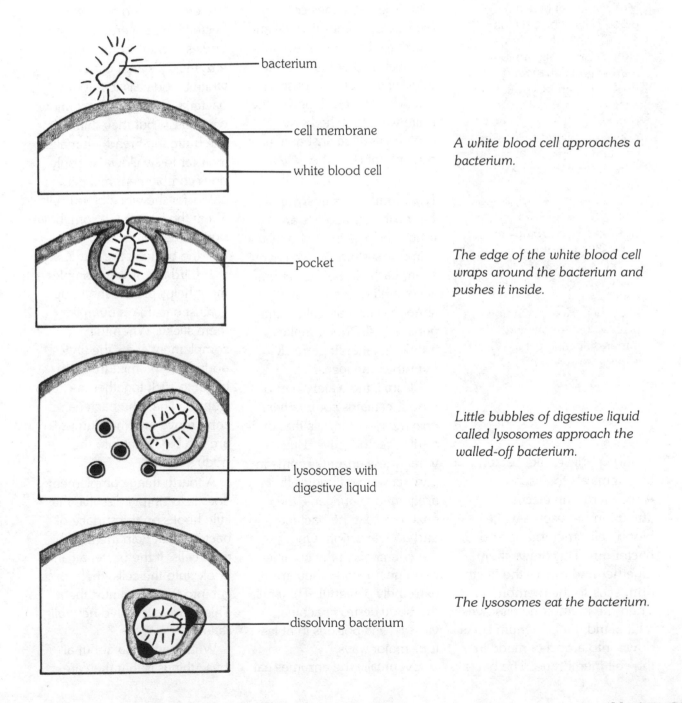

bacterium

cell membrane

white blood cell

A white blood cell approaches a bacterium.

pocket

The edge of the white blood cell wraps around the bacterium and pushes it inside.

lysosomes with digestive liquid

Little bubbles of digestive liquid called lysosomes approach the walled-off bacterium.

dissolving bacterium

The lysosomes eat the bacterium.

Antibody-antigen games

Take two interlocking pieces of an old jigsaw puzzle. One piece represents an antibody, the other an antigen, like a bacterium or virus. Once the antigen is stuck to the antibody, it can't hurt anyone anymore.

Make a model of a white blood cell eating bacteria or a virus. Roll a ball of Play-Doh or Silly Putty up to a marble and right over it. Push the marble into the center of the Play-Doh and cover it completely. This is how white blood cells cure you and keep you well—by phagocytizing bacteria or viruses.

Here's a way to see how the chemical called complement makes it easier for white blood cells to eat viruses and bacteria. First, chew up a plain piece of bread and swallow it. Now take another piece of bread, put a lot of butter on it, and eat it. Which is easier to swallow?

strange particles like bacteria by chemicals they send out. Also, there's an electrical attraction between a white blood cell's membrane and a bacterium. This draws them together and makes the bacterium stick to the membrane. Then the membrane dissolves a little and the bacterium sinks down into a pocket made in the cell membrane. The bacterium keeps on sinking until it is surrounded by the cell membrane's pocket, which closes in on top of it. The hole in the outside membrane closes and the pocket breaks off and moves deep inside the cell. Then little sacs called *lysosomes* move toward the bacterium's pocket and attach to it. The lysosomes contain digestive enzymes that kill and digest the bacterium. Anything left over is taken back to the edge of the cell and pushed out. This process is one of the main ways that the body protects itself against dangerous substances.

How antibodies destroy bacteria Antibodies are crucial helpers in the body's immune system. As we have seen, each kind of bacterium is covered with specially shaped chemicals called antigens, and the body makes antibodies that fit perfectly over these antigens.

Plasma, the watery part of blood, contains *complement enzymes*—chemicals that ordinarily are not active. But, when these enzymes come in contact with antibodies that are joined to antigens, the enzymes coat the bacteria and go into action. Once the chemicals in the complement get to work, they are extremely powerful. They help the body destroy bacteria, viruses, and poisons in at least four major ways.

Eventually the enzymes eat little holes in the surface of a bacterium. Then salt and water from the plasma rush into the bacterium. Pressure builds up and the bacterium explodes! This process is called *lysis*. It comes from the Greek word for dissolving.

Another thing that complement enzymes do is make bacteria easier to eat. When bacteria are covered with antibodies *and* the complement enzymes, it's a lot easier for white blood cells to eat the bacteria. Scientists don't know why this is, but they think it's like buttering bread—it makes it easier to swallow. Not only does complement make it easier for the white blood cells to eat the bacteria, it somehow signals the white blood cells that the bacteria are there.

A third major way complement helps protect the body against bacteria is by making them sticky. When the complement coats the antibody-bacteria mixture, they begin to stick together in clumps. Then the bacteria can't move and the clumps are too big to get into the body's cells.

A fourth thing complement does is to simply dissolve the little hooks on the surface of bacteria that help them grab onto cells. If the bacteria can't hook onto the cells, they can't get into them and hurt them. This process is called *neutralization*.

What's amazing about all these things is that they are

Bacteria are surrounded by anti-bodies, the body's own protective proteins.

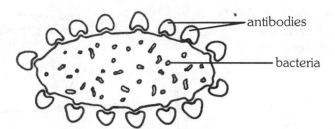

antibodies

bacteria

Bacteria and antibodies are coated with a digestive fluid from the blood, called complement.

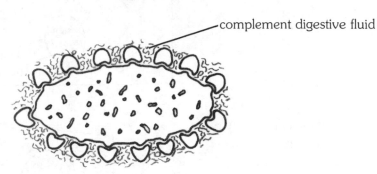

complement digestive fluid

The complement dissolves and explodes the bacteria.

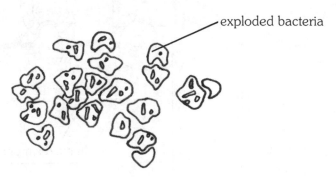

exploded bacteria

happening all the time in your body without your even being aware of them. But doctors are finding that these anti-body-complement reactions work best when people are happy and relaxed.

The body's school for lymphocytes

The body has special white blood cells called lymphocytes that help fight disease. There are two different types of

lymphocytes. The first type, *B-lymphocytes,* make anti-bodies, the chemicals that attach to the surface of viruses and bacteria and help kill them. The B-lymphocytes themselves do not hurt the bacteria; the antibodies do (*see* page 238).

The second kind of lympho-cytes are *T-lymphocytes.* They don't make antibodies; they themselves recognize and grab onto bacteria. Sometimes they shoot out lysosomes, the little sacs of digestive enzymes that

dissolve the bacteria (*see* page 127). More often the T-lymphocytes send out a chem-ical that attracts thousands of macrophages, the *giant* white blood cells which surround bacteria and *eat* them.

B- and T-lymphocytes are made in the marrow in the center of bones. When the lymphocytes are first made, they are called *stem cells.* Amazingly, these stem cells can't make antibodies or recognize bacteria. To do this, they have to go to "school"

In the thymus gland, white blood cells called lymphocytes are taught to recognize one kind of germ.

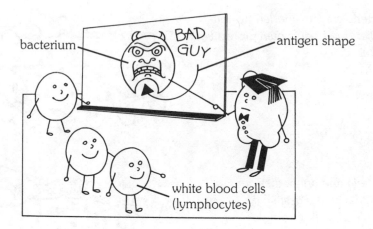

The lymphocytes change so they can "lock onto" the germ when they see it.

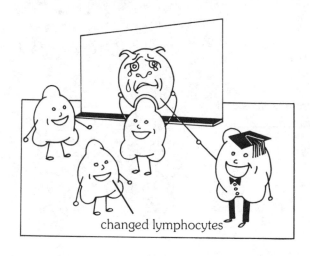

outside the bone marrow where they were made. The stem cells travel to one of two "schools" in the body. The T-lymphocytes go to the *thymus,* a gland located in the chest between the lungs. The B-lymphocytes are thought to go to school in the liver. In school, the lymphocytes are taught to recognize the bacteria and viruses by the antigens that cover them.

The lymphocytes actually become changed so that they can deal with an antigen. The T-lymphocytes grow shapes on their outside so they will fit like puzzle pieces over antigen shapes on the outside of the bacteria. The B-lymphocytes are changed so that they can make antibodies that will fit onto antigens. Each group of lymphocytes is taught to recognize only one kind of antigen. And there are thousands of different antigens on different bacteria and viruses. It's as if each child in a class were taught to look for just one particular number. One child would look for number 26s, one for number 27s, and so on.

After the lymphocytes go to school, they are sent out into the blood to watch out for "their" bacteria, like a police officer on a beat. When all is quiet, they just watch and wait. But, when a lymphocyte finds the bacteria it's trained to look for, it goes into action. It grows and splits again and again, making an army of thousands of trained lymphocytes. These lymphocytes are called *clones* because they are all exactly like the first one. If they are B-lymphocytes they make antibodies; if they are T-lymphocytes they attack and eat bacteria or viruses.

Chapter 7

Stress, nutrition, and exercise

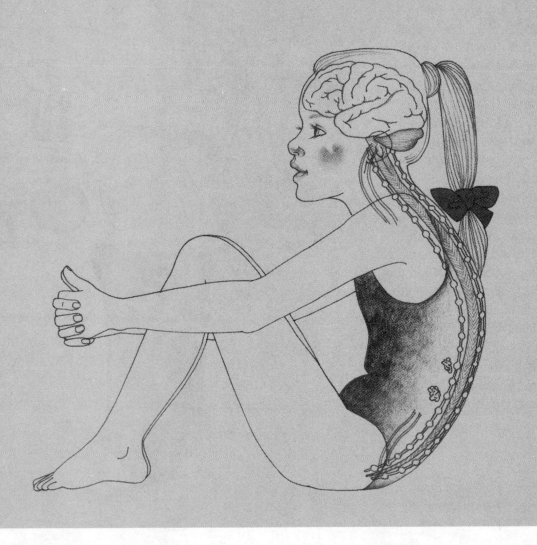

The whole environment

Children's health is affected by their whole world. Their minds are happy or scared depending upon what goes on around them. Their bodies take in air, food, and water and grow from these materials. They run and play, stretch and balance. And all these things affect their health.

When children are happy and relaxed, their brains send out messages to their organs to grow and stop infections. When children are scared, tense, or unhappy, their bodies can't do this as well. Then they are more likely to get sick or have an accident. When children eat food that has material for making energy and new cells, they grow and stay healthy. When they don't get enough food with building blocks like protein and vitamins, they don't grow as well and can get sick easily. When kids breathe fresh air and drink pure water, they keep healthy. When they breathe polluted air and drink water filled with dangerous chemicals, they eventually become sick. When children move their bodies and get lots of exercise, their heart, lungs, muscles, and bones grow big

Your body is affected by everything you do and by everything in the environment around you.

and strong. When children get little exercise their bodies are weaker and more likely to become ill.

Children themselves can do a lot to keep healthy. They can learn to relax and do things that they enjoy. They can learn what foods are good for their bodies, and avoid foods that aren't. And they can realize that exercise strengthens them, and can make it a part of their lives.

Thinking healthy

Doctors have found that people who think of themselves as healthy tend to be healthy, and people who think of themselves as getting sick all the time get sick more often. Doctors found this out in a special experiment. They sprayed cold viruses into the throats of a lot of healthy young people. Most of the people who thought they

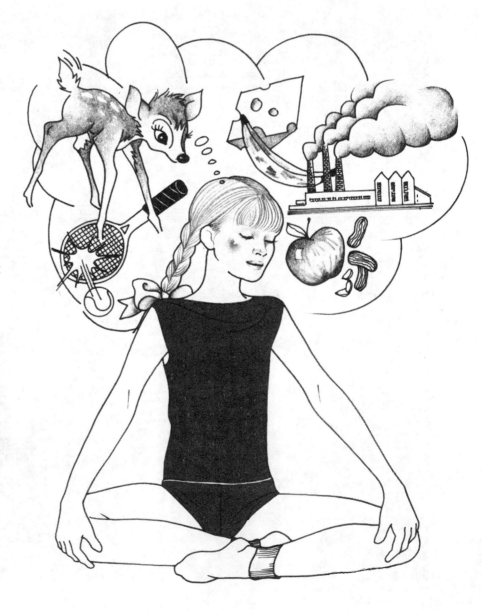

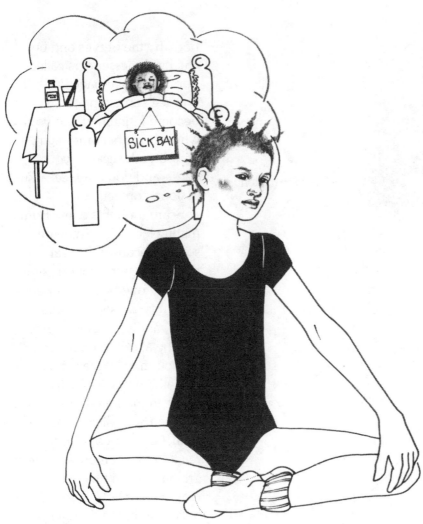

How you think affects how healthy you are. People who always think about being sick tend to get sick more often.

never got sick and had *few worries did not* get sick even though the germs were put right in their throats. Many of the people who thought they always got sick, *did* get sick.

Another experiment was performed on the people who always got sick. The doctors sprayed plain water in their throats, but told them the water had cold viruses in it. Over one-quarter of the people immediately got colds with runny noses, coughs, and fevers. Their minds made them sick! It's important to realize that you can't be healthy if you think sick.

Friendly coexistence is the rule We're surrounded by bacteria and viruses all the time. Millions of bacteria live on our skin, in our mouths and throats, and in our intestines. There are also bacteria and viruses in the air, in the soil, on our food, and in our houses.

Most of the bacteria don't hurt us, and some even help us. Bacteria enrich the soil, break down dead plants and animals, and help to make cheese and yogurt. In our bodies, good bacteria make our mouths acid so bad bacteria won't grow there. In our intestines another kind of bacteria makes vitamins that we can't live without. On our skin, helpful bacteria eat other kinds of bacteria that would give us infections.

Most people even have some bad bacteria or viruses in their body at any given time. But they aren't made sick by them. People only get sick when there are too many

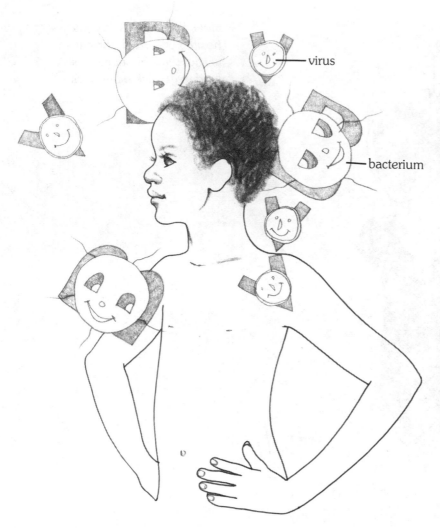

virus

bacterium

We're surrounded by bacteria and viruses all the time and don't get sick because most bacteria help the body, and the disease-causing ones don't usually hurt us.

body by the nerves and by chemical messengers called hormones (see page 206). If you see something scary, you become frightened and your whole body becomes tight, your breath sticks in your chest, and you may feel a knot in your stomach.

Scary thoughts come from many places. You may be scared because of a real danger like a poisonous snake in a tree overhead. Your eyes send this message to your brain, and your brain sends out the alarm to your body. Or you may be scared by something that looks like a snake in the tree, but turns out to be a rope coiled in the branches. Yet your body reacts in the same way. The "thing" doesn't have to be real to scare you. If you believe in it, the thought is real. And your body still gets the alarm—it can't tell the difference between the two thoughts. Even a movie of a snake can be scary, although a part of your mind knows there is no snake there.

Sometimes people even think scary thoughts for days *after* something that has happened, or *before* something that is going to happen —although nothing scary is really going on at the moment. Kids can get worried or upset about tests, about baseball games, about how their friends treat them, or about their parents' fighting.

Whenever people are upset

of a particular kind of disease-producing bacteria. Bacteria only *overgrow* like this when a person's body allows them to. The healthier a body is to begin with, the better it can control the number of bacteria that might harm it.

How stress affects the body

What you think affects how your body feels. Thoughts take place in the brain, which is connected to all parts of the

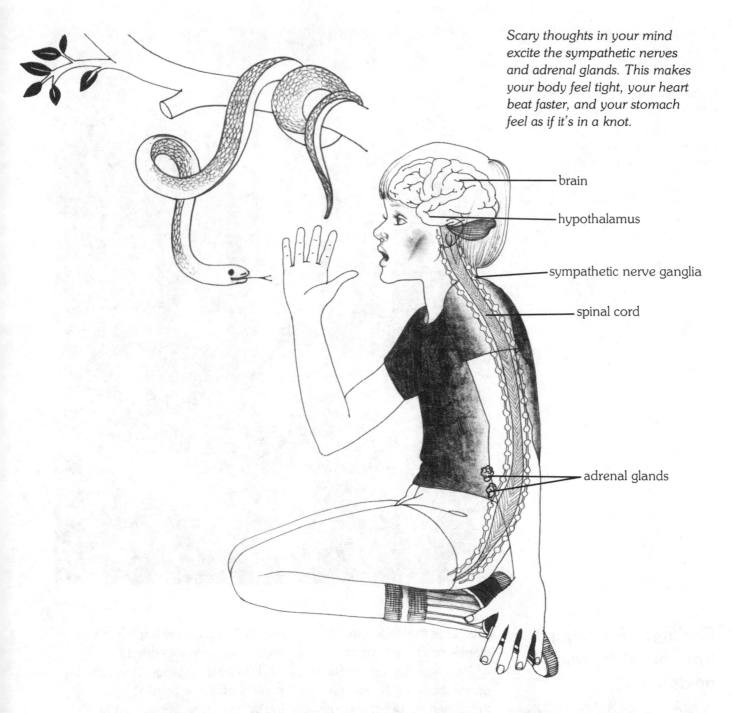

Scary thoughts in your mind excite the sympathetic nerves and adrenal glands. This makes your body feel tight, your heart beat faster, and your stomach feel as if it's in a knot.

brain

hypothalamus

sympathetic nerve ganglia

spinal cord

adrenal glands

or worried, a whole series of things happen inside their body. Some of these things they can easily feel; some they aren't even aware of. When people think, tiny bursts of electricity race from nerve cell to nerve cell in the brain. Some of these bursts go to the part of the brain called the hypothalamus (see page 190). The hypothalamus makes two things happen. First, it sends electrical messages down the sympathetic nerves (see page 190). These nerves make the heart speed up, which is why it pounds. They make the digestive system slow its working, which is why people feel flutters or a knot in their stomach when they are worried. The sympathetic nerves also go to the sweat glands, which is why people perspire when they are nervous. At the same time, the hypothalamus makes

When people are frightened, blood goes to their big muscles so they can fight or run.

Delacroix, Eugène. Arabs Skirmishing in the Mountains. *1863. Oil on canvas. 36⅜ × 29⅜". National Gallery of Art, Washington. Chester Dale Fund, 1966.*

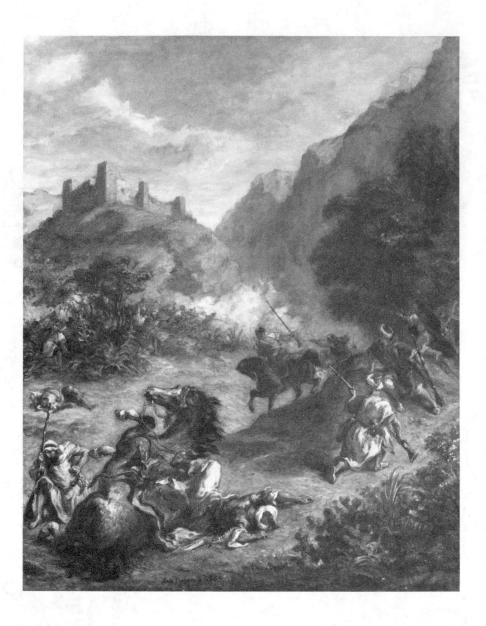

Feelings kids can get from being tense and anxious

Stomachaches

Headaches

Having to urinate frequently

Tiredness

Pains in feet and legs

Accidents of all kinds

several of the endocrine glands produce hormones, which have the same effects on the body as the sympathetic nerves, but they work more slowly and last longer.

All these body reactions are good if you need to run away from a snake. But they're not helpful if they happen too often or over a long period of time. Eventually they will even make you sick. Your heart will work too hard and your blood pressure will be too high. Your food won't digest properly. And your white blood cells will get less and less good at fighting germs. In a constant state of alarm or worry, the body doesn't direct its energy toward making new cells, repairing damaged cells, or healing. That's why it is so important for kids to learn to handle things that worry them. This will actually help to keep them healthier.

How relaxation affects the body

When people have peaceful or happy thoughts, they feel warm and their muscles feel loose. Their whole body feels very comfortable. In general, they feel healthy. People feel this way because peaceful thoughts actually set off a series of changes inside their bodies.

When people have peaceful or happy thoughts, bursts of electricity race from cell to cell in the brain's thinking center and to the hypothalamus, which lowers the number of alarm signals to the sympathetic nerves. Because few alarm signals are going out, the brain also tells the muscles of the body to rest and loosen up. At the same time the parasympathetic nerves send messages to the heart to beat slower and to the digestive system to work harder. All these things mean that the body runs smoothly. Food is digested and energy is put into building new cells, replacing old cells, and keeping healthy. When people are relaxed and calm, they're better able to fight germs and heal injuries.

People are relaxed or calm when they're having fun,

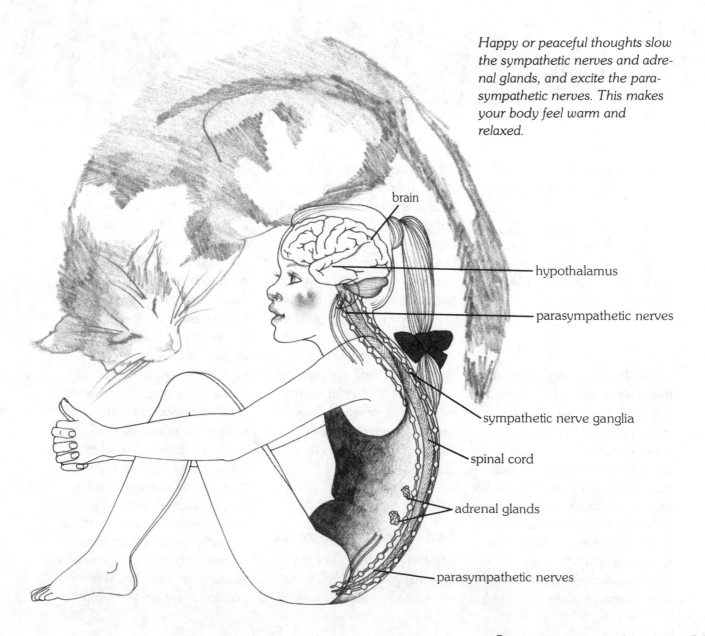

Happy or peaceful thoughts slow the sympathetic nerves and adrenal glands, and excite the parasympathetic nerves. This makes your body feel warm and relaxed.

brain

hypothalamus

parasympathetic nerves

sympathetic nerve ganglia

spinal cord

adrenal glands

parasympathetic nerves

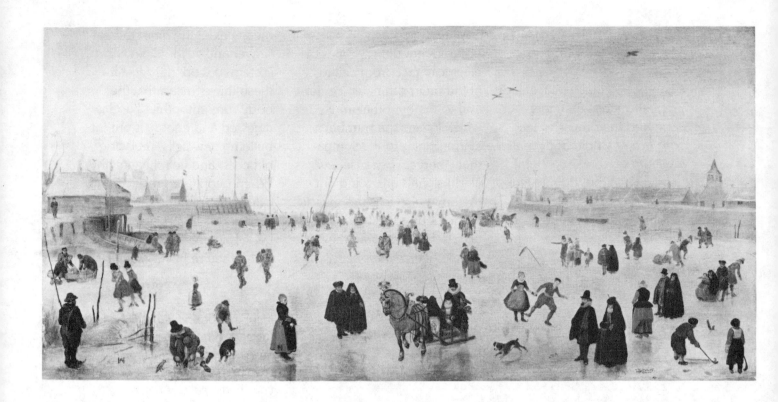

People's bodies are calm and relaxed when they are having fun.

Avercamp, Hendrick. A Scene on the Ice. 17th cent. Oil on wood. 15½ × 30⅜". National Gallery of Art, Washington. Ailsa Mellon Bruce Fund, 1967.

when they're doing something they like or when they're resting. Some people seem to be more relaxed than others. This is not necessarily because better things happen to them, but because of how they look at things. For example, some kids may be happy because they think they still have half their vacation left to play. Other kids may be unhappy or upset because they think their

vacation is already half over. Both groups of kids still have the same amount of time left, but one group is happy, the other is not. Lots of times being happy or not being happy is a matter of how people look at things. People can decide to be happy and then look at the world in this way. They will tend to see the good things, and pass over things that aren't fun or interesting. With practice, anyone can learn to pick out and concentrate on things they enjoy.

Learning how to relax

Children can learn to relax and make their bodies healthier by giving their muscles

instructions to relax. This may sound silly, but it actually works. The muscles that attach to bones and move the body always get their instructions from the mind. When you want to raise your arm, you think, "raise my arm," and your muscles do it. The mind sends signals down the nerves to your arm telling certain muscles to squeeze or tense. In the same way, if your mind sends messages to your muscles to relax, they will.

Most kids aren't used to sending messages to their muscles to tell them to relax. So people have figured out a way to help kids do this. It is a relaxation exercise or game. All that kids have to do is sit or lie down in a comfortable position. Then in their minds they repeat instructions to each area of their body to relax (see page 253).

The first step in learning to relax is learning what tension feels like. Relaxation is the opposite of tension. Muscles tense when they are working, but relax when they're at rest. Tension means a muscle is getting shorter and using lots of energy to do it. Relaxation means a muscle has let go and is using very little energy. Sometimes muscles remain a little tense even when they're not working. This kind of tension wastes energy and can

even make a person sick. If kids learn how tension and relaxation feel, they can relax more easily and make themselves healthier.

Here is an easy exercise to show the difference between how tension and relaxation feel. Sit comfortably and rest your arm on the side of a chair or table. Raise your hand *slightly* by bending up your wrist. Hold your arm in that position and feel the tension in your forearm. The muscle feels as if it's pulling—it's a little hard, a little hot, and a little bit uncomfortable. When

you do this, you can see the muscle move in your forearm and you can even feel it harden with your other hand.

Now let your hand drop and go totally limp. The muscle in your forearm will relax. You will feel as if you're resting instead of working. Your arm will feel comfortable and a little warm.

You can tighten or contract any muscle in the body to see how it feels when it's tensed, as compared to how it feels when it's relaxed. Often people don't even notice when their muscles are a little

You can feel tension in the muscle of your forearm when you bend up your wrist, and relaxation when you let your hand drop.

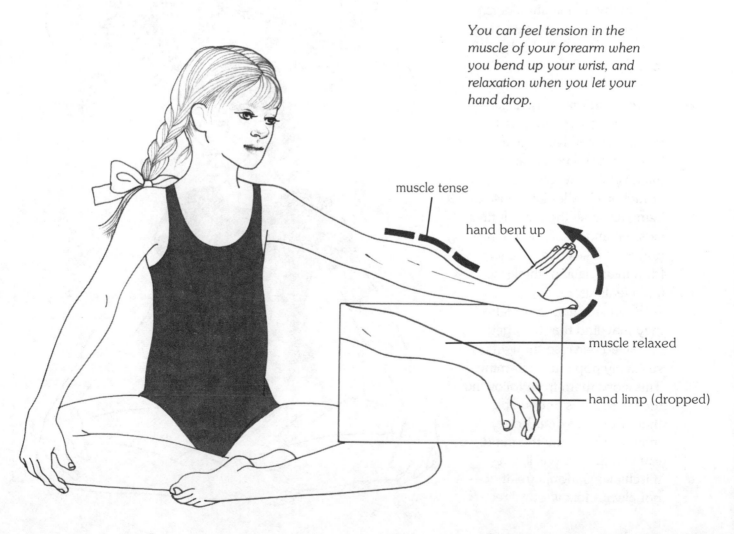

muscle tense

hand bent up

muscle relaxed

hand limp (dropped)

tense. But with practice you can learn to recognize the different feelings.

If some area of your body feels uncomfortable, chances are that area is a little tense. Many times when kids are angry or upset for any reason, their whole body or some parts of it become tense. They may not even be aware of it. If the tension goes on for a long time, kids may develop ways of holding their bodies that make it harder for them to move freely and to keep healthy. Some kids always bend their head forward, some "cave in" their chest, some hunch their shoulders. When kids learn to relax, they can loosen up their body and lose these bad habits.

Concentration Just as kids can learn to let their muscles relax, they can learn to let their minds relax. When the mind is full of worrisome thoughts, it's a lot like muscles being tense all the time. It tires kids out and wears down their bodies. It takes energy away from their playing, thinking, and creating.

When kids first try to relax they may find that they get distracted because thoughts suddenly pop into their mind. This stops them from following the instructions and keeps them from relaxing. Yogis, Indians who study the mind, say that the mind is like a mischievous monkey—it does not always follow our direc-

tions. Say you are trying to concentrate on relaxing your muscle, but thoughts come into your mind about your bicycle, the test coming up tomorrow, or a movie you want to see this weekend. All of a sudden you realize you've forgotten about relaxing. Kids often have the most trouble controlling their thoughts

when they are worried about something. Once you understand what's happening, you

Thoughts come into a person's mind and then disappear like birds flying across the sky. You can learn to watch your own thoughts come and go, the way you watch birds come and go.

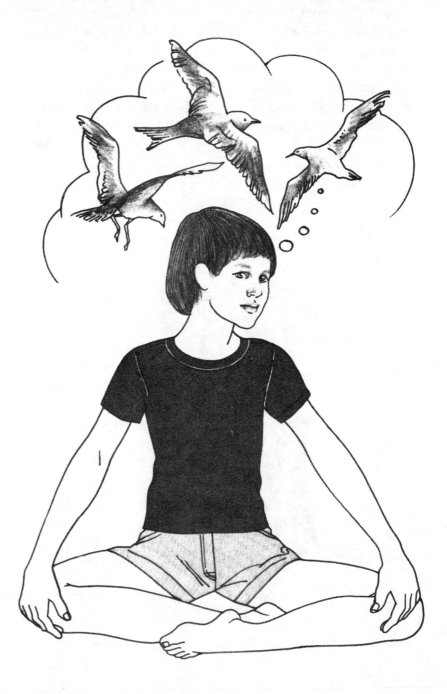

can begin to control your thoughts with practice. Although the mind is like a mischievous monkey, it can be tamed.

Here is an exercise to show you how your mind works and to help you control it. All the exercise involves is counting your breaths. It may sound simple, but it's not easy. Sit in a quiet, comfortable place. Close your eyes. Breathe in and out slowly through your nose. Let your tummy go in and out as you breathe. Count to yourself 1 as you breathe in, 2 as you breathe out, 3 as you breathe in, 4 as you breathe out, and so on up to 10. When you reach 10, start all over again. Concentrate as hard as you can on just breathing and counting up to 10.

You will find that no matter how hard you try, you'll suddenly be thinking of something else. Chances are, you won't even realize you've stopped counting for some time; you'll find yourself in the middle of some long, complicated thought. This shows how little control most people —kids and adults—have over their own thoughts. As soon as you realize what's happening, start counting again. Don't worry about stopping, just go back to the count. The more you practice this, the sooner you'll catch your mind wandering.

With practice, many people find they can "see" thoughts come into their mind like birds going across the sky. If they don't pay attention to the thought, but go back to counting, the thoughts will pass just as birds disappear after they cross the sky.

It's amazing, but few people can count for more than a minute without other thoughts entering their mind. Kids who practice counting their breaths begin to find that they can stop worrisome thoughts. And they will find that if they're trying to learn something new or study for a test, they can concentrate much better. This ability to concentrate also makes it easier to follow all the instructions in this book for relaxation and visualization.

A relaxation exercise Sit or lie in a quiet place. Have someone read the exercise to you or read it and then repeat it to yourself. You don't have to use the exact words. First get into a comfortable position, close your eyes, and breathe in and out slowly. Let your tummy go in and out as you breathe. As you breathe slowly and evenly you will start to relax. Now tell your feet to relax. Say to yourself, "My feet are relaxing." Rest and let your feet relax. Then tell your lower legs to relax. Say to yourself, "My lower legs are relaxing." Rest. Tell your thighs to relax. Rest. Tell your hips to relax. Rest. Tell your tummy to relax. Rest. Tell your chest to relax.

Rest. Tell your whole back to relax. Rest. Tell your upper arms to relax. Tell your lower arms to relax. Rest. Tell your hands to relax. Rest. Now tell your neck to relax. Rest. Tell your jaws to relax. Rest. Tell your face and eyes to relax. Rest. And finally tell your head to relax. Stay in this relaxed state as long as you want to.

When kids relax deeply they say that their body feels floppy, loose, tingly, and warm all over. Some kids say they feel light as air; other kids say they feel heavy as a rock. As kids become used to relaxing they find that they can become relaxed almost instantly as soon as they start breathing slowly and thinking about relaxation. But if they're upset or sick, it may help to repeat the whole exercise very slowly or do a longer exercise, like the following one.

Get in a comfortable position, close your eyes, and breathe in and out slowly. As you breathe slowly and evenly you will start to relax. Let your feet relax. Feel them getting heavier and heavier. Feel them getting a little tingly. Let your lower legs relax. Feel the tingliness spreading up to your legs. Let your thighs relax. Feel the tingliness spread further. Let all the muscles around your hips relax. Let your hips drop and become heavy. Let your tummy relax. Let it sink down each time you breathe out. Let your chest relax. Feel your heart beat

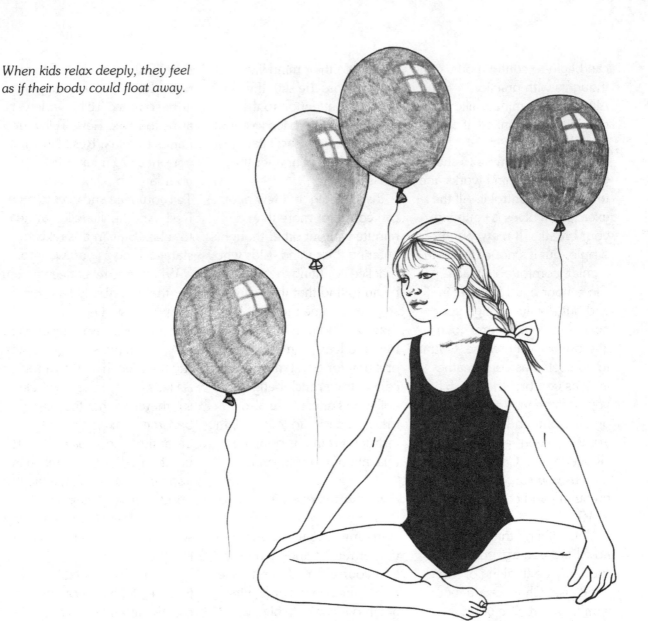

When kids relax deeply, they feel as if their body could float away.

slowly and steadily and your chest rise and fall evenly. Let your lungs sink down every time you breathe out. Let your upper arms relax. Feel them get heavier. Let your lower arms relax. Let them hang loosely. Let your hands relax. Feel them getting a little tingly. Let your neck relax. Feel your head drop and your throat widen. Let your jaw relax and drop. Your mouth will open and your cheeks will stretch. Let your eyes relax. Your eyes will feel as if they're flattening out. Let your forehead relax. It will feel as if it's sliding down over your eyes. Let your whole head relax. You will feel as if you are wearing a warm cap. If any area of your body still feels tense, let relaxation spread to it. Allow the calm, peaceful feelings of relaxation to spread all over your body.

Exercises for deepening relaxation After kids have learned to tell their muscles to relax, they can learn to deepen this comfortable feeling. There are several kinds of deepening exercises. The basis of most of these exercises is to count backward from 10 to 1. As people say each number they also repeat to themselves the instruction that they are getting more relaxed. When kids deepen the relaxation they reach a point where they may be hardly aware of their bodies. Their minds may feel as if they are floating in a dream. This is a special, pleasurable sensation that is very different from the hustle and bustle of school or playing. It's like the inner world of daydreams and is a deeper level than everyday thought.

Before doing the deepening exercise, first relax your whole body (page 253). Breathe in and out several times. When you feel quite relaxed, begin counting backward. Say to yourself, "10 . . . I am feeling very relaxed. Rest. 9 . . . I am feeling more relaxed. Rest. 8 . . . I am feeling even more relaxed. Rest. 7 . . . I am feeling deeper and more relaxed. Rest. 6 . . . more and more relaxed. 5 . . . even more relaxed. Rest. 4 . . . deeper and deeper. Rest. 3 . . . deeper and deeper. Rest. 2 . . . still deeper. Rest. 1 . . . very relaxed. Rest. 0 . . . I am now in a very relaxed place. My body feels healthy. My mind feels peaceful and open. I can stay in this relaxed place as long as I want. I can return to it easily. To return to my everyday world, all I have to do is gently wiggle my fingers and open my eyes."

Some people find they relax better if they picture the numbers as they go down. One way is to imagine that you are in an elevator that starts on the 10th floor and goes down to the main floor. Imagine the feeling of the elevator dropping and the numbers lighting up. When you get to the main floor, you will feel very relaxed.

When to relax

When you're nervous, scared, tired, crying, hurt, before a test or game, doing homework, at bedtime.

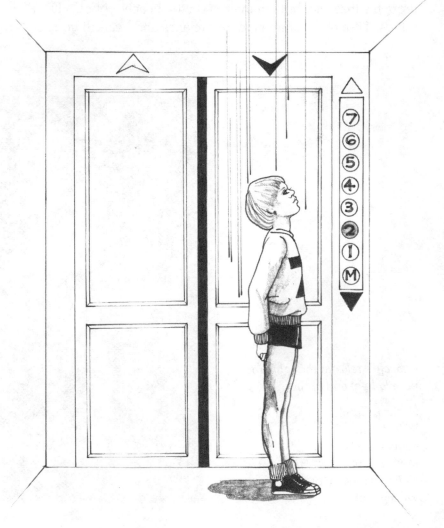

One way to relax very deeply is to imagine you are in an elevator and watch the floor numbers light up as you go down.

Visualization and imagery

Whatever thoughts children hold in their minds affect their bodies. Peaceful or relaxed thoughts help make people heal, grow, solve problems, and create. Upset or scary thoughts make people's bodies tighten up and get ready for action. This is fine if some action really does take place. But if the scary or upset thoughts stay in the mind and nothing happens, this will eventually make people sick.

Many kids don't realize it, but they can choose the thoughts that they hold in their minds. Thoughts in the mind are like pictures and sounds and feelings. If you close your eyes and "see" your bedroom, you can look around in your mind's eye and see where your bed is, where the doors are, and where you keep your clothes and toys. It's different than seeing with your eyes. It feels more like using your imagination.

When you're picturing a scene in your mind, like your room, your body doesn't know if you're really seeing it or just imagining it. If you picture a peaceful happy scene in your mind, like lying on the beach, your body relaxes and heals. If you picture a scary scene, like a train coming at you, your body gets tense and your heart speeds up. Doctors have found that if you picture in your mind that there's an ice cube in one hand, that hand will actually get colder. If you picture your hand in hot water, it will actually get warmer.

Kids can learn to picture calm, peaceful scenes when they want to get rid of scary thoughts, stop something from hurting, or heal themselves if they are sick. They can picture running fast if they're about to run a race or picture getting a high grade if they are about to take a test.

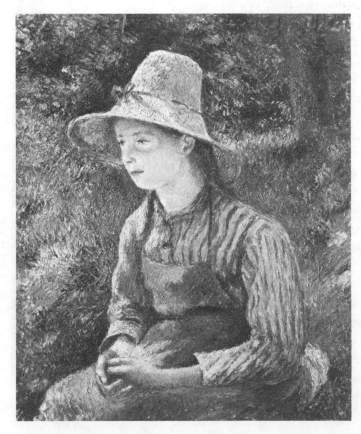

Peaceful, relaxed thoughts make people heal and grow.

Pissaro, Camille, Peasant Girl With A Straw Hat. *1881. Oil on canvas. 28⅞ × 23½". Ailsa Mellon Bruce Collection, 1970, National Gallery of Art, Washington.*

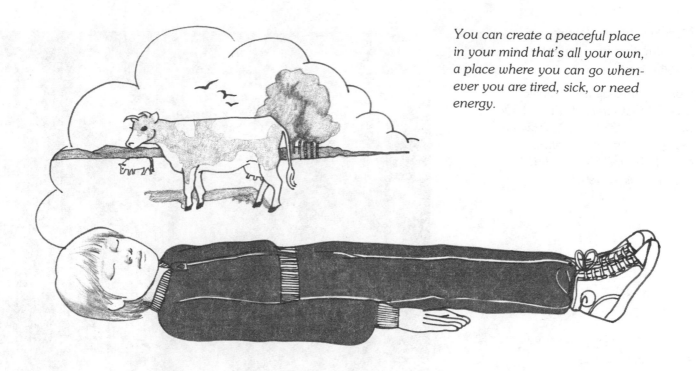

You can create a peaceful place in your mind that's all your own, a place where you can go whenever you are tired, sick, or need energy.

Like relaxing, kids can picture scenes in their mind by doing an exercise or game. All you have to do is sit or lie in a comfortable place, close your eyes, and relax. Then you can picture whatever you want to see.

Imagining a peaceful scene Most kids are very good at picturing things in their minds. In fact, they do it all the time. They may daydream about hitting a home run or becoming class president. What many kids don't realize is that they can daydream on purpose. You can imagine something whenever you want to, to make you feel good, be healthier, or do better at school or sports.

You can practice helpful daydreaming by doing the following exercise. Sit or lie in a quiet place. Have someone read the exercise to you or read it and then repeat it to yourself. You don't have to use the exact words. Get in a comfortable position, close your eyes, and breathe in and out slowly. Let your tummy go in and out as you breathe. As you breathe slowly and evenly you will become more and more relaxed. Now picture in your mind the most peaceful scene you can think of. It may be a familiar place you've been to often, a place you've only been to once or twice, or a place that you make up in your imagination. It may be a warm, sunny beach that you love, a place high in the mountains where you camped, or a country meadow with a cow grazing on grass. It

may be your own bedroom, or a workshop or studio you've been to. Or it may be a totally imaginary place like an underwater cave or a faraway planet with a cool purple sky. When you can picture a peaceful scene, look all around. Notice the color of things. What is right around you, what is far away? How do things feel? Imagine that you are really there. Listen to the sounds of the place, smell the air. Spend as much time as you want in this peaceful place. And remember you can easily return whenever you want. This can even be a special private place that only you can go to. You can use it whenever you are tired, sick, or need energy. You can also use it when you just want to relax.

Most kids have a favorite peaceful scene that they can return to in their mind.

Corot, Jean-Baptiste-Camille. *The Eel Gatherers.* 19th cent. Oil on canvas. 23¾ × 32". National Gallery of Art, Washington. Gift of Mr. and Mrs. P. H. B. Frelinghuysen, 1943.

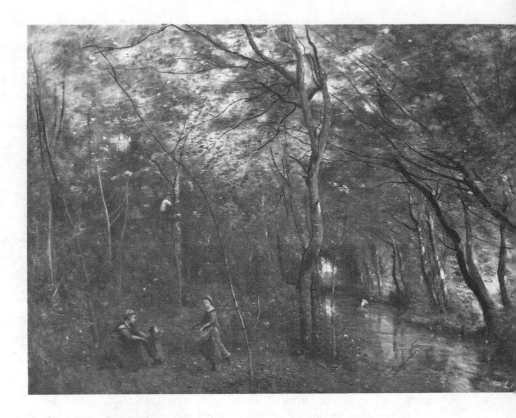

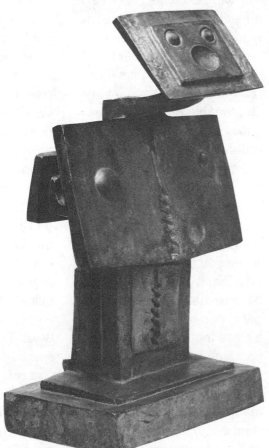

Kids often feel nervous or have scary thoughts.

Ernst, Max. *Anxious Friend.* 1944. Bronze. Height: 26⅜" Collection, The Solomon R. Guggenheim Museum, New York. Gift of Dominique and John de Menil, 1959.

Dealing with stressful scenes Kids often have scary or worrisome thoughts or daydreams. They may be concerned about a test or an important game or recital. Pictures may pop into their minds of past scenes that scared them. They may remember when a dog chased them and barked loudly. They may remember when they took a bad fall. Or they may remember a TV show or movie that was especially upsetting. Sometimes these thoughts keep coming back. Then they make it hard to study or play, keep kids from doing certain things, or even give them headaches or stomachaches.

Often kids don't even know

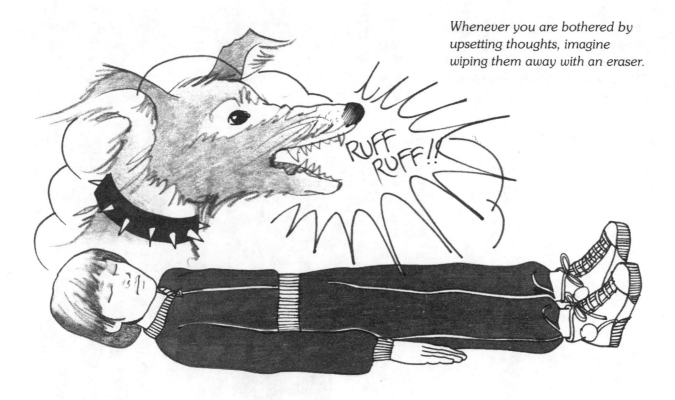

Whenever you are bothered by upsetting thoughts, imagine wiping them away with an eraser.

RUFF RUFF!?

that they are having such thoughts. They just suddenly realize that they feel uncomfortable. If they "look at" what they were thinking about, they understand that this is what made them uncomfortable. Most kids don't realize it, but they can stop upsetting thoughts if they want to. All they have to do is relax, erase the bad scene, and imagine a good scene on purpose.

Whenever you're scared or worried, get in as comfortable a position as you can. (You can do this exercise anywhere, anytime.) Breathe in and out slowly. As you breathe slowly and evenly, you will start to relax. Let the bad scene appear again, if it has gone away. Remember the scene is

just in your mind, so it really can't hurt you. Now imagine a giant eraser rubbing out the scene like a picture on a blackboard. Or imagine ink dripping down and covering the whole scene. You can even imagine tearing the scene in half like a photograph. Once the bad image is gone, put a good image in its place. Think of the most wonderful thing that could happen to you or the most peaceful place you've ever been. Be there. As you picture this good scene you will feel better and better.

Being able to get rid of bad images gives you tremendous power over your own life. It doesn't matter how you get rid of them. There are many ways to remove a bad scene. Other

examples are letting the wind blow it away, watching it fall apart like pieces from a puzzle, or changing the channel as on a TV set. The best way may be the one you think up yourself. Doing this is a little like getting rid of ghosts—the important thing is to realize that you can do it yourself.

Imagining a blank screen
One of the best ways for many kids to picture things in their minds is to imagine a TV set. Most kids are used to seeing all kinds of pictures on a TV screen and they are used to changing the pictures and shutting them on and off.

Picturing things on an imaginary TV screen is especially good for solving prob-

One of the best ways to use mind pictures to get ideas or solve problems is to imagine a blank TV screen onto which your ideas come as pictures.

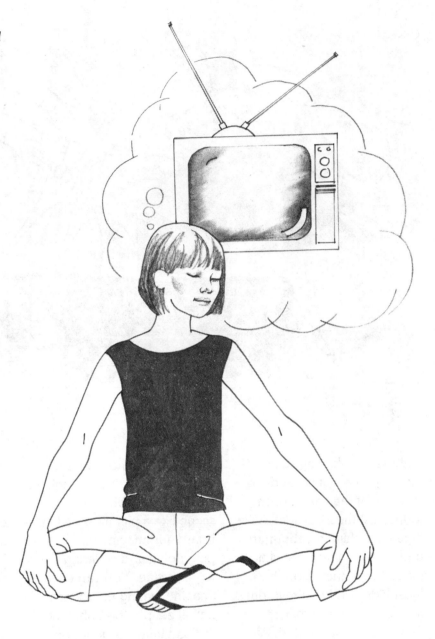

lems and getting ideas. To do this, simply imagine a blank screen, ask yourself a question, and wait for a picture to appear. The pictures that appear come from a deeper part of your mind that you may not be aware of.

Sit in a quiet place where you will not be disturbed. Get in a comfortable position and close your eyes. Breathe in and out slowly. As you breathe slowly and evenly you will start to relax. When you are quite relaxed, picture a magic television set. Look at the box and the control knobs. Imagine the screen is blank. Think of something you're trying to make a decision about or a situation that you don't know how to handle. Picture yourself solving the situation, making a decision, or handling a problem. Imagine that you do just the right thing to make everything work out right. Picture exactly what you say to someone, exactly what a scene that you're drawing will look like, exactly what you want, or what is bothering you. Pictures will come to your imaginary screen like thoughts popping into your mind. If you still have questions, repeat them to yourself and see what other pictures appear on your magic screen.

Let's say that you have to make up a story about traveling to the moon and you don't know what to write. Think of the homework assignment and imagine what it would be like to fly to the moon. Let your imagination run free. Picture the rocket ship, the controls, and what might happen. Teachers have found that students who try this kind of exercise get more interesting and creative ideas.

Another time to use the blank screen is when you have a problem. Let's say some kids at school are making fun of the way you talk. Usually you get so upset you don't know what to do. Picture this happening on a blank screen. Then imagine that you suddenly know just what to do or say to solve this problem. You might see yourself walking away and playing with someone you don't know very well. Or you might see yourself saying, "Do you want to repeat that in front of the teacher!" Next time you are teased, try doing what you saw on your imaginary screen.

Imaginary sports   One of the best ways to use mind pictures is in sports. Many coaches who train famous athletes use mind pictures to

When to use mind pictures or visualizations

When you're scared, nervous, or hurt, picture a favorite peaceful scene.

When you're tired, picture yourself resting and filling up with energy.

When you're upset and crying, picture your feelings smoothing out like waves flattening out when the wind stops.

Before a test or a big game, picture yourself doing well.

When you can't go to sleep, picture a still, quiet scene.

When you're being teased, picture the words bouncing off of you.

When you feel really angry, picture all the anger coming out of you like steam blowing out of a boiling tea kettle.

When you're feeling sorry for yourself, picture the thing you do best.

How to use mind pictures to solve problems and get ideas

Picture a blank screen or stage and imagine something appears . . . .

The idea for a story or drawing

The answer to a test problem

The part that's needed to finish something you're building

The people who could help you with a special project

The way you could make up after a fight

How you'd feel if you were the other person

What you could do to make a certain part of your life better

You can get better at sports just by imagining yourself doing the motions.

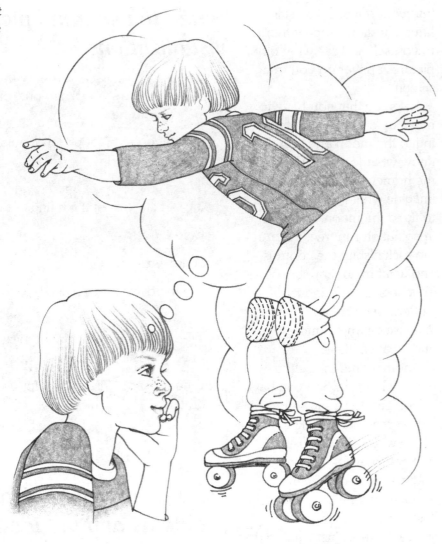

help them get better at their sport. When kids picture doing a sports movement in the right way, their real performance improves. Coaches discovered this by dividing a basketball team into two groups. Both groups practiced shooting baskets at school, but one group practiced shooting baskets in their mind. The group who did mind-practice as well as real practice did much better.

Mind pictures are actually another way of practicing. Even though you may not feel it, the same nerve cells in the brain and muscles that are excited by hitting a baseball, for example, are excited by *imagining* hitting the ball. Scientists have detected tiny amounts of electricity in the nerves and muscles of people who were sitting still, but imagining a movement. Each time a series of nerve cells is excited, it makes a loop or path; and each time the path is used, it gets smoother and more efficient.

To try using mind pictures in sports, sit in a quiet place, in a comfortable position. Close your eyes. Breathe in and out slowly. As you breathe slowly and easily, you will start to relax. When you are quite relaxed, picture yourself practicing the sport at which you want to improve. Imagine the kind of clothes you usually wear, and the place where you practice. Feel the bat or ball in your hands or the roller skates or skis on your feet. Feel and smell the air around you. See the people you play with and the goal you're aiming for. See yourself actually making the series of movements you're working on. *Feel* the movements in your muscles as you do it. Make those perfect movements over and over in your mind. If something doesn't feel quite right, make corrections in your mind. Bend more, lean more, or jump higher—whatever you need to do to make your mind picture just right. The clearer your pictures and the more often you do them, the better you'll become.

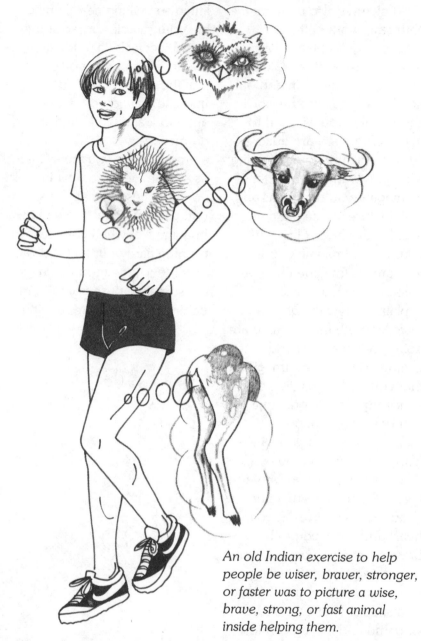

An old Indian exercise to help people be wiser, braver, stronger, or faster was to picture a wise, brave, strong, or fast animal inside helping them.

Picturing body helpers Kids can work at improving any part of their lives with mind pictures. Just as you can improve your performance at sports with mind pictures, you can improve your grades at school, your strength, or even your courage. It is just like rehearsing for a play. The more often you ''see'' it, and the clearer and more detailed your picture, the more you will improve. Kids who practiced giving a speech in their mind spoke better and were less nervous than kids who didn't do any mind-practicing. Kids who, in their mind, practiced reading smoothly or doing well on tests, actually did better.

Mind pictures work best if they are done many times and if they are backed up by hard work. But they do make people less scared and more confident in their own abilities.

Mind pictures also make nerve pathways work better.

Sit in a quiet place in a comfortable position. Close your eyes. Breathe in and out slowly. As you breathe slowly and evenly, you will start to relax. When you are quite relaxed, picture yourself doing what you want to be better at.

Imagine you're wise as an owl. Picture a wise old owl who is your helper living in your mind. Imagine you are very smart. Imagine that you enjoy learning and like explaining new things you have learned. Imagine you are doing well in school and getting good grades. Imagine that you find it easy to concentrate for a long time, that you have a good memory, and that you can learn new things easily. . . .

Imagine you are as brave as a lion. Picture a calm, courageous lion who lives in your heart and helps you to be braver. Imagine yourself trying something new and feeling proud. Imagine yourself going to a special after-school class or game and feeling comfortable right away. Imagine yourself telling a large group of older kids not to make fun of someone. Imagine yourself having a good time hiking a steep trail that scared you last year. . . .

Imagine you are as strong as an ox. Picture a powerful ox inside your muscles who helps you to be stronger when you need to be. When you are lifting something heavy, imagine your muscles are so strong the object feels light. Imagine that in a tug-of-war you easily pull the rope to your side. Imagine that you can work and work and work, and still do more. . . .

Imagine that you are as fast as a deer. Picture a deer in your leg muscles that helps you when you need to be fast. Imagine that when you are running hard your feet almost don't touch the ground. Imagine someone pushes you from behind when you are running up a hill. Imagine that your lungs can send more and more oxygen to your muscles. Imagine that you can run long distances without becoming tired.

Letting words pass by   All kids have times when they are surprised or hurt by things people say to them. Parents may yell at you, friends may tease, a teacher may scold you. Whether what they say is right or wrong, it can hurt your feelings or upset you. When they're hurt or upset, people

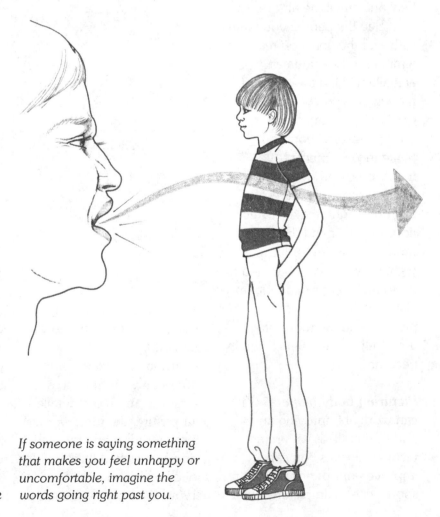

If someone is saying something that makes you feel unhappy or uncomfortable, imagine the words going right past you.

don't usually think about what's been said, they just react. This means that they can't learn from what's happened or even explain if a mistake has been made.

When people are upset by something that's been said, they feel uncomfortable and a little bit shaky. Their muscles tense, they feel a knot in their stomach, their eyes may sting, and their voice may sound funny. Their mind has heard something alarming and their brain puts their body on alert. It's like the flight-or-fight response in which someone runs from a dangerous situation.

Most kids don't realize it, but they can control these kinds of uncomfortable feelings through mind pictures and relaxing. And they can do this while the person is still talking to them. In fact, if they practice the exercise at home, they'll be able to do it automatically the next time someone makes them feel uncomfortable.

As soon as you start to feel upset, take several deep breaths. As you breathe slowly and evenly, you will start to feel relaxed right away. Picture yourself covered with an invisible protective shield. Words that are said to you just slide right by this shield like a wind. The words can't come inside, but you can hear them. Remember you are still yourself. Feel strong and calm. If it will help, picture yourself doing something that you are good at. While you are in this strong, protected place, you can listen to what's being said without being upset by it. You can sort out what's true and what isn't and you can answer calmly.

Being able to deal with upsetting moments can help all kids and even adults. When kids become very upset for long periods of time, they are much more likely to become sick or have accidents. The stronger and happier people feel, the better their bodies work.

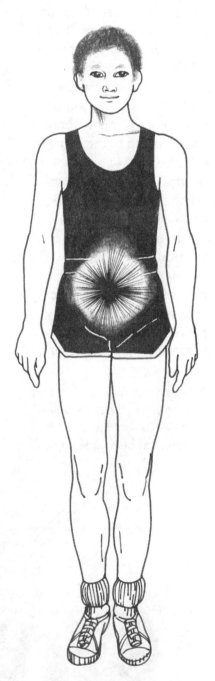

Feeling your center Feeling your own center helps make you feel calm, solid, and powerful. It's like being balanced or getting in harmony with the world around you. The center of your body is the part you would balance on if you were a seesaw. The center of your weight is just below your navel, or belly button. This center doesn't change. The center of your height is around your belly button when you are a baby, and drops as your legs grow longer. By the time you're ten or so, your height center has dropped down to where your legs meet your body.

Because kids' bodies are growing and changing so much, it's especially important for them to be aware of the center that doesn't change.

Concentrating on the center of your body makes you feel calm, solid, and powerful.

On a physical level, centering makes all movements smoother and easier. On another level, it keeps us in touch with ourselves and makes our lives easier.

Sit or lie in a quiet place. Get in a comfortable position, close your eyes, and breathe in and out slowly. Let your tummy go in and out as you breathe. As you breathe slowly and evenly you will start to relax. Picture your breath going to the center of your body. As you breathe in, picture energy from outside going to your center. Soon you will begin to feel more aware of this area, and it will be more real to you. It will feel heavy and connect you to the ground. It will feel full of energy and give you new power and strength. As you breathe out, let this feeling of strength and power spread over your whole body. Stay in touch with these feelings as long as you want.

Centering is very healthy and very useful before taking a test, giving a speech, or playing an important game— or anytime that you might feel a little uncomfortable. It brings your energies together and focuses them.

Picturing healing energy

Mind pictures can actually help kids get better when they're sick because they affect nerve cells in the brain that control the rest of the body. Healing pictures relax the muscles, slow the heart and breathing, and bring white blood cells and food to all parts of the body to help repair and grow new cells.

Mind pictures not only help the body heal itself, they can also do other things, like help to numb an area and take away pain when it's hurt, help stop bleeding from a cut, or help make breathing easier.

Sit or lie in a quiet place. Get in a comfortable position, close your eyes, and breathe in and out slowly. Let your tummy go in and out as you breathe. As you breathe slowly and evenly, you will start to relax. Picture your body surrounded by glowing light. Imagine your whole body is filled with healing energy. With each breath you take in, imagine the energy gets stronger and the light glows more brightly. With every breath you let out, imagine that all the tiredness, sickness, and hurt goes out of your body. If any area of your

Whenever you are sick or hurt, picture your whole body filled with healing energy and surrounded by a glowing light.

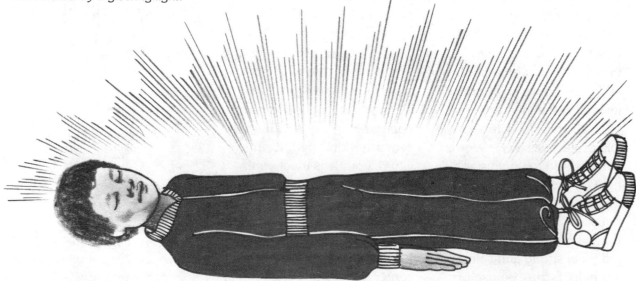

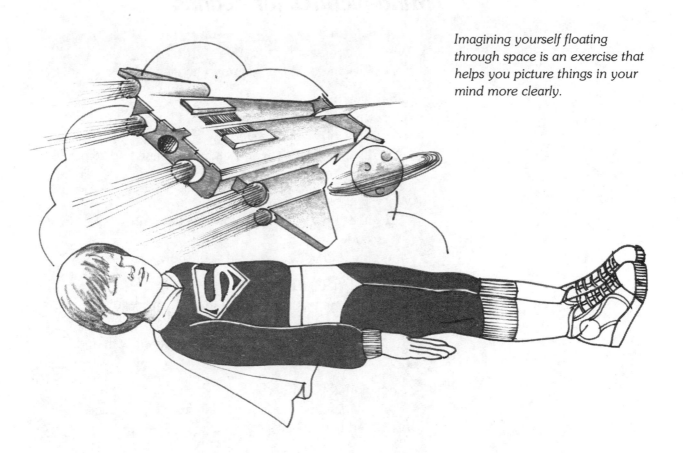

Imagining yourself floating through space is an exercise that helps you picture things in your mind more clearly.

body is bothering you, let extra healing energy go to that part. If any area hurts, picture the pain as dark smoke and let it flow out of your body. Picture your body working to heal you. Picture yourself as healed and healthy. Imagine you're as strong as you've ever been.

Visualization deepening exercise After kids have learned to picture things, they can learn to go deeper into their minds. This helps to make their mind pictures feel sharper and more real. Then kids concentrate better and are less bothered by outside noises and funny feelings in their body. This kind of deepening exercise is a lot like the exercise for deepening relaxation (page 255). When kids get deeply relaxed, they sometimes have daydreams of floating or traveling through space. This exercise uses those natural daydreams.

Get in a comfortable position, close your eyes, and breathe in and out slowly. As you breathe slowly and evenly, you will start to relax. Picture yourself floating through space. Imagine you are weightless and you float without any effort. See the deep blue-black color of space all around you. As you look around, you will notice that space goes on forever in every direction. All around are stars and planets. As you move, you'll see the stars and planets pass by you. With every star that passes by, you will feel more and more relaxed. Now picture an area of light ahead of you. Imagine yourself traveling into the light until it's all around you. This is a special relaxed place where you can imagine anything you want to and figure out answers to questions you have. When you want to return to your ordinary world, move your fingers, rest a minute more, and then open your eyes.

Imagining a spirit guide workshop All people have in their mind a picture of a special private place and a

Mind pictures for healing

When you're afraid
 . . . imagine being in your favorite place.

When you hurt
 . . . imagine the pain coming out of your body and blowing away like smoke.
 . . . imagine that the pain is a thin red line and snip it off with scissors.

When you have a fever
 . . . imagine a cool wind blowing over your whole body.
 . . . pretend you're covered with snow.

When you have a cut
 . . . imagine that the sides of the cut get sticky, then join together, and the bleeding stops.
 . . . imagine that the line of the cut gets smooth and disappears.

When you have a nosebleed
 . . . imagine the blood is coming from a tiny faucet and you slowly shut it off.

When you get a bruise
 . . . imagine the swelling disappearing the way air goes out of a balloon.
 . . . imagine the black-and-blue mark turning into tiny dots and then gradually disappearing.

When you get an insect bite or sting
 . . . imagine the hurt going out of the stinger hole in a thin red line.
 . . . imagine the swelling slowly going back into the rest of your body and disappearing.

When you get a burn
 . . . imagine the burned area feeling as if it's in ice water.

When you have a broken bone
 . . . imagine the bones being stuck together with glue and being stronger than ever.

When you have a rash
 . . . imagine your skin feeling as smooth as silk.
 . . . imagine the redness disappearing as though it's being erased.

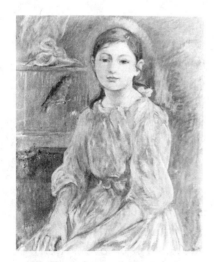

When kids picture healing energy, blood goes to parts of the body that need repair.

Morisot, Berthe. The Artist's Daughter With A Parakeet. 19th cent. Oil on canvas. 25¾ × 20⅝". National Gallery of Art, Washington, Chester Dale Collection.

When your skin itches
   . . . imagine your skin feeling as if a cool breeze were
       blowing over it.
   . . . imagine you're floating in cool water.

When you have a skin infection
   . . . imagine the area feeling warm and tingly, and
       pulsing like your heartbeat.

When your eyes itch or burn
   . . . picture a black cat or a dark room.
   . . . picture a distant horizon at dusk.
   . . . imagine your eyes feeling cool, like stones.

When you have a runny nose
   . . . imagine the lining of your nose shrinking and
       becoming dry.
   . . . imagine a faucet at the top of your nose being
       shut off.

When you have a sore throat
   . . . imagine cold ice cream sliding down the back of
       your throat.

When you have an earache
   . . . imagine the pain turning into a thin red line, and
       cut it into little pieces until it goes away.

When your ears are stuffed up
   . . . imagine that the tubes that go from your ear to
       the back of your throat pop open.

When you have a cough
   . . . imagine your chest becoming warm.
   . . . imagine that the sticky stuff in your throat
       becomes thin and watery.

When you have trouble breathing (from asthma or
allergies)
   . . . imagine a calm, peaceful scene.
   . . . imagine the tiny tubes in your lungs becoming
       wider and air sliding in and out more easily.

When you have a stomachache
   . . . imagine that your stomach becomes calm like a
       smooth lake.
   . . . imagine a little bit of the ache going away with
       each breath.

You can have your own helper who you can visit anytime in your imagination.

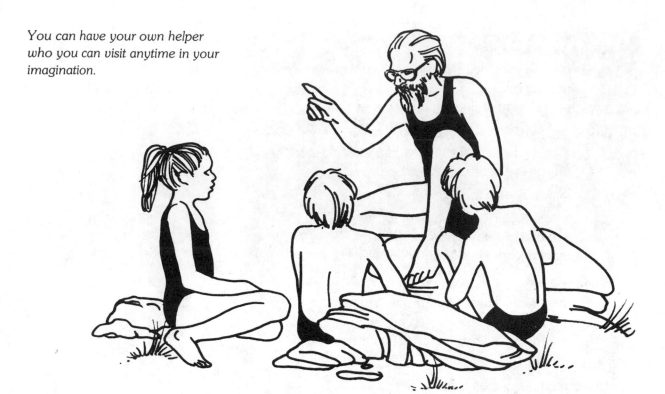

private helper. Although the place and person are in the imagination, they can be very helpful in everyday life. The place is like a secret hideout where you can go whenever you like. And because it's in your imagination, you can go there any time, no matter where you are. The imaginary helper may be someone you know, someone you've never met, a space creature, or a magic talking animal. Your helper is someone you can always speak with, someone who listens well and gives good advice. Many kids who've done an exercise like this have found that their special place is very restful and the helper is really useful in solving problems. Some doctors are even using imaginary places and helpers to

treat people when they are sick.

Get in a comfortable position, close your eyes, and breathe in and out slowly. As you breathe slowly and evenly, you will start to relax. When you feel quite relaxed, begin counting backward. Say to yourself, "10 . . . I am feeling very relaxed. Rest. 9 . . . I am feeling more relaxed. Rest. 8 . . . I am feeling even more relaxed. Rest. 7 . . . I am feeling deeper and more relaxed. Rest. 6 . . . more and more relaxed. Rest. 5 . . . even more relaxed. Rest. 4 . . . deeper and deeper. Rest. 3 . . . deeper and deeper. Rest. 2 . . . still deeper. Rest. 1 . . . very relaxed. Rest. 0 . . ." You are now in a very relaxed place. Your mind feels peaceful and open. As you look

around you will see a special place. A place where you can rest and think and work. It may be a new place or one you already know. It may be outdoors or indoors. It may be a meadow or a treehouse. As you explore you will see special things—the ground or the floor, rocks or walls, plants or shelves. And as you look around more, you will see your helper. Notice what your helper looks like and how big the helper is. Then ask the helper's name and whether he or she will come to your special place whenever you have questions or need help. If you have some questions now, ask them before leaving. When you are ready to return to the ordinary world, gently move your arms and legs, and open your eyes.

Healthy foods

You are what you eat. Your whole body is made of molecules that come from the food that you eat. Food is used to make energy, to grow, and to replace old cells. Three-quarters of the food we eat is used just to make heat.

There are five basic kinds of food. Each is needed by the body and each does a different job. If the body doesn't get the right amounts of them, growth can be affected or the body can become sick. Getting enough of the right foods is called *nutrition*.

The body needs energy for everything it does. It needs energy to move, to make the nerves and glands work, and to make the heart pump. Scientists measure energy in terms of calories. One *calorie* will raise the temperature of 1 kilogram of water by 1° Centigrade. Different foods have different amounts of energy in them. For example, a hamburger has 350 calories, a glass of milk has 166 calories, and an apple 101 calories. And different jobs that the body does require different amounts of calories. Walking uses 200 calories an hour, running 570 calories an hour, and sleeping 65 calories an hour.

The amount of calories people need in a day depends on (1) how big they are, (2) how fast they're growing, and (3) how much exercise, or work, they're doing. An average 7- to 10-year-old, weighing 60 pounds, needs 2000 calories a day. If children can't get enough calories, they will grow less, lose weight, and run out of energy. If children get more calories than they need, they get fat.

The body gets its energy from *carbohydrates* and *fats*. Fats are found in butter, oil, meat, cheese, and potato chips. Fats feel greasy, don't dissolve in water, and can be melted into a liquid. Fats come from both animals and plants.

Carbohydrates include bread, cereal, potatoes, spaghetti, fruits, corn, and desserts. Carbohydrates contain sugars and starches. They are made of molecules of many different kinds of sugar.

The building blocks for the

How much energy certain activities take

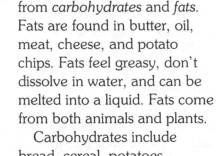

Activity	Energy (calories per hour)
Sleeping	65
Sitting	100
Standing	100
Making dinner	175
Cleaning your room	200
Walking	350
Walking upstairs	1100

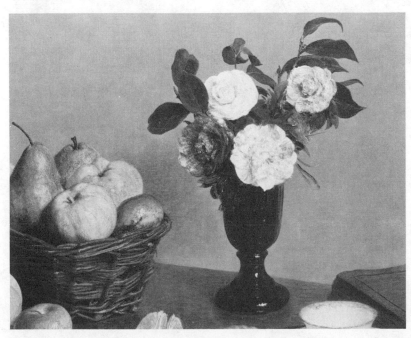

Fresh, natural foods provide the best nutrition.

Frantin-Latour, Henri. Still Life. 19th cent. Oil on canvas. 24³⁄₈ × 29¹⁄₂". National Gallery of Art, Washington. Chester Dale Collection, 1962.

body come from *proteins, vitamins,* and *minerals.* All the cells in the body, as well as antibodies, hormones, and digestive enzymes, are made of protein. Protein is found in milk, cheese, nuts, eggs, fish, chicken, red meat, and corn, beans, wheat, oats, and rice. Proteins themselves are made up of tiny parts called *amino acids.* Amino acids combine in many different ways to make different kinds of proteins. Protein that we eat is digested or broken down into its amino acid parts. Then when the body makes its own proteins it puts the parts together in special ways. Animal proteins like fish, meat, and milk have all the amino acids that people need to build their own proteins. Plant proteins like corn, beans, and rice don't have all the proteins the body needs, so they have to be combined with each other if people eat no meat.

Vitamins are chemicals that the body needs tiny amounts of in order to do special jobs. Vitamin A, for example, is used by the eyes to see light. Other vitamins also help to digest food and are needed to make hormones and digestive enzymes. The body has to get vitamins from its food because it can't make them itself.

Minerals are chemicals found in rocks. The body can't make minerals and can't live without them. It uses them in very tiny amounts for certain jobs. For example, calcium and phosphorus are used in making bones and teeth. The average 8-year-old body has 2 pounds of minerals inside, including mostly calcium, sulphur, and salt. Minerals regulate the body fluids, help in digestion, make nerves and

Recommended daily amounts of proteins, calories, vitamins, and minerals (1980)

	4–6 yrs.	7–10 yrs.	11–14 yrs.	Sources
Calories (cal.)	1300	2400	2200–2700	
Protein (gm.)	30	34	46	Milk, eggs, beans, cheese, peanut butter
Vitamins A (I.U.)	2500	3300	5000	Liver, greens, carrots, apricots, squash, cantaloupe
B_1 (mg.) (thiamin)	.9	1.2	1.4	Soy, liver, asparagus, greens, beans and peas
B_2 (mg.) (riboflavin)	1.0	1.4	1.6	Milk, dairy products, meats
B_6 (mg.)	1.3	1.6	1.8	Milk, meats, grains, beans, bananas
B_{12} (mg.)	2.5	3.0	3.0	Liver, cheese, fish, eggs
Niacin (mg.)	11	16	18	Meat, poultry, liver, beans, dairy products

	4–6 yrs.	7–10 yrs.	11–14 yrs.	Sources
Folacin (mg.)	200	300	400	Liver, leafy vegetables, oranges
C (mg.)	45	45	50	Oranges, grapefruit, cabbage, greens, strawberries
D (I.U.)	400	400	400	Milk, cheese
E (I.U.)	6	7	8	Enriched cereal, beans, greens, liver, meat, eggs, prunes

Minerals

	4–6 yrs.	7–10 yrs.	11–14 yrs.	Sources
Calcium (mg.)	800	800	1200	Milk, cheese, egg yolks
Phosphorus (mg.)	800	800	1200	Dairy products, meat, legumes
Iron (mg.)	10	10	18	Liver, dried peas and beans, fortified cereals
Zinc (mg.)	10	10	15	Seafood, meat, peas and beans
Magnesium (mg.)	200	250	350	Nuts, soybeans, grains, legumes, shellfish
Iodine (mg.)	90	120	150	Iodized salt, milk, seafood
Sodium (mg.)	450–1350	600–1800	900–2700	Salt
Chloride (mg.)	700–2100	925–2775	1400–4200	Salt
Copper (mg.)	1.5–2.0	2.0–2.5	2.0–3.0	Shellfish, organ meats, legumes
Manganese (mg.)	1.5–2.0	2.0–3.0	2.5–5.0	Nuts, whole wheat, grains
Fluoride (mg.)	1.0–2.0	1.5–2.5	1.5–2.5	Seafood, tea
Chromium (mg.)	.03–1.2	.05–.20	.05–.20	Yeast, animal meat
Selenium (mg.)	.03–1.2	.05–.20	.05–.20	—
Molybdenum (mg.)	.06–.15	.10–.30	.15–.50	—

Adapted from the Food and Nutrition Board, National Academy of Sciences–National Research Council, 1980 figures.

muscles work, help red blood cells carry oxygen, and help make certain hormones and enyzmes.

In addition to food, the body needs water. Water is used to carry food all over the body, and it helps to regulate body temperature and to remove waste products. In fact, the human body is over *half* water.

The body works perfectly if it is fed the right amounts of protein, carbohydrates, fats, minerals, vitamins, and water.

Healthy foods compared with empty foods

Food	Energy* (KCal.)	Protein (grams)	Fat (grams)	Carbo- hydrate (grams)
Milk, 1 cup	160	9	9	12
versus				
Cola, 1 can	145	0	0	37
Cheddar cheese, 1 inch cube	70	4	6	trace
versus				
Gum drops, 1 oz.	100	0	0	25
Pizza, 1 slice	185	7	6	27
versus				
10 pretzel sticks	10	0	0	2
1 orange	65	1	trace	16
versus				
1 orange popsicle, 3 oz.	70	0	0	18
1 carrot	20	1	0	5
versus				
Hard candy, 1 oz.	110	0	25	0
Recommended daily allowance for kids 7–10	2400	34	†	†

* KCal. equals 1,000 calories.

† Indicates unknown value.

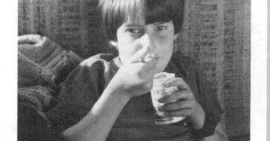

But if the body gets too much or too little of any of these things, the balance is upset and the body isn't healthy.

Right now many kids in the United States aren't eating the healthiest diet that they might. Children, and adults as well, have gotten into some bad eating habits. First, people are eating many foods that don't have much in the way of proteins, minerals, or vitamins. Nutritionists call these "empty foods." Some empty foods like candy bars are mostly sugar. They give you energy, but they don't make you grow. And some foods, like white bread, lack vitamins and minerals because their ingredients have been ground up and heated so much in the making. That is, they've been *processed* so much that their vitamins and minerals have been lost or destroyed. As opposed to a candy bar, an apple or a peach contains not only sugar, but also vitamins and minerals. As opposed to white bread, whole-wheat bread has more complete proteins and more vitamins and minerals. Unfortunately, your stomach fills up just as much on empty foods as it does on foods that are rich in building blocks. Your stomach can't tell the difference, so it stops sending hunger signals. If you eat junk food all day, you won't be hungry any more for the good foods, and you'll be low in protein, vitamins, and minerals.

Two other things are bad about junk foods or highly processed foods. First, unlike natural foods like fruits, vegetables, and whole-grains the processed foods have very little *roughage*. That is, they are very finely ground up and they don't have much *cellulose*, the tough, indigestible part of fruits and vegetables. Roughage and big chunks are needed to help the intestines work well. Without them the intestines work slowly and without much energy. Some

Calcium (milligrams)	Iron (milligrams)	Vitamin A (international units)	Thiamin (milligrams)	Vitamin C (milligrams)
288	.1	350	.07	2
0	0	0	0	0
129	.2	230	.01	0
2	.1	0	0	0
107	.7	290	.04	4
1	0	0	0	0
54	.5	260	.13	66
0	0	0	0	0
18	.4	5500	.03	4
6	.5	0	0	0
800	10	3300	1.2	40

Values from Home and Garden Bulletin No. 72, 1971; United States Department of Agriculture.

In general, the more candy you eat, the fatter you become and the more cavities you get.

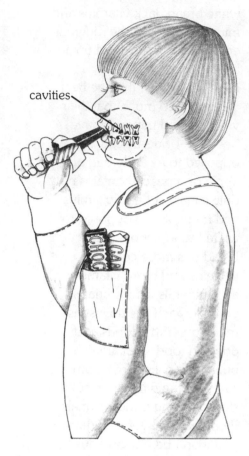

cavities

doctors think this may eventually lead to cancer of the intestines.

Second, processed foods usually contain lots of chemicals that have been added. Food coloring chemicals are put in to make foods look more appealing, and preservatives are put in to make foods last longer without becoming rotten. Some of these chemicals can make kids nervous or allergic and some are thought to cause cancer. None of these chemicals is needed by the body.

Some foods actually can make people sick if they eat too much of them. Too much sugar makes people fat and gives them cavities (see page 310). Too much salt can give certain people high blood pressure when they get older, and can lead to heart attacks eventually. Too much fat, especially fat from animals, also increases people's chances of having heart attacks when they are older. What kids eat when they are young actually affects how healthy they will be when they are grown up and how long they will live.

Eating empty foods or too much of foods that aren't

Amounts of sugar in foods that kids eat

Food	Tablespoons of sugar
Chewing gum, 1 stick	½
Gingersnap, 1	1
Marshmallow, 1	1½
Syrup, 1 tablespoon	2½
Brownie, 1 2″ × 2″	3
Cocoa, 1 cup	4
Doughnut, 1	4
Canned fruit cocktail, ½ cup	5
Ice cream, ½ cup	5
Chocolate bar	7
Soda, 1 can	9
Cherry pie, 1 large slice	14
Chocolate cake, with icing, 1 slice	15

From the American Dental Association

Nutritional value of common foods

Protein foods		Protein (grams)
Yogurt	½ cup	3.7
Hamburger	2 oz.	15.4
Chicken drumstick		12.2
Peanut butter	1 tbsp.	4.0
Egg	1	5.7
Bologna	1 oz.	4.6
Tuna	¼ cup	11.5
Hot dog	1	5.6
Cheese	1 oz.	7.1
Milk (whole)	1 cup	9.0

Combining proteins	Protein (grams)
¾ cup oats + milk + soy	8
½ cup potatoes + milk	4
½ cup macaroni and cheese	7
½ peanut butter sandwich	4
2 tortillas, ¼ cup beans	4

Fat foods		Fat (grams)
Mayonnaise	1 tbsp.	11.5
Butter	1 tsp.	3.8
Cheese	1 oz.	7.1
Peanut butter	1 tbsp.	8.1
Hot dog	1	11.5
Hamburger	2 oz.	15.4
Potato chips	10	8.0

Carbo-hydrate foods		Carbo-hydrates (grams)
Whole-wheat bread	1 slice	13.0
Cornflakes	½ cup	10.7
Potato chips	10	10.0
Spaghetti	¼ cup	8.0
Rice	½ cup	10.0

Vitamin C		(milli-grams)
Broccoli	1 spear	22
Cantaloupe	¼ cup	27
Grapefruit	½	37
Orange	1	66
Orange juice	½ cup	62
Strawberries	1 cup	88
Tomato	1	42

Vitamin A		(inter-national units)
Beef liver	1 oz.	15,112
Canned apricots	¼ cup	1,125
Peaches	1	1,330
Carrots	¼ cup	3,808
Sweet potatoes	¼ cup	5,038
Spinach	¼ cup	3,645

good for you is like building a house with rotten lumber or running a car on bad gasoline. It just can't last long. So make sure that what you eat not only tastes good, but is good for you.

A good diet includes lots of fresh fruits, vegetables, and whole-grain breads and cereals. It includes some meat, fish, and chicken, milk, eggs, and cheese. And a good diet includes *little* fat, salt, and white sugar.

How long certain activities take to burn up your food

Activity	Bread and butter (2 slices)	Milk (1 glass)	1 hamburger
Lying down	1 hour	2 hours	4 hours
Walking	15 minute	½ hour	1 hour
Running	4 minutes	9 minutes	18 minutes

You are what you eat! Go toward fruits and vegetables, whole grains, lean meat, and fish. Leave behind junk foods and foods that are very salty, sweet, or greasy.

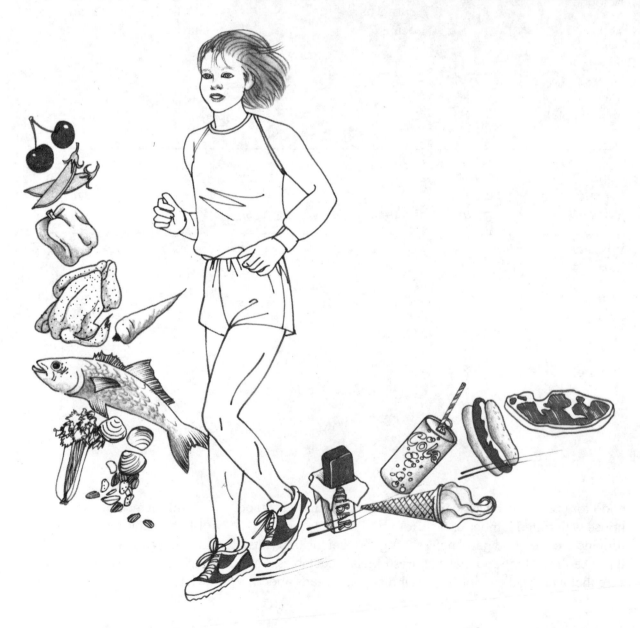

Pollution

Many chemicals in the environment have been found to be harmful to our bodies. These chemicals are found in some of the foods we eat, the beverages we drink, the air we breathe, and in cigarettes. The chemicals irritate the body's cells, make it harder for them to function, and eventually cause many diseases, including cancer.

Chemicals in *cigarette smoke* enter your lungs and get stuck in the tiny air sacs. The cilia, the little wavy arms that line the throat and passages to the lungs (see page 164), try to push out these chemicals, but finally they get stuck and stop working. Then your body can't protect itself as well against colds and lung diseases. Cigarette smoke also causes the lining of the lungs to swell, which means less air can come in with each breath. Cigarette smoke contains carbon monoxide, the same poisonous gas that is in car exhaust. Carbon monoxide is taken up by the red blood cells, which prevents them from picking up

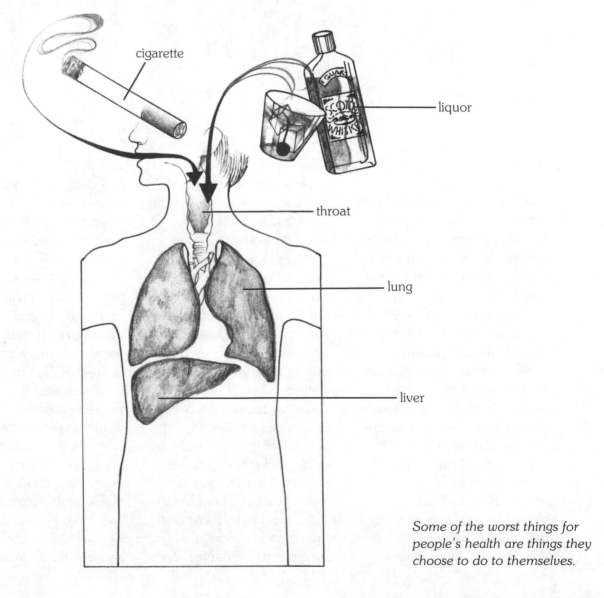

cigarette

liquor

throat

lung

liver

Some of the worst things for people's health are things they choose to do to themselves.

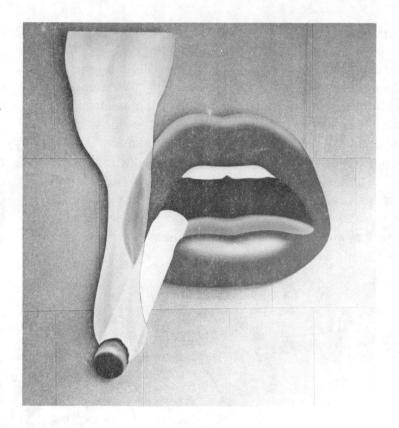

Smoking is a leading cause of early death from cancer and heart disease.

Wesselmann, Tom. Smoker, I (Mouth) 12. 1967. Oil on canvas. In two parts, overall, 9'7⅞" × 7'11". Collection, The Museum of Modern Art, New York. Susan Morse Hilles Fund.

the oxygen the body needs. Carbon monoxide stays attached to the red blood cells for almost a day. So when smokers exercise, they can't get enough air in—their blood carries less oxygen, and their heartbeat speeds way up. This is why athletes don't smoke: Nonsmokers can do ten times more work than smokers.

Smoking is responsible for almost half of all forms of cancer. Not only are smokers hurt by their smoking, everyone around them is, too. If you can smell smoke in a room you're inhaling that smoke. Sitting all day in a smoky room is like smoking half a pack of cigarettes.

Somewhat like cigarette smoking, *air pollution* makes the lining of the lungs swell and stops the cilia from getting rid of tiny particles in the lungs. Air pollution comes from car exhaust and from factories that burn things. It's made up of dust, smoke, carbon monoxide, and several other poisonous gases. In a smog alert, there is so much carbon monoxide in the air that people can't see or think as well as normal. Air pollution or smog also makes all illnesses of the nose and lungs worse, including colds and asthma. Air pollution is a major problem of our big cities and certain other areas that have many factories. For example, in 1974, New York had significant air pollution on 257 days out of 365 days in the year. And it had 36 days when the pollution was so bad it was considered unhealthy just to be in the city.

Alcohol is a powerful drug that is found in liquors, beer, and wine. In small amounts it makes people relax and feel happy. In large amounts it makes people unsteady, confused, and sometimes sick to their stomachs. Heavy drinking is associated with a very large number of all car accidents. This is because people can't coordinate their movements very well when they have alcohol in their blood. Drinking too much is also bad for people's bodies.

Large amounts of alcohol kill the cells lining the stomach and it takes several days for them to grow back. Alcohol is broken down in the liver. In heavy drinkers the liver actually gets fat and begins to work less and less well. People who drink very heavily for many years are killed eventually by this habit.

Scientists are beginning to find that some of the chemicals that people use in the normal course of a day at work or at home are dangerous. A hundred years ago there were few chemicals around to worry about. Now we have invented so many chemicals that we can't avoid contact with them: They are in building materials, furniture, paints and cleaning products, bug sprays and weed killers, even in foods and medicines.

Some chemicals are immediately poisonous if they are accidentally eaten. These include oven cleaners, bleaches for washing clothes, and even an excessive dose of vitamins that have iron.

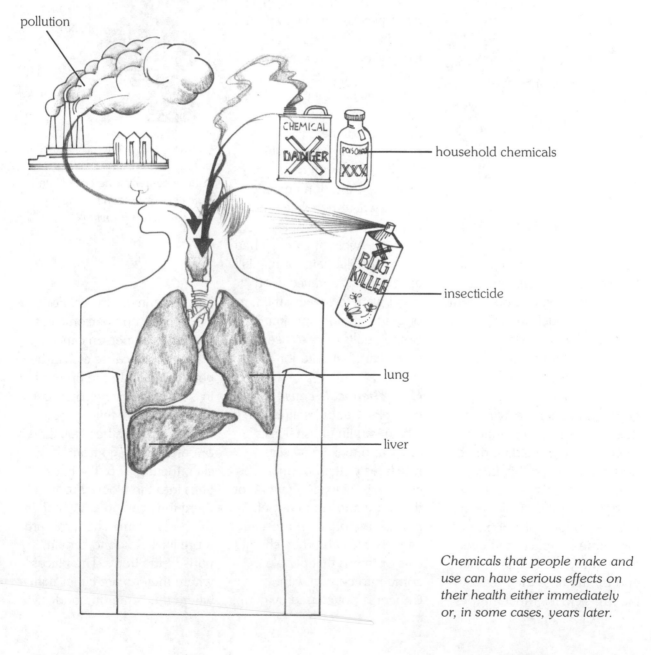

pollution

household chemicals

insecticide

lung

liver

Chemicals that people make and use can have serious effects on their health either immediately or, in some cases, years later.

Avoid these chemicals to be healthy

Chemicals in cigarette smoke

Chemicals in air pollution

Alcohol

Chemicals from factories or dumps

Chemicals in insect sprays

Chemicals in paints

Chemicals in cleaners

Food colorings

Cosmetics

Almost any medicine can be poisonous if too much is taken at one time. Some chemicals, like paint removers, are caustic; that is, they can burn your skin if you touch them. Others, like bug killers, can cause an allergic reaction. Some chemicals are dangerous even to breathe: Many glues can make the liver sick; dust from sanding paint or sawing certain building materials can damage the lungs themselves.

Many chemicals take years to make people sick. For a long time people aren't even aware they are becoming ill, and by the time they realize they're sick, it's much harder

to heal their bodies. Miners who breathe in coal dust can develop black lung disease. People who work in cotton factories can develop brown lung disease from the cotton dust. And both groups of people are more likely to get sick if they also smoke cigarettes. People who work or live near chemical factories or oil refineries are more likely to get certain kinds of cancer. Even people who buy and use the chemical products are more likely to get cancer.

A good rule for kids is to be extremely careful using chemicals or being around them. Follow safety instructions exactly. Never use smelly chemicals without opening windows. And don't go into places where people are working with chemicals unless you have to. Avoid any area where chemicals like paint or bug killers are being sprayed. You don't want to breathe them in or get them on your skin. Some adults have to use these chemicals, but you don't.

How chemicals cause cancer
Cancer is a disease in which certain unusual cells grow and make new cells much faster than normal. The cells they make don't work for the body and aren't a useful part of any organ. Almost all cancers are caused by chemicals or things that people come into contact with. Cancer is not caused by germs

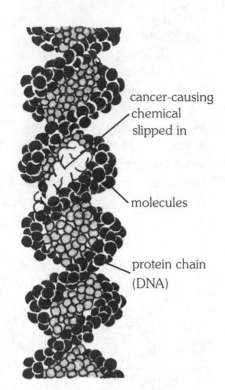

cancer-causing chemical slipped in

molecules

protein chain (DNA)

Cancer-causing chemicals lock onto proteins in the nucleus, the control center of the cell. Then new cells are made incorrectly and can't stop growing.

like bacteria or viruses. For that reason one person can't give another person cancer.

Chemicals cause cancer by getting right into the proteins in a cell. These chemicals get into the body because they have been breathed, touched, or eaten. They go from the skin, the lungs, or the intestines into the blood. From there they can go anywhere in the body. Some chemicals are more likely to go to certain parts of the body. The places where they go are either right where they enter the body (skin, nose, throat, or lungs) or where they are broken down or stored (liver, intestines, and bladder).

Once a cancer-causing chemical gets inside a cell, it goes to the nucleus or control center. There it locks onto the *DNA chain,* the protein that tells cells what to do and how to make new cells. Then when new cells are made, they are not made correctly and can't stop growing.

Sometimes the cell itself can cut out that part of the DNA chain that is cancerous and put in a new healthy piece. If this doesn't happen, the body's defense system usually spots the sick cell and immediately sends out white blood cells, which eat the whole sick cell. White blood cells do this all the time.

But sometimes the body either doesn't find or can't eat all the sick cells. Then the sick cell makes a lot of cells like itself and keeps on making them. When enough sick cells grow, they start using food that the body needs. Eventually, if the clump of sick cells gets big enough, it starts to squeeze healthy organs and makes it hard for them to keep working as usual. Finally, the person becomes ill and must go to a doctor to have the cancer treated. Most chemically caused cancers are found in older adults and don't show up until many years after exposure to the chemicals.

Aerobic exercise

When kids run, ride bikes, or swim, they are getting exercise. They are using their big muscles again and again, making them tighten and relax in a cycle. When a muscle tightens or contracts, microscopic fibers inside slide past each other, grabbing hold as they slide (see The muscles, page 153). To do this work, the muscle fibers need oxygen and glucose, a special kind of sugar that the body makes. When the fibers use the oxygen and glucose, they have waste products that must be gotten rid of. These wastes, carbon dioxide and lactic acid, are carried away by the blood.

If the blood doesn't bring new oxygen and glucose and carry away the carbon dioxide and lactic acid, the muscle becomes "tired" and can't do any more work. The amount of blood that comes to working muscles depends on how hard the heart can pump, how much air the lungs can take in, and how well the blood vessels can get the blood to the muscles.

When kids exercise rather than sit still, their bodies work very differently. Their heart pumps faster, sending out more than 4 times as much blood. Their breathing speeds up and their lungs take in 20 times as much air. And their blood vessels widen in the big muscles, bringing in 20 times as much blood. When muscles

The best aerobic exercises for kids

Hiking
Running
Biking
Swimming

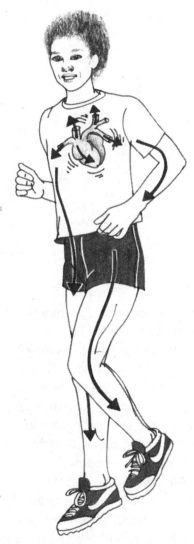

Exercise that makes your heart pound hard is called aerobic exercise. It makes your heart, lungs, and blood vessels grow bigger and work better for your whole life.

Running is excellent aerobic exercise.

Klee, Paul. Runner at the Goal. *1921. Watercolor and gouache on paper, mounted on paper. 11⅞ × 9″. Collection, The Solomon R. Guggenheim Museum, New York. Photograph by Robert E. Mates.*

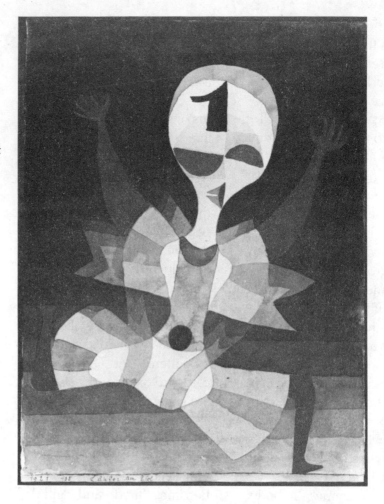

squeeze or contract, they not only use up to 20 times as much energy, they force blood to return to the heart. This helps to keep the whole cycle going. The more kids exercise, the bigger and stronger their heart, lungs, blood vessels, and muscles become.

All kids have a certain distance they can run before they get tired. This distance depends upon how much exercise they usually get. Kids who get little exercise get tired quickly because their hearts, lungs, muscles and blood vessels can't do as much work. If they keep on doing a little more all the time, their bodies will get stronger and stronger, and they'll be able to do more and more because their bodies will grow and adjust to the new level of exercise. This whole process is called *aerobic training.*

With training, *anyone* can and will get stronger. This is why athletes exercise every day. There is no such thing as kids who are born weak; they just don't get enough exercise. If they do a little more each day, they'll get stronger, too. Their hearts will get stronger and be able to pump out more blood with each beat. The amount their lungs can breathe in will go up. The size of their muscle fibers will get bigger. And extra blood vessels will grow into those larger muscles. Their bones will actually get thicker and stronger.

When kids train seriously over a period of time, their bodies actually grow differently. And the changes stay with them throughout their lives! Adults who trained as kids will always be able to do more exercise than adults who never trained as kids. Adults can train, too, but the biggest changes can be made only while kids are still growing.

Developing the parts of the body that bring air to the muscles is called building *aerobic power*. All kids can build up their aerobic power by exercising 20 minutes a day, 3 or 4 days a week. Certain kinds of exercise are best for increasing aerobic power because they involve steady work for the whole time. Fast walking, running, swimming, bike riding, or basketball are all excellent aerobic sports.

Complete breathing Good breathing is important all the time to maintain a healthy body. Breathing is automatic, but people can learn how to breathe more deeply, which gets more oxygen to all their cells with less work. Then they won't tire as quickly. Deep breathing is especially important for kids with health problems like asthma or allergies and for kids who are interested in strenuous sports like soccer and basketball.

As people breathe in, the

With the complete-breathing exercise, you can learn to breathe in more deeply. As you breathe in, (1) let your stomach stick out, (2) let your chest expand, and (3) let the top of your chest rise.

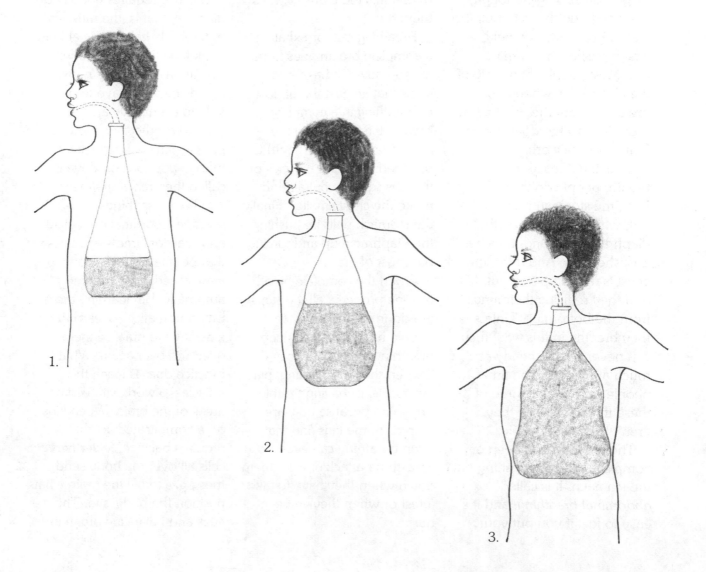

1.

2.

3.

muscles around the chest make the chest bigger. The diaphragm, the big flat muscle under the lungs, drops down, and the muscles between the ribs pull them up. When the chest expands, it creates a vacuum and air is sucked into the lungs.

Most of the time people breathe in only a little air—about two cups. This only partly fills their lungs. But it's possible for people to breathe in as much as seven cups by purposely making their lungs bigger. Surprisingly enough, the way to do this is to pull the diaphragm down strongly, which pushes the stomach out. Most people think only of the chest rising when they breathe in, but the diaphragm dropping is what does three-fourths of the work.

In taking a really deep breath, people do three things. First, the stomach is pushed out, which drops down the diaphragm. Second, the chest is pushed out. And third, the chest is raised up and out. It's as if they're filling their lungs from the bottom up. Unless they breathe in this way, they can never take in nearly as much air. Most of the time people don't do all three of these things because they aren't breathing deeply.

The first part of a deep or complete breath is pushing out the stomach. It is called *abdominal breathing,* and it's easy to feel if you put your hand on your stomach when you're lying down. Babies and sleepers breathe abdominally, because it's very relaxing and efficient. The second part of the complete breath, when the chest expands, is called *chest breathing.* The third part, when the chest rises, is called *high chest breathing.* You can practice this by pretending to pant like a dog. High chest breathing is a lot of work, and it doesn't bring in much air. People breathe this way when they're nervous, scared, or out of breath. And it quickly tires them out.

Breathing out, or exhaling, a complete breath goes from the top down. It has three steps that are just the opposite of breathing in a complete breath. First the top of the chest (near the collarbone) is dropped. Next the muscles of the ribs squeeze out air and make the chest smaller. Finally the stomach pulls in, pushing the diaphragm up and forcing out most of the air.

When the complete breath is done properly, all the steps are done smoothly. Once people have practiced deep breathing a little, they can do it when they are running, playing sports, or having trouble breathing because they are scared. Some kids find that deep breathing can even stop an asthma attack or calm them down when they have to take a test or when they've been hurt.

Balance

Balance is the body's ability to stay in different positions without falling. The better a person's sense of balance, the more smoothly he or she is able to do any exercise. Certain kinds of balancing skills are necessary for many complicated movements. These are balancing on your toes, balancing on one foot, balancing with your eyes closed, hopping, and walking on a balance beam.

Balance requires good *coordination;* that is, the muscles of the body have to be able to work together in harmony. To stay in balance while moving means muscles have to be able to act quickly and easily. This is called *agility.* How fast people can change their muscle positions or move is called their *reaction time.*

All of these things—balance, coordination, agility, and reaction time—are skills that people learn. Once they are learned, they become automatic. But learning them isn't automatic. To learn them, kids have to practice them over and over again. What practice does is teach the muscles to work with certain areas of the brain. When kids do a complicated act that requires balance, feeler nerve cells all over the body send messages to tell the brain what position the body is in. The eyes and balancing organ in

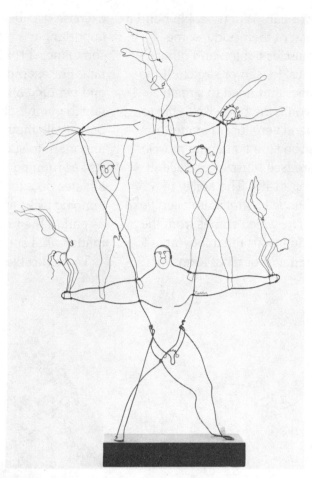

the inner ear (see page 202) also send messages to the brain about the body's position in space. All these messages go from one area of the brain to another until the brain figures them out and sends signals out to doer, or motor, nerves, telling each muscle what to do. Areas in the brain also "look" at the movements the body is making and correct them if they are not quite right. This is what is happening when kids' movements are jerky, as they learn a particular new skill. Once the body has gotten through a whole series of movements, it can do them again more smoothly because all the nerve cells in the brain that passed the messages along have now formed a circle called a *circuit.* Once a circuit has been formed, the brain remembers it, and it's easier for the electrical signals to go around again. It's like making a path in the woods—every time it's walked on it becomes a little clearer and easier to follow.

There is even an area in the brain whose job is to remember patterns of muscle movements. Once a particular pattern has been stored here, it can be repeated quickly and automatically. This is how a baby learns to walk. First it learns to totter and fall, then to balance, then to balance and walk. Once people have learned to do one complicated pattern, then they can learn to do something even more complicated that uses the first pattern. For example, kids first learn to catch a ball, then they learn to catch a ball while running. This is called *nerve-muscle learning.*

Nerve-muscle learning lasts for people's whole lives. The best time to do this kind of learning is while kids are still young. Adults generally have a harder time learning a new kind of nerve-muscle skill than kids do. People who have established many nerve-muscle circuits have an easier time developing new circuits than people who know just a few.

Flexibility

As kids grow up, their muscles stretch less easily. Adults often can't bend into positions that kids can. When people bend a part of their body, some muscles tighten and others must loosen or stretch. If the ones that need to stretch won't, the body isn't able to bend very far no matter how strong the tightening muscles are (see Muscle contraction, page 149). The ability of a muscle to stretch is called *flexibility*, which comes from the Latin word meaning "able to bend." For most forms of exercise, flexibility is just as important as strength, and sometimes it is more important. For example, *stretching* and *bending* are very important in gymnastics, skiing, and basketball; they are even important to such a basic exercise as running. That is why all athletes do exercises like jumping jacks and knee bends as part of their training, no matter what sport they play.

To be flexible, muscles have

Shaking your whole body stretches muscles and releases pent-up energy.

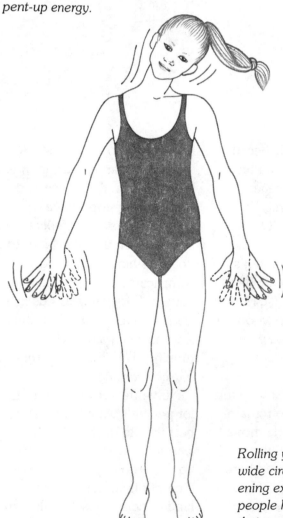

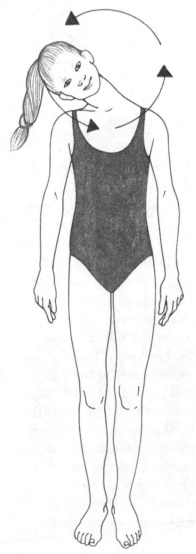

Rolling your head around in a wide circle is an important loosening exercise because most people have lots of tension in their necks.

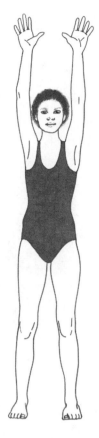

Stretching and bending exercises help to keep the body flexible.

to be loose. For muscles to be loose, they have to be relaxed and used to stretching. Muscles that are not regularly stretched become tight all the time. Many adults aren't used to moving around very much, and this is why kids can bend in ways that most adults can't.

As all kids grow, their bodies get accustomed to being in certain positions much of the time. Some kids sit hunched over, some never stand up straight. These are called *habit postures*. When kids worry, their muscles tend to tighten up, often in one area, like the neck. All these things tend to make kids less flexible, and they affect the way in which kids' bodies work. They slow down blood flow and keep muscles from getting fresh oxygen and food.

Constant tension in an area even affects how organs work and that can make people sick. For example, tight muscles in the neck can cause a headache.

People who study yoga positions believe that when an area of the body is tense all the time, it uses up extra energy and it blocks energy from getting to other areas of the body. They believe that stretching exercises release tension and make the whole body work better. Energy isn't wasted on tensing and can flow to the whole body more easily. In fact, when people stretch out tense muscles, they not only have more energy, they feel happier. The worries that made the muscles tense go away when the muscles loosen up.

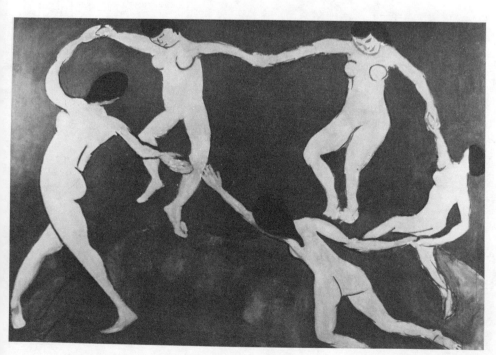

Dancing helps to keep muscles flexible.

Matisse, Henri. Dance (First Version). 1909, early. Oil on canvas, 8' 6½ × 12' 9½". Collection, The Museum of Modern Art, New York. Gift of Nelson A. Rockefeller in honor of Alfred H. Barr, Jr. Photograph by Eric Pollitzer.

Common illnesses and accidents of childhood— for parents and children

When the dog bites,
When the bee stings,
When I'm feeling sad,
I simply remember my
    favorite things,
and then I don't feel so bad.

—Richard Rodgers and Oscar
    Hammerstein II,
    "My Favorite Things," The Sound
    of Music

How to use this section

This part of the book is for parents and children to use together. It describes common illnesses and accidents in simple, nonfrightening terms and is designed to help children take part in their own health care.

The diseases are arranged by the part of the body they affect: *skin, head, allergies, abdomen,* and *childhood diseases.* So if a child has a rash, look at the skin diseases to see which description fits. The accident section is arranged in alphabetical order. The chart on page 340 helps to locate information quickly.

Each disease discussion is divided into five sections: *signs and symptoms, what's happening, helping yourself, the doctor,* and *prevention.* Signs and symptoms are listed to the side—they tell in one or two words what is wrong. "What's happening" tells the story of the illness or accident more completely. "Helping yourself" tells what can be done at home. "The doctor" tells when to go to the doctor and what the doctor will do. "Prevention" tells what can be done to keep from spreading the disease or getting it again.

Chapter 8

Common illnesses

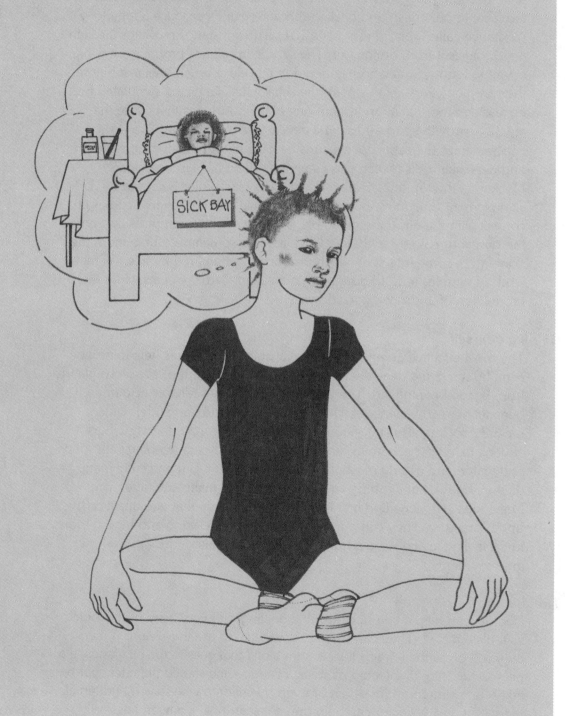

The skin

Acne

What's happening

Acne is a skin problem that many young people have sometime between the ages of 8 and 18. In fact, more than three-fourths of all children develop acne at some point. Acne is really just oil glands in the skin that have become plugged. Most of the oil or sebaceous glands are located on the face, upper chest, and back. Sebaceous glands produce a fatty, oily substance called *sebum* (see page 131). This substance moistens the skin and protects it from drying out. The sebaceous glands produce the waxy covering found on newborns, then don't produce much until just before the teen-age years. At this point the sebaceous glands are stimulated by increasing amounts of androgen, one of the hormones that cause the teen-age growth spurt and sexual development (see pages 216–20).

Sometimes the sebaceous glands become plugged with excess sebum and dead skin cells, which causes pimples. If an oil gland becomes blocked at the top, a *blackhead* forms. The black color is caused by dark skin pigment (*melanin*), not dirt. The melanin darkens when it comes in contact with the air. If the gland plugs up at the bottom, it puffs up under the skin and makes a *whitehead.* Whiteheads sometimes burst under the skin and become infected, which produces a painful red pimple. All these kinds of pimples tend to disappear in the later teen-age years when the production of androgen goes down.

Helping yourself

The most effective creams that are available in drugstores help improve acne by removing dead skin cells. This tends to keep the sebaceous glands from becoming plugged. The creams contain either retinoic acid or benzoyl peroxide (Benoxyl, Desquam-X, Pan Oxyl Vanoxide). Until recently doctors also suggested cutting down on certain foods such as chocolate, nuts, cola drinks, and seafood, and advised washing with soap and water, and getting reasonable amounts of sun. But presently many doctors doubt that washing and dietary changes make any difference. Many kids with acne find it always gets worse when they are upset or under pressure. They can improve their acne by relaxing and having more fun. Healing in acne is generally slow. It usually takes a month to show improvement.

The doctor

Doctors can help if you have trouble dealing with your acne or if it looks as if it's infected. They can suggest how often to use the creams. Often they will prescribe tetracycline, an antibiotic that goes to the oil glands, if a person has a lot of infected pimples. (Tetracycline should definitely *not* be taken by children under seven or even by children who haven't gotten all their teeth in.) A doctor can help prevent scarring if a person has really bad acne.

Pimples (whiteheads, blackheads) on the face, back, and chest

Oily skin

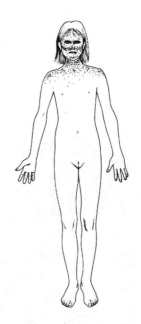

Acne pimples most often occur on the face, upper chest, and back.

Prevention

Some doctors believe that it's good to eat foods that are high in vitamins A and B, and clean the skin well. But acne does seem to be an almost unavoidable part of growing up.

Eczema (atopic dermatitis, rough skin patches)

What's happening

Sometimes kids have little patches of sensitive skin that may be itchy, rough, and red. If the patches are scratched a lot, they sometimes ooze, get crusty, or even bleed. When the patches become swollen and inflamed, they can be uncomfortable or cause pain.

Usually these patches of sensitive skin are first noticed when kids are babies. In many children they disappear by two, but some kids continue to have the rash until they are grown up. Most of them notice that the rash is sometimes better, sometimes worse. Many kids find that warm weather, very cold weather, and some kinds of fabric make the rash worse.

Among kids 6 to 12 the most common places to have rough skin patches are the hands, elbows and knees, corners of the mouth, behind the ears, and on the back of the neck. Such kids tend to have dry skin as well because they have fewer oil glands in their skin than normal. This means they have less protection for their skin and water evaporates more easily from it. That's what makes the top layers of their skin get little cracks —especially around the rough areas. These kids also tend to sweat more, which makes them more likely to be itchy.

Doctors call this kind of skin condition *eczema,* or *atopic dermatitis.* Sometimes kids with eczema or members of their family have allergies or asthma. But doctors are not sure whether eczema is an allergic reaction.

Helping yourself

Two things help to heal or prevent eczema. The first is keeping the skin moist. The second is avoiding anything that makes the patches worse. The area can be kept moist by rubbing on oil-and-water creams or lotions such as Alpha-Keri, Nutraderm, or Nivea. These creams are all slightly different, so kids need to find out which one agrees best with their skin. Generally, it is good to avoid lotions that contain perfumes, lanolin, preservatives, or alcohol. Kids should bathe in plain water for a few minutes to let it soak into their skin. It may be good to add a pure bath oil after soaking and avoid strong soaps or shampoos. Some doctors also suggest avoiding common allergic foods and rough fabrics (see chart, page 331).

The doctor

If the eczemic patches are very uncomfortable, kids should see a doctor for help. The doctor can prescribe steroid creams that will reduce the

Signs and symptoms

Itching

Dry skin with cracks

Red rash with crusts and thickened skin on hands, corner of mouth, elbows, or knees

Rough skin patches

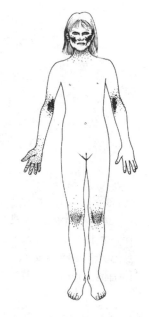

Patches of rough skin occur most commonly on the hands, elbows, and knees, and around the mouth, ears, and neck.

Basic eczema treatments

Moistening treatment

Put on moistening cream or lotion three or four times a day.

Bathe two or three times a day for a few minutes in water, then add bath oil; when you get out, don't dry completely, and put moistening cream on.

Use special soaps such as Basis or Neutrogena.

Avoid moistening agents with perfume, preservatives, or lanolin.

No water treatment

Do not bathe with water except to use a washcloth for armpit and crotch areas.

Wash with Cetaphil lotion two times a day.

General eczema guidelines

Use food allergy diet (see food allergy).

Use household allergen control (see allergy).

Avoid rough clothing such as wool.

Avoid clothing that does not breathe and makes you sweat, such as tight nylon.

Wash new clothes before wearing.

Avoid harsh detergents on clothes.

Deal with stress and tension.

swelling and redness. If a patch is infected from scratching, the doctor may prescribe an antibiotic cream to kill the bacteria causing the infection (see Impetigo, page 301). If kids are really bothered by itching, the doctor may prescribe antihistamines. If the antihistamines make kids feel sleepy, they should tell the doctor so he or she can change the prescription (see Drugs, page 379).

Prevention

Since the exact cause of eczema is still unknown, no one knows how to prevent it. However, when children understand what makes it worse for them they can usually prevent it from flaring up.

Blisters

What's happening

A blister is the result of unusual, continuous rubbing on some area of the body. The most common places for blisters are the soles of the feet and the palms of the hands. People get blisters on their feet from shoes that don't fit or from a long walk. They get blisters on the hands from working with a tool like a rake or a hammer for too long a time.

The friction from constant rubbing actually splits the top layer of skin from the middle layer. The areas between the separated layers fill with clear fluid that gives the blister its puffy look. The body may reabsorb the fluid or, if rubbing continues, the blister may pop and the fluid may ooze out. Blisters can be very uncomfortable, but they heal by themselves. Sometimes the skin layers rejoin, sometimes the top layer dries out and falls off. Then new skin grows over the moist, tender middle layer. For the blister to heal, the rubbing must stop or the area must be protected.

If the rubbing continues for several days but isn't extreme, the skin cells in the top skin layer, which are hard and flat, increase in number and form a thick, protective, leathery layer. This is why people who ordinarily walk a lot or work with their hands don't get blisters on the feet and hands.

Helping yourself

If you notice that an area of skin hurts and is red when you are walking or working, stop the rubbing. The redness and soreness are the first signs of a blister. Stopping the rubbing may prevent a blister from forming or will allow the body to heal the blister while it is still small. You can stop rubbing on your feet by putting on a Band-Aid, by changing socks or shoes, or by stopping the walk. You can stop rubbing on your hands by putting on a Band-Aid, by switching hands or changing position, by wearing gloves, or by stopping your work.

Signs and symptoms

A puffy area of skin with clear fluid under it

A patch of skin peeling off

Painful red skin patches

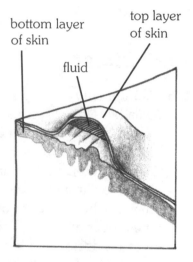

bottom layer of skin

top layer of skin

fluid

When you get a blister, the top layer of skin separates from the bottom layer, and the space in between fills with fluid.

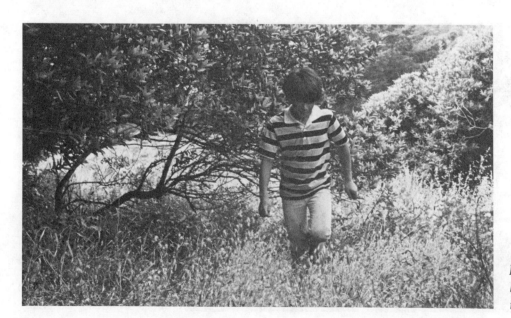

Kids often get blisters after a long hike or when breaking in new shoes.

The doctor

Children rarely need to see a doctor for a blister.

Prevention

You can prevent most foot blisters by wearing sturdy, comfortable shoes for hikes and long walks. New shoes, especially leather ones, should be taken off as soon as they feel uncomfortable, until they are soft and "broken in." Hand blisters can be prevented by starting slowly and not working too long at a completely new job.

Flea bites

What's happening

Flea bites look like small red bumps, about one-eighth of an inch wide, and can be extremely itchy. For this reason, there are often scratch marks around them and they may have scabs if they have been scratched hard enough to break the skin. Occasionally flea bites that have been scratched become infected. Generally there is more than one flea bite, although they may not be near each other. Fleas can bite anywhere on the body, but they especially seem to like the scalp, the abdomen, or the back. For reasons doctors don't understand, some people seem to be especially susceptible to flea bites and react strongly to them.

Flea bites are often the cause of an itchy rash. This is particularly likely if the pets in your house have fleas. Occasionally you may see a flea on you or in your bed, as well as on your pet. Fleas, and therefore flea bites, are most plentiful in late summer and early fall.

Signs and symptoms

Tiny red areas like bumps, on the scalp, abdomen, or back

Itching

Crusts and pimples and scabs

Scratch marks

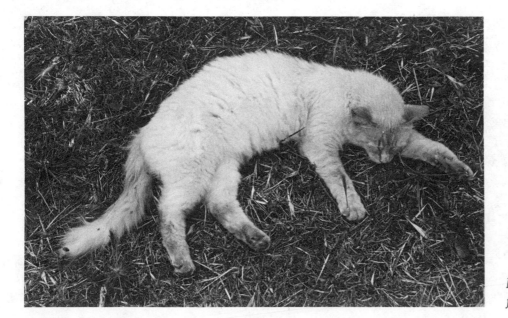

Most flea bites come from fleas on household pets.

Helping yourself

You can get some relief from the itching by applying calamine lotion or taking a cool bath. Some kids find they think less about the bites and scratch them less if they wear clothing that covers them.

If the scabs appear oozy or swollen, it is important to wash them daily with warm water and soap. This will help to keep them from becoming infected.

The doctor

It is not usually necessary to see the doctor about flea bites. Doctors often see flea bites because parents don't know what is causing a rash and are concerned.

Prevention

Generally fleas prefer animals to people, but when there are lots of fleas and not enough animals to go around, they begin to bite people as well. Shampooing and combing animals tends to help control low numbers of fleas. But when the numbers get too large, more has to be done. There are organic flea powders at health food stores; brewer's yeast added to pet food may also help to repel fleas. If flea collars or powders or shampoos that contain pesticides are used on animals, they should be kept outdoors. Such pesticides can affect people, too.

If fleas are in your bed, the sheets and blankets should be laundered and a plastic cover can be placed over the mattress. Your pet should not be allowed to sleep with you until the fleas are under control. Couches, rugs, and pets' beds should be vacuumed frequently to remove flea eggs.

Head lice

What's happening

Head lice are tiny insects that live and breed in people's hair. In fact, they are so tiny they can't be seen without a powerful magnifying glass or a microscope. In very bright light you can see their egg cases (*nits*), which are shiny, white oval sacs. They are the size of dandruff flakes, but they are stuck firmly on the hair shaft. The egg cases are most commonly found at the hairline around the back of the neck and the ears.

The lice lay their eggs at the base of a hair. The egg is attached to the hair and moves outward as the hair grows. The eggs take one week to hatch. In another two weeks, the lice are grown and ready to produce their own eggs. Away from people's bodies, the lice will die in less than a day. But the egg cases can live away from people until they hatch.

The lice spread easily from one person to another. They hop from head to head when people are close to each other, and even from one jacket or

Signs and symptoms

Itching on the head and scalp

Pimples and scabs near hairline and behind ears (sometimes)

Tiny white egg cases on the hairs that look like small rice grains

hat to another on school coatracks. For that reason many children in a class or a school will get head lice at the same time.

Head lice do not make people sick and they do not carry any serious diseases. But they are a real nuisance and they do itch terribly. In fact, one of the first signs of head lice is children scratching their heads frequently. The itching occurs because the body has a mild allergic reaction to the lice.

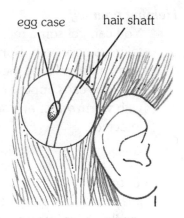

egg case   hair shaft

Head lice are too small to see, but their shiny white egg cases are visible sticking to hairs close to the head.

Helping yourself

Children who are scratching their heads a lot should be checked for head lice. Finding the egg cases requires a slow, careful look in very bright light. If egg cases are found, everyone in the family, as well as close friends, should be checked. The school nurse should be informed since it is likely other children in the class will have them.

Head lice are treated fairly easily by washing the hair with a nonprescription shampoo like RID or A-200. These contain pyrethrum, a natural insecticide made from chrysanthemum flowers. It is important to follow the instructions on the shampoo and leave it on the hair for the required length of time or the egg cases may not be killed. Some of the dead egg cases can be removed with a very fine close-toothed comb. Otherwise, they will eventually grow out and be cut along with the hair. If egg cases are found more than one-half inch out from the scalp after shampooing with an insecticide, they are probably dead egg cases that have remained attached. But if egg cases are seen close to the base of the hair, they may be a new group of head lice and the person should reshampoo.

Clothes and sheets need to be washed in *hot* (120°F) water for 10 minutes to kill the lice and the egg cases. Or clothing can be put in a hot dryer for 20 minutes. Things that can't be washed or dried, like hats or stuffed animals, can be put away in a closed plastic bag for at least three weeks to insure that all the eggs have hatched and died.

The doctor

Many doctors prescribe an insecticide called Kwell shampoo in place of RID or A-200 because they think it works better. However, some doctors now avoid Kwell or caution people about using it repeatedly or for more than four hours because in large amounts it affects the nervous system and can make people sick. One of the chemicals in Kwell is also known to cause cancer in animals.

Prevention

Frequent shampooing, clothes washing, and vacuuming may make it less likely a person will catch lice. When other children have lice it's important not to share clothes or put heads close together.

Impetigo

What's happening

Impetigo is a skin infection caused by staph or strep bacteria. Many people have *some* of these bacteria living in their body from time to time, yet they don't necessarily get impetigo. An infection occurs only when the bacteria greatly increase in number and overpopulate. This sometimes happens when the bacteria get into a cut or scratch on the surface of the skin. A cut is a warm, moist place with "food" from the body—just the kind of place where bacteria like to grow.

Children tend to get impetigo more often than adults. Doctors think this is because kids get more scrapes, play in dirtier places, and don't usually wash as carefully. Impetigo frequently appears around the nose, mouth, arms, or legs. The nose is the most common site because bacteria live in the fluid in the nose. Impetigo starts with one pimple, then spreads out into a little red patch with yellowish brown crusts on it. These crusts are made up of dead white blood cells that were fighting the bacteria.

Impetigo patches are frequently itchy or bothersome. If kids scratch the patches they can become even bigger and the bacteria can get under their fingernails and spread to different areas. It's also easy for other children with cuts and scratches to get catch impetigo—especially brothers and sisters or kids who play together a lot.

Helping yourself

The best way to cure impetigo is to wash the bacteria off. This makes it easier for your body to fight the infection. The little crusts should be scrubbed with soap and water until they come off. The scrubbing should be done two or three times a day. Washing in the bathtub is fine, but kids with impetigo should use their own washcloths and towels. After scrubbing, rub on an antibacterial cream like Bacitracin or Neosporin. Kids with impetigo need to make a real effort to keep extra clean, washing their hands and face often with soap. It may also keep impetigo from spreading if fingernails are cut short. Clothes that touch the infected area should be washed frequently.

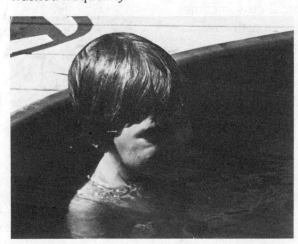

Impetigo is a disease that is cured with soap and water. Washing becomes especially important when people around you have impetigo.

Pimples with yellow or honey-colored crusts around the mouth and nose, or on the arms and legs

Itching

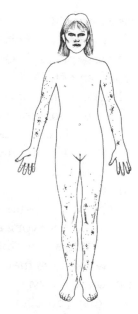

Impetigo is a skin infection most commonly found around the nose, mouth, arms, and legs.

The doctor

The doctor should be seen if the child runs a fever, if the infection starts to spread, or if it lasts more than a week. The doctor will probably want to prescribe an antibiotic to kill more of the bacteria (see Antibiotics, page 380) and to prevent the rare possibility of kidney damage caused by strep bacteria.

Prevention

The best way to keep from getting impetigo is to wash often with soap. This is especially important if a friend or family member has the condition.

Poison ivy (contact dermatitis)

What's happening

Poison ivy and poison oak are skin rashes that develop after touching one of these plants. These rashes are the most common skin diseases among children between 2 and 20. The rash, which often occurs as a line of blisters, is an allergic reaction to one of the chemicals in the plant's oils. Once the body's white blood cells (lymphocytes) have learned to recognize the oil, they quickly come to the area and produce antibodies that combine with the molecules of oil and neutralize it. At the same time the body produces chemicals that cause the redness, swelling, and blisters of the rash.

The rash appears between 18 and 72 hours after the plant has been touched. The worst of the rash generally occurs 4 to 7 days after exposure. At this point the blisters may pop and ooze plasma (body fluid) and the whole area may be intensely itchy. The plasma will not cause the poison ivy or oak to spread, but scratching it may further inflame the area and may cause it to become infected. Poison ivy and poison oak can be picked up in any season from the leaves or stems of the plants. But spring, when the leaves are unfolding, is usually the worst time. Pets sometimes bring home the oil on their fur, but usually a person gets a rash after walking or playing in the woods. Smoke from burning the leaves can also give a person poison ivy or poison oak.

Not all children are allergic to poison ivy or oak. Once in a while a child will get a similar-looking rash from other substances that they are allergic to such as soaps, shampoos, cosmetics, glues, nickel jewelry, or zippers.

Helping yourself

If you have touched poison ivy or oak, wash immediately with strong soap and lukewarm water. Use a nail brush to carefully clean under your fingernails—oil under your nails is the most common way people spread the

Signs and symptoms

Very itchy rash

Red areas, blisters with clear fluid or dry crusts, often in lines

Red swollen skin

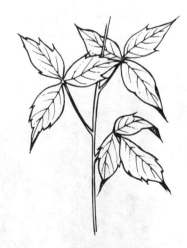

Poison oak and poison ivy have three shiny reddish-green leaves that come off a single stem.

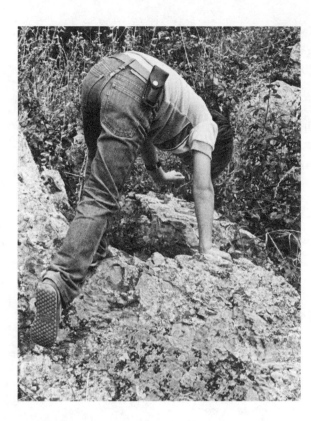

Kids need to learn to recognize poison oak and poison ivy and be on the lookout for the plants when they play in country meadows or woods.

rash. Keep cool because overheating and sweating make the itching worse. Wear loose, comfortable clothes. Try not to scratch; it only makes it worse! It may help if you wear long-sleeved shirts or clothes that cover the rash. Calamine lotion, which is available at drugstores without a prescription, may help to relieve itching. The lotion cools as it evaporates and dries. You can do almost the same thing by wetting the rash with cold water or by taking a cool bath or shower. Some skin doctors suggest that people may feel more comfortable if they apply Burrow's solution (1 Domeboro tablet in 16 ounces of water) or witch hazel compresses called Tucks. These are both available without a prescription.

The doctor

The doctor should be seen if a child is very uncomfortable or has significant swelling around the eyes, nose, or genital areas. The doctor may prescribe a cream containing steroids, a hormone produced by the adrenal glands. This will reduce the redness and swelling by keeping white blood cells from coming into the area to neutralize the oil.

In severe cases of poison ivy or poison oak the doctor may prescribe steroid pills. The drug is given for a week's time, starting with a big dose and gradually tapering down. It is important to take steroids in the recommended doses because suddenly stopping steroids can make a person sick or cause the rash to return in a *rebound effect* (see page 380).

Prevention

The best way not to get poison ivy or poison oak is to learn to recognize the plants and avoid touching them. This is especially important if you have had bad cases of poison oak. If you even *think* you have touched a plant, *wash carefully* (see "Helping yourself") as soon as you can. If you can wash off the oil before it has penetrated your skin, you are much less likely to develop a rash. Don't fail to wash even if you can't get home for several hours. Also, handle your clothes as little as possible when you take them off, and wash them in hot, soapy water.

Ringworm

What's happening

Ringworm is an infection of the top layer of the skin. It isn't actually caused by a worm, but by a kind of plant called a *fungus*. Fungi are unique plants because they lack chlorophyll, the green substance in other plants that enables them to make their own food. Mushrooms are one kind of fungi.

The ringworm fungi make a toxic substance that the skin reacts to by developing a circle of red pimples with a clear center. This circle is very characteristic of ringworm and helps to distinguish it from other kinds of skin rashes. Ringworm can also appear in the hair. In that case it appears as a red scaly patch with broken-off hairs. In either case, ringworm may be quite itchy.

Generally, ringworm is spread from one person to another by touch, but sometimes it may be picked up from a dog or cat who has it. Ringworm is fairly contagious; that is, it's easy to catch. For that reason, it's important to treat it before it spreads to other areas or other people.

Signs and symptoms

Skin
Raised, red, scaly ring about 1″ around with clear center

Itching

Hair
Patchy, scaly area with hair loss

Dull hairs broken off above the skin

Red skin on scalp

Helping yourself

Ringworm of the skin is easily treated with a skin cream called Tinactin (Tolnaftate). It is available at drugstores without a doctor's prescription. Small amounts of Tinactin should be applied to the area two or three times a day. The area will look better in six or seven days, but the cream should be put on for another seven days after the circle has disappeared.

Ringworm of the scalp does not respond to the skin cream because not enough of the medicine enters the hair to get to the fungus. It must be treated with a drug prescribed by the doctor.

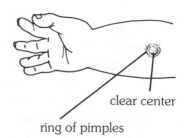

clear center

ring of pimples

The doctor

A doctor uses a special ultraviolet light to diagnose ringworm of the scalp. Under this light the fungus glows greenish white. The doctor can also see the spores (seeds) of the fungus under the microscope.

Ringworm is a skin infection caused by a fungus. It appears as a circle of red pimples with a clear center.

If a person does have ringworm of the scalp, the doctor will prescribe pills called griseofulvin, which are taken for six weeks. The hair should be shampooed frequently to remove loose hairs and any spores of the fungus. However, griseofulvin is believed to cause cancer in animals, and therefore it may be better to use the old treatment, which was Whitfield's ointment—a mixture of benzoic and salicylic acid.

Prevention

The best way to prevent ringworm is to avoid close contact with people who have it and to treat new cases right away. People who have ringworm should bathe frequently and should use only their own clothes and comb and brush.

Sunburn

What's happening

When people are in the sun, their skin becomes tanned. Ultraviolet rays from the sun cause changes in pigment, the chemical in skin cells that gives them a black-brown color. The pigment, called melanin, begins to darken after only a few minutes in the sun. Increased amounts of melanin are made when people are in the sun for days. The tan caused by the increased melanin protects lower layers of cells from being burned by ultraviolet light.

When untanned people are exposed to *very* hot sun for more than a half hour their skin can actually become burned. In severe cases the burned areas will turn red, swell, and blister just as if the skin had been scalded by hot water or touched by a heater or stove. The redness is caused by a widening of the blood vessels under the skin, which brings more blood to the skin's surface. Meanwhile, the burned skin cells release a chemical that triggers the pain nerves under the skin. The discomfort caused by this can last for several days.

After burning, cells in the middle layer of the skin change their shape and lose their attachments to each other. The result is that the top layer separates from the middle layer and causes blisters to form. The blisters swell and become puffy when body fluids come in to protect the area and wall it off. If large areas of people's bodies are sunburned, they may feel very tired, have a headache, or even run a fever in addition to the blisters. Three or four days after the blistering, large white scales may peel off from the blistered areas. These scales are made up of five to ten layers of dried skin cells. By this time the body has formed new healthy skin underneath the peeling layers. Sunburn almost always heals by itself without scarring or any other problem.

Signs and symptoms

Red, hot, swollen skin

Pain and burning

Blisters and peeling skin

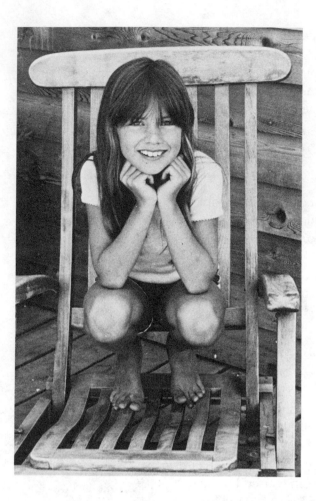

Untanned people need to guard against sunburn whenever they are out in bright hot sun for long periods.

Helping yourself

At the first sign of sunburn, people should cover up or get out of the sun. People often feel more comfortable if they apply cool, wet towels, wet their clothing, or soak in a cool bath. In severe cases of sunburn, aspirin may make people feel less uncomfortable, especially if it is taken early. Moisturizing creams like Vaseline or colloidal oatmeal lotion help to keep the burned area from drying out. Benzocaine sprays, available at drugstores, give only brief relief and sometimes cause other problems.

Loose-fitting, light, airy clothing will make people feel the most comfortable. Going back out in the sun should be avoided except for very brief periods. It's also good to wear clothing that covers the sunburn even on cloudy days or when swimming. Sunblock lotions or ointments containing zinc oxide may be put on for comfort and protection against further sunburn and drying.

The doctor

It is usually unnecessary to see a doctor for sunburn. But if a child develops a rash on areas that have been exposed to the sun (mostly the arms and face), the doctor should be seen. The rash is an allergic reaction to the sun. The doctor may prescribe a steroid cream and a sunblock lotion. If people are very uncomfortable because of itching, the doctor may prescribe an antihistamine. Antihistamines often make people drowsy (see page 379).

Prevention

Sunburn is totally preventable. Parents and children should watch for possible sunburn whenever they go out in very hot sun or are out in the sun for very long periods of time. Paying attention to the sun is especially important on the first few days at the beach or around pools or lakes. It is crucial in the tropics where almost any child out in the sun for more than an hour, at midday, unprotected, will become sunburned. Children with fair skin are most likely to become sunburned. Parents should limit the time children spend in the sun and certainly see that the children put on lightweight clothing if their skin begins to look pink. Parents, or children themselves, can check for sunburn by pushing on different areas of the skin. If the area you press turns very white, and the area around it looks very pink, it's time to get out of the sun or cover up! Most skin doctors recommend that people put on lotions like Pabanol that screen out only those ultraviolet rays of the sun that cause sunburn (2900–3200 angstrom units). These doctors believe that too much time in the sun is not good because it makes it more likely people may someday develop skin cancer. So they advise against getting a dark suntan.

Warts

What's happening

Warts are little lumps on the skin with scaly surfaces. They can occur alone or in groups. Warts actually are an overgrowth of skin cells caused by a very small virus made up almost entirely of DNA, the material in a cell's nucleus (see page 129). Sometimes the virus doesn't stimulate the cells much and you get a small, flat wart; sometimes the virus makes the skin cells grow a lot and you get a big (one-quarter-inch) wart with a rough surface that looks like a miniature cauliflower. The rough, irregular surface is caused by the skin folding over on itself. When warts occur on the bottom of the foot (the plantar surface), they get pressed into the skin, so they appear flat. Like an iceberg, most of a *plantar wart* is below the surface. Plantar warts are the only ones that can cause severe discomfort, because of the pressure put on them from walking.

It's important to know that warts generally go away by themselves. Little ones disappear in a few months, big ones may take a year. Just as your body heals itself of a viral cold, it will heal viral warts.

Signs and symptoms

Small growths with rough surfaces and black specks on the skin

May appear on bottoms of feet or flat hard areas

May hang from a stalk

Helping yourself

The best treatment for most warts is to let them go away by themselves. But many people want to speed up the process, especially if the warts are uncomfortable or if they look ugly. Several medicines are available without a prescription at the drugstore. They all contain salicylic acid, which burns the wart cells and destroys them. Salicylic drops must be applied twice a day for two to four weeks. The crust that forms can be removed gently every few days until all of the wart is gone. This process works more than half the time, although the warts do grow back in some cases.

It has also been found that warts respond to hexing. That is, if a person "tells" the wart to go away and believes it will, the wart will often go away. Sometimes it helps to paint a colored solution on the warts at the same time. Hexing is a fascinating example of the body's ability to direct the healing power of its immune system with a thought or visualization. Even doctors sometimes use hexing with young children. Kids have vivid imaginations, so hexing works well with them.

The doctor

Doctors have more powerful means of killing the wart cells and the virus causing them. Over the years they have used a number of different methods. Some, such as X-rays, have been discontinued due to the danger of too much radiation; others, such as electric burning, have been discontinued due to the scars it left and the high chances the warts would grow back.

The most popular methods now are freezing with liquid nitrogen and burning with acid. In the first method, a Q-tip dipped in liquid nitrogen ($-195°C$) is touched to the wart for 20 seconds, which freezes the wart to ice. A blister forms over the wart one to two days later and the blister usually falls off by itself in a week. This is successful eight out of ten times. Some doctors paint the wart with a chemical called Cantherone and cover it with a Band-Aid. This treatment is repeated if necessary.

Prevention

There is no known way to prevent warts. The virus is very difficult to grow in the laboratory, so doctors haven't found out why people get warts or what makes them go away.

Eye infection (conjunctivitis)

What's happening

Conjunctivitis is an infection of the lining of the inside of the eyelids. This lining, called the mucous membrane, is normally moist and pink, and helps to spread tears over the eye and keep it lubricated. (It is similar to the linings of the nose and throat.) When the lining is infected, a watery or greenish-yellow fluid gathers at the corner of the eye. Doctors call this fluid a discharge. The fluid sometimes causes the eyelashes to stick together especially after a night's sleep. That can be scary and uncomfortable, but it is not at all serious. Often an infection makes your eye feel sore or itchy; sometimes it feels as if something is *in* your eye. If you pull down your eyelid, the edges will look bright red and swollen.

Several different things can cause eye infections. Blowing dirt or smog can irritate eyes so badly that they get red, swollen, and oozy (inflamed). This is not really an infection, but it acts the same way. A true infection is caused by either bacteria or viruses. It often comes with a cold or the flu, but can happen without your feeling sick in any other way. In a sense, conjunctivitis is a cold that has settled in the eyes instead of the nose. A bacterial conjunctivitis usually has a greenish-yellow discharge that looks like pus or mucus. A viral conjunctivitis usually has a more watery-looking discharge.

Helping yourself

Your body usually cures an eye infection by itself in a week or so. But you can help speed this up by not rubbing your eyes when they itch. A cool rinse will make your eyes less itchy. Washing your eyes three or four times a day with warm water will keep your eyelashes from becoming sticky. The doctor should be seen if a conjunctivitis doesn't seem to be getting better in four to seven days and the child has large amounts of yellowish-green pus.

The doctor

The doctor treats bacterial conjunctivitis with eye ointments or drops that contain an antibiotic that will lower the number of bacteria. These are put in the eyes three or four times a day for several days. The infection usually gets better quite rapidly.

The ointment is an oily kind of cream that comes in a tube. It is easy to put in the corner of the eye because it doesn't roll out as drops do. But the ointment may make a film over the eye that makes things look blurry. Eye drops are harder to put in because they roll out if you move your head. Also, some people find that the drops burn their eyes a little for a few seconds. The best way to put in drops is to have children lie down or tilt their heads back. Since it's hard not to blink, some doctors suggest closing the eyes first. A drop is put in the inner corner of each eye, then the children can open their eyes, and the drops should roll in.

Prevention

Children should avoid getting dirt or sand in their eyes. Since bacterial and viral conjunctivitis are easy to catch, it's a good idea to wash your hands and face more often than usual if you are around anyone who has red, runny eyes.

Signs and symptoms

Lining around eye is red

Feeling of something in the eye

Watery or yellow fluid at the corner of the eye

Sticky eyelids

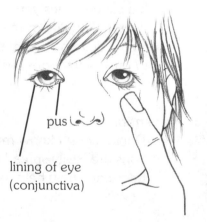

pus

lining of eye (conjunctiva)

Conjunctivitis is an infection of the lining of the eye that causes tearing or pus at the corner of the eye.

Sty

What's happening

A sty is really a little infection like a pimple on the eyelid. The body keeps it from spreading by making a wall around it. When the sty is on the outside of the eyelid, it means a tiny oil (sebaceous) gland at the bottom of the hair follicle is infected. When the sty is on the inside of the eyelid, it means another kind of gland is infected. The infection is caused by staph bacteria. Sties usually last for several days or more, and can be quite uncomfortable at their peak. Often they develop a white head, which may pop and drain by itself. Unfortunately sties do tend to come back again.

Helping yourself

Place a hot, moist washcloth over the sty three or four times a day. The heat helps to increase blood flow to the area, which means more white blood cells come to fight the bacteria. Also the hot, moist washcloth will make you feel more comfortable if the sty is really hurting. Such "hot compresses" work much better if they are left on for 15 minutes or more. Make sure to use your own washcloth and change it frequently.

The doctor

If a sty becomes very big or uncomfortable, or just doesn't go away, see a doctor. The doctor may prescribe an eye ointment or drops that have an antibiotic to help fight the infection. (See page 309 for instructions on how to put in eye drops easily.)

Prevention

Doctors don't know much about preventing sties. But since staph infections are easily spread to other people, washing with soap and water frequently may help to keep the problem from passing on.

Signs and symptoms

A pimple or red swollen area on the lining of the eye

Tender area on eye lining

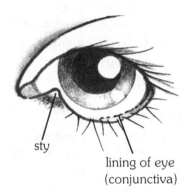

sty

lining of eye
(conjunctiva)

A sty is a little infected gland on the eyelid that looks like a pimple.

Cavities

What's happening

A cavity is a hole in a tooth. This hole is made by acid in your mouth that dissolves the calcium in the hard outer layer of the tooth (the enamel). The acid is made by bacteria that normally live in your mouth. These bacteria are relatives of strep throat bacteria, but they don't cause sore throats. Just like strep throat bacteria, these bacteria are a kind of infection. In that sense, cavities are the most common disease people get.

The bacteria eat and digest the same things that we eat—and they especially like sugar! One of the things that is left over after they digest

Signs and symptoms

Brown spots on teeth that do not brush or scrape off

sugar is acid. The bacteria like to live on a thick, gluelike stuff that builds up on teeth when they aren't cleaned. This sticky stuff is called *plaque* (rhymes with black). Plaque gives a home to acid-forming bacteria and allows them to "digest" the surface of your tooth more easily.

At first you don't even feel a cavity because there are no nerves in the enamel layer of your tooth. But when those acid-making bacteria dissolve the tooth all the way into its center, the *pulp,* then you do feel it. The pulp contains pain nerves that connect with your brain.

The whole cavity process happens so often that over *half* of all three-year-old children in the U.S. have cavities already! By the age of five, most kids have over six fillings. But cavities don't *have* to happen. Eskimos, for example, don't have any cavities because all they eat is meat, fish, and plants. They do not eat ice cream, candy, cookies, and so on. As soon as Eskimos start eating these things, they get cavities, too.

How many cavities you get not only varies depending on what you eat, it varies with how "hard" or "soft" your teeth are. Some kids definitely get cavities more easily than others. Dentists say that those kids are more *susceptible.* Being susceptible is something you get from your parents — you inherit it in your genes. What if one of your parents is susceptible to tooth decay, but the other isn't? What will you be? Unfortunately, there's no real way to tell until you start to get cavities. But if your baby teeth were susceptible, your permanent teeth will be, too.

Sugar products and even bread and rice tend to stick to your teeth. Keeping anything like candy or gum in your mouth for a long time is really bad. This gives the acid-making bacteria food to grow on all the time. Even frequent snacks tend to give the bacteria food all the time. Another thing that helps the acid-forming bacteria is if food is already broken down a little. So it's worse for your teeth to eat cookies and crackers that are made of flour that's been ground until it's very fine.

When cavities aren't filled, even in baby teeth, they can get so deep they can give you a toothache. A tooth that is too rotten may even have to be taken out. And you don't want to lose a baby tooth too early, because it holds the proper space open for the permanent tooth to come in.

Helping yourself

There's really nothing you can do at home once a cavity has started. You should see your dentist as soon as possible.

The dentist

Regular checkups allow your dentist to spot any cavities while they are still small. The dentist can tell a cavity by the fact that that area of the tooth is brownish and a little soft when pushed on with the sharp point of a dental probe. The dentist may take X-rays, which will show how deep a cavity is

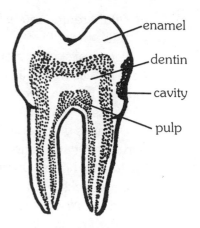

A cavity is a hole in the enamel of a tooth. It is caused by bacteria eating sugar. This forms an acid that actually dissolves the enamel.

and if there are any hidden cavities between the teeth that can't be felt with the probe.

The dentist cleans out the cavity with a tiny drill. If drilling will take place near nerves that will hurt, the dentist will first give you a shot of Novocain in the gum near the tooth. You may feel a brief pinprick when this happens or you may feel nothing at all. Within a few minutes the Novocain makes your tooth feel numb. It does this by blocking the tooth's nerve so it can't send pain messages to your brain. Novocain usually lasts for several hours. During this time you should be careful not to bite your lips or cheeks. You won't feel it when you do it, but it may hurt later. When the Novocain starts to wear off, your gum may feel funny and tingly for a half hour.

To clean out a cavity the dentist will probably use a high-speed drill at first. It makes a high, whining kind of noise. Then the dentist may switch to a slow drill that can only clean out rotten or decayed spots, not a healthy tooth. After all the bacteria and decay are out, the dentist will fill the clean hole with silver (*amalgam*) or a white plastic. This protects the inside of the tooth and keeps out new food and bacteria.

Prevention

Cavities *can* be prevented. The more susceptible your teeth are, the more important prevention is. But all kids should learn good dental habits.

Brushing

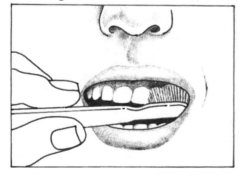

Brushing

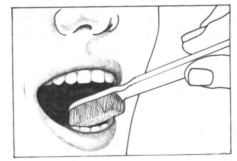

With proper brushing and flossing, you may never have to lose a permanent tooth.

Flossing

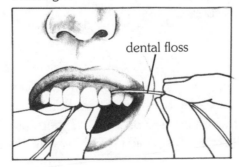

dental floss

Preventing cavities

Avoid foods sweetened with sugar—especially sticky ones.

Avoid food sweetened with honey and molasses, and very sweet dried fruits.

Avoid sticky processed foods.

Avoid drinks that have sugar added.

Avoid any between-meal snacks with sugar added.

If you eat any sugar-sweetened foods, eat them once a day after a meal.

Eat lots of rough fruits and vegetables that clean your teeth and make you produce more saliva to rinse your teeth.

Don't eat right before you go to bed because you make less saliva during sleep.

Eat nonsweet food for snacks—cheese, yogurt, vegetables, fruits.

Brush and floss every day.

Use a fluoride rinse or go to the dentist for fluoride treatments.

There are several things that will help to prevent cavities. *First, eat less sugar.* Avoid the kinds of food that stick to your teeth or sit in your mouth. The more sugar you eat, the more cavities you are likely to get. (During World War II people in Norway could get almost *no* sugar and the number of cavities people got dropped remarkably. After the war, when they could get more sugar, they again got more cavities.)

Second, don't eat sugar between meals. Studies show that people get fewer cavities if they eat the same amount of sugar *with* their meal, like dessert, instead of separately, like a snack.

Third, learn to brush and floss properly, and do it every single day. Brushing and flossing remove food particles and plaque. To test how well you brush, ask your dentist for a "disclosing" tablet that stains any plaque you missed with food coloring.

Fourth, see your dentist for regular checkups and cleanings. It is much easier and more comfortable to treat cavities when they are small.

Fifth, use fluoride. Children raised with fluoride in their water supply have less than half the cavities of children in nonfluoridated areas. Fluoride is also available in vitamins and toothpaste, and your dentist can paint it on your teeth.

Of all the diseases that kids get, cavities are the most common and the most preventable. And kids really have the greatest role in cavity prevention both by what they eat and how they brush.

The common cold (acute nasopharyngitis, inflammation of the nose and back of the throat, rhinitis)

What's happening

The common cold is an infection of the nose and throat, which is the upper part of the breathing, or respiratory, system. There are over 100 different viruses that can cause a cold and a number of different bacteria. Probably nine out of ten colds are caused by viruses. Bacterial colds tend to make people sicker; they sometimes start after you already have a viral cold.

Colds are the most common childhood disease. Almost everybody has had a cold sometime, but some kids seem to get colds all the time. These kids are just more susceptible; that is, they seem to get colds more easily. All kids seem more likely to get sick when they are overtired, under pressure, or not eating well.

Younger kids from one to six years old tend to get the most colds. They may get as many as six colds a year and have each one anywhere from three days to two weeks. Most colds start about two days after people are exposed to a particular virus or bacterium.

How a cold begins. A cold usually begins with a runny nose or a sore throat. Doctors call these *local symptoms* because they involve just one part of your body. A fever is a *generalized symptom*—it takes place all over your body.

A runny nose means there are lots of viruses or bacteria growing in that part of your body. The runny nose and sneezing are your body's way of trying to get rid of the organism causing your cold. When the infection starts, your body sends extra white blood cells to the area in order to produce antibodies and round up and get rid of the dead viruses or bacteria (see page 238). When you blow your nose, you are actually helping your body. Dead germs, plus white blood cells that have been killed in the fight, are in the mucous discharge that comes from your nose. In order to clean up the dead cells, your body needs lots of liquids. Liquids make the mucus from your nose thinner and more watery, which makes it easier to blow your nose.

If your throat becomes infected, you get a sore throat and a cough. Cells in the lining of the windpipe produce a mucous discharge called phlegm, the thick, yellowish discharge that comes up when you cough. A cough is your body's natural way of getting rid of all the dead germs and white blood cells. If you don't drink enough liquids, the phlegm tends to become thick, sticky, and hard to cough up. A "tight" cough not only slows down healing, it hurts.

Your body may run a fever when the cold is at its worst. Your temperature goes above the normal 98.6°F and you feel hot and flushed. Often you feel achy all over and have very little energy. Most people tend to stay in bed with a fever, which is probably just what your body needs to help

Signs and symptoms

Running nose, sneezing

Fever

Sore throat

Cough

Tiredness

Muscle aches

Crankiness

Loss of appetite

fight the cold. The hotter your body is, the more you tend to dry out, and the more you need extra liquids. With a severe cold, the fever may last from one to six days. Often the fever will go up at night, and be lowest in the morning. When a fever is very high (102°F to 104°F), a person's eyes may be sore and sensitive to light. People with a cold also tend to be crankier and less hungry than normal. There is nothing dangerous about a normal fever. In fact, a fever is just another way your body tries to fight the cold. Doctors believe that a higher body temperature may make it harder for the viruses or bacteria to live and may make the body's own chemicals work better.

Complications of a cold. A runny nose, sore throat, cough, and fever can all be part of a regular, uncomplicated cold. A more serious or complicated cold begins in the same way, but it does not start to get better after five or six days. Instead it gets worse. The fever returns or goes up and new symptoms appear.

Sometimes the cold spreads to a new area; sometimes people get a bacterial infection in addition to the viral one that started the cold; or they get infections of the ears, the tonsils, the vocal cords *(laryngitis),* the bronchial tubes, or the lungs *(pneumonia).* All of these areas have the same kind of lining (mucous membrane) and connect with one another. This makes it easy for the virus or bacteria to spread from the nose and throat to these other areas.

Helping yourself

There are two things to do when you have a cold. One is help your body to do its job of healing; the other is to make yourself feel as comfortable as possible.

Rest is one of the most important steps in treating a cold. When you're sick, your body has to work harder than usual to deal with the bacteria or virus. So it's important to find quiet things to do, rather than things that tire you out like hiking. Keeping reasonably warm but not hot helps to save your energy; sleeping gives your body a chance to build up energy. When you have a cold, go to bed early and perhaps even take naps.

Drinking extra liquids is extremely important because they help to thin out mucous congestion and flush out dead cells. Plain water and apple juice are the liquids most commonly recommended. Some people feel that milk and milk products tend to be mucous producing and therefore should not be eaten in large quantities during the early stages of a cold. If your stomach is upset as well, small amounts of noncola sodas may be the best.

Another way to increase the amount of liquid you take in is to use a *vaporizer.* Moisture sprayed into the air by the vaporizer enters your lungs and is absorbed by your body. Vaporizers are particularly important in helping to loosen a tight, painful cough. As the phlegm becomes thinner, you can cough it up more easily. Extra moisture in the air is most impor-

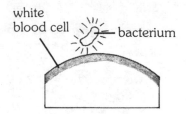
white blood cell — bacterium

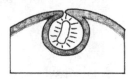

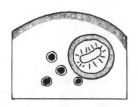

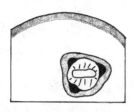

You cure colds by yourself when your body's white blood cells eat the viruses or bacteria causing the cold.

Treatment for a cold

Helping your body heal itself

Rest
Sleep as much as you like, do quiet peaceful activities—read, play games, build models, or watch TV.

Avoid staying up late, going out shopping, playing games and sports, playing with friends.

Warmth
Wear what feels comfortable, take off clothes when you feel hot, put on clothes when you feel cold.

Food
Eat what you like, drink a lot of liquids such as juice, water, soda.

Relieving symptoms

Fever
Do nothing if it doesn't bother you.

Take clothes off, drink fluids.

Sponge yourself off with warm water and let it dry.

Aspirin or acetaminophen (Tempra or Tylenol) can be used if you are very uncomfortable.

> **Aspirin dose:** over 5 years—1 adult aspirin (15 gr.)
> every 4–6 hours for not more than 2 days.
> **Acetaminophen:** 3–6 years—1 tablet (120 mg)
> Over 6 years—2 tablets (240 mg)

Cough
Coughing helps your body by bringing up mucus.
At night, if coughing isn't bringing up mucus, a cough suppressant can be used.

Liquids, honey, or cough drops can slow a cough.

Sore throat
Warm milk or tea with honey, or cough drops will ease the soreness.

tant in the winter months when central heating systems tend to dry out the air in the house.

Sometimes you feel so miserable with a cold that you want to treat its symptoms, or signs. Of course, this won't make the cold go away and probably doesn't even speed up your recovery, but it *might* make you feel a little better. And that may make you get better faster.

A high fever can be very uncomfortable and even upsetting. Your thinking may become "fuzzy" or confused and your feelings very sensitive. This is perfectly normal and you shouldn't worry about it. When your fever goes down, you will feel like yourself again. In the meantime, wear light clothing as long as you do not have the chills. If you're extremely hot, you can even take a lukewarm bath or sponge yourself off. The water evaporates as you dry off and this cools you down. Aspirin tends to bring down a fever, and will also help to relieve a headache and muscle aches; but it is not *necessary* to take aspirin when you have a cold.

Some cough medicines are designed to "suppress" or stop a cough. They tend to keep you from getting the phlegm out, which doesn't help you to get better. Suppressant cough medicines should only be taken at night if you are being kept awake by shallow spells of coughing that you can't stop and that don't bring up any phlegm. There are other cough medicines that are designed to *bring up* phlegm. They are called *expectorants.* They may be helpful, but the first and most important thing is to increase the amount of liquids you are getting.

Nose drops may be taken if you have a very stuffy headcold, although they are generally not very effective. Again, the most important thing is to drink more liquids.

The doctor

The doctor should be called if parents are worried, if a child has a fever over 101°F or 102°F, if the child is extremely listless, or if the child doesn't seem to be getting better after several days. Generally the doctor will advise rest, lots of liquids, a vaporizer, and possibly aspirin, cough medicine, and/or nose drops. The doctor may want to see the child if he or she is concerned about the possibility of strep throat, ear infection, or some other complication of a cold. The doctor will do a regular physical exam, including listening to the lungs with a stethoscope, looking at both eardrums with an otoscope, and possibly taking a throat culture to rule out a strep infection. To do a throat culture the doctor simply rubs the child's throat with a cotton swab to get a sample of the phlegm. This is sent to the lab to see if strep bacteria grow from it. If the doctor thinks the infection is bacterial, he or she may start the child on antibiotics right away.

Prevention

Cold viruses are communicable ("catchable") from a day before the cold begins until about five days afterward. The time it takes for the cold to develop after you have been exposed can vary quite a bit—anywhere from 12 hours to a week or more. Colds are very easily passed on to other people by spreading around the virus. Both coughing and sneezing send viruses into the air, landing on anyone or anything nearby. When you have a cold, cover your mouth when you cough and your nose when you sneeze. Mouth or even hand contact can also spread the virus. It's good not to get too close to or spend too much time with someone who's sick. It also helps to wash your hands and not use the same utensils or glasses and so on.

A particular kind of virus can spread rapidly from one person to another in a family, a school, or a town. When lots of people get the same cold, doctors call it an *epidemic*. Each time you get a cold, your body learns to make antibodies against that particular virus. From then on, you are better able to fight off that virus. Doctors call this developing immunity to the virus. Young children tend to get more colds than older children because they have not yet developed immunity to many viruses.

The healthier you are in general, the less likely you are to get a really bad cold or to get any complications of a cold. When a particular virus is going around, some kids don't get it. In fact, as doctors know, some kids almost never catch colds, while other kids seem to get sick with *every* virus that comes around. Part of being susceptible may be inherited, but probably most of it has to do with your environment. If you eat nutritious foods, get enough sleep, gets lots of exercise, and are basically happy, you are likely to be healthy. All of these things strongly affect how susceptible you are to colds and how sick you'll get from one.

Another important way to lower the number of colds you get and to keep colds from becoming severe is to pay attention to your body's signals. Be alert if you notice a slight sore throat, start sneezing, or feel like coughing. If you treat these *first* signs of a cold, you may never develop the cold. For example, if you always get sick when you get cold and wet, change your damp clothes as soon as you can. Even if you just feel really tired or cranky, go to bed early. Your parents can notice if you seem to be getting sick, but you know your own body best. And you can make yourself healthier.

Strep throat

What's happening

Strep throat is an infection of the back of the throat caused by *streptococcus* bacteria. Almost one-fourth of all kids have small amounts of this bacteria in their throats at any given time, but they don't necessarily get sick. Kids only become sick when the number of bacteria gets high.

The sick child's throat is very red, sore, and quite swollen, and may be covered with patches of white pus. When the bacteria start growing in large numbers, they begin to hurt cells in the lining of the throat. The

Signs and symptoms

Very sore throat

Swollen glands in the neck

Fever

Tiredness

damaged cells and other nearby cells send out lots of fluid, which causes the throat to swell and keeps the bacteria from spreading. The redness is caused by additional blood coming into the area. This blood brings extra white blood cells to fight the infection. The white blood cells kill bacteria and make special antibodies that can "lock up" the bacteria. Then the white blood cells get rid of all the dead bacteria and throat cells. This is what makes the patches of white pus.

With a strep throat, glands in the neck may also become swollen and tender. These glands are actually lymph nodes that run in a chain on either side of the neck (see page 175). The lymph nodes drain much of the fluid made by cells lining the throat. As the fluid passes through, the nodes filter out the dead bacteria and dead cells and digest them. The nodes also grow the special white blood cells that make antibodies against the strep bacteria. The fact that the nodes are swollen shows how hard the body is working to heal itself.

Children with strep throat usually become sick fairly suddenly and may be sicker than with a virus-caused sore throat. The children run a fever and sometimes vomit. They are usually very tired and have little energy. Kids begin to feel better in 3 or 4 days and are well by 10 to 14 days.

It is uncommon, but sometimes kids get a rash like a sunburn on their armpits and belly on the second day. This rash is called *scarlet fever*, because kids look red and have a high fever. It is caused by a poison given off by certain kinds of strep bacteria.

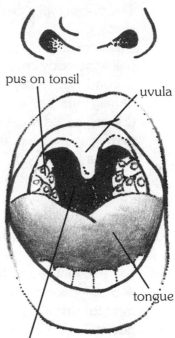

pus on tonsil

uvula

tongue

back of throat (pharynx)

When a person has a strep throat, the back of his or her throat is swollen, sore, and may be covered with patches of white pus.

Helping yourself

Children with strep throat will feel best if they rest in bed at first. This allows the body to concentrate all its energies on healing. The sore throat may be helped by sucking on cough drops, drinking apple juice or warm tea with honey, or by eating ice cream or sherbet. Most kids' throats are too sore for them to eat regular meals for the first several days. Lots of liquids and soft foods are best. The swollen nodes in the neck may be made more comfortable if kids put on warm wet towels or use a hot water bottle. If children are very uncomfortable from the fever or muscle aches, they can take aspirin in appropriate doses.

The doctor

The doctor can tell if children have strep throat by doing a culture. To make a culture, the doctor simply touches a cotton swab to the back of the throat and then rubs it on a dish filled with a Jell-O-like substance. If strep bacteria are present, they will grow rapidly on the "food." In 1 or 2 days the doctor will see little dots if bacteria are growing.

A culture is the only way to absolutely tell whether a sore throat is caused by strep. Doctors treat all proven strep throats with antibiotics. Penicillin works best against strep and is used unless a child is allergic to it.

The doctor will either prescribe ten days of pills or give one long-acting shot.

Doctors treat strep throat with an antibiotic for two reasons. First, it helps the body cure the sore throat and may make kids feel better faster. Second, penicillin prevents the rare possibility of heart disease or kidney damage that sometimes follows an untreated strep throat. The heart disease, called *rheumatic fever,* is due to the body's own strep antibodies damaging the heart muscle. One study showed there were three cases of rheumatic fever out of 1,000 cases of untreated strep throat, and those who contracted rheumatic fever all had an inherited family likelihood of getting the disease. It's been found that 10 days of penicillin are necessary to prevent rheumatic fever. The kidney damage is due to an infection called *glomerulonephritis,* in which the body's own strep antibodies get stuck in the glomerulus of the kidney (see page 178). The type of strep bacteria that causes this to happen is extremely rare.

Some doctors don't bother to culture for strep throat, but go ahead and treat for strep if the child has a fever, pus on the throat, and swollen lymph nodes. Unfortunately this means they are treating a large number of kids with viral sore throats. Antibiotics do nothing for a virus-caused sore throat and may have side effects, including rare allergic reactions. Moreover, following a course of antibiotics, helpful bacteria in the intestine that make vitamins are destroyed. (Eating yogurt will introduce more of these bacteria.)

Prevention

Kids with strep throat readily spread the disease by coughing, sneezing, and touching. The bacteria can actually travel through the air in droplets as well as be passed hand to hand. For this reason some doctors culture everyone in the family of a child with strep. Children with strep can pass the bacteria around before they get symptoms and for a day after they start treatment. They should be kept home until they have started antibiotics and feel better.

Ear infection (acute otitis media)

What's happening

Acute otitis media is an infection of the middle of the ear, a special closed area behind the eardrum. The walls of this area are the eardrum and the bones of the skull. When the ear is infected, nearby cells make lots of fluid just the way the nose gets runny with a cold. The only way for fluid to get out of the middle ear is through a tube that goes to the back of the nose and throat (the Eustachian). In an ear infection, the lining of the tube becomes swollen, fluid can't go from the middle ear to the back of your throat, and pressure builds up. As fluid accumulates in the middle ear, it presses on your eardrum, which has lots of sensitive nerve endings. Fluid presses on the nerves and causes pain. That's what an *earache* really is.

The warmth and wetness of the fluid trapped in the ear is an ideal place for viruses or bacteria to grow. As more and more bacteria or viruses grow, the body brings more white blood cells to the area to engulf or eat them. This causes more pressure. And the *dead* bacteria and white blood cells that have been used up in the fight and are now trapped also add to the pressure.

For many kids, an earache is the longest, sharpest pain they have ever felt. The pain begins to go away as soon as fluid starts to drain out of the middle ear and the pressure drops. Three things can cause the pressure to drop: (1) The eardrum actually pops and fluid comes out of your ear; (2) the lining of the swollen Eustachian tube starts to shrink back to normal; and (3) the body begins to get ahead of the infection and begins to sponge up or absorb some of the fluid in the middle ear. Bursting of the eardrum only happens occasionally (one in ten times), but it is not necessarily serious. The split normally heals by itself within 2 weeks. During this time hearing may be a little fuzzy in that ear.

Helping yourself

Generally earaches come on very suddenly, with a sharp, intense pain. Often kids are awakened in the middle of the night by an earache. There are several things that can help to ease the pain. You can hold a heating pad or a hot water bottle against your ear. Sometimes the pain will get better if a little warm oil is put in your ear. And aspirin may ease the pain even if it doesn't make it go away entirely. Nonprescription nose drops or ear drops with pain medication rarely help much.

Pain in the ear

Fever (often)

Pus or watery fluid coming out of the ear

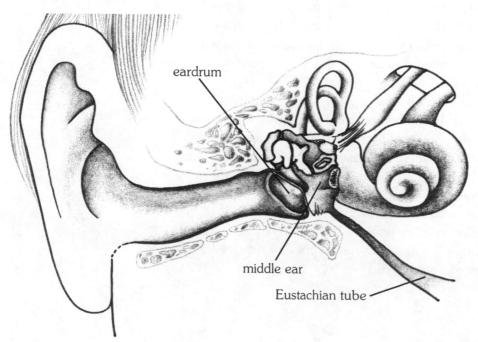

eardrum

middle ear

Eustachian tube

When you have an ear infection, the middle ear becomes plugged up with fluid because the Eustachian tube swells shut. This makes nerves in the eardrum hurt.

The doctor

In order to tell if you have an ear infection, the doctor looks into your ear with a special little machine called an otoscope. This machine shines a bright beam of light into your ear. If the ear is infected, the eardrum will look bright red and may be swollen. A healthy eardrum is a silver-gray color and the light from the otoscope flashes back from it somewhat as it would reflect from a mirror. Sometimes people have just one infected ear, sometimes both.

Since the middle ear is closed to the outside, there is no way the doctor can take a culture (see page 200) to tell if an ear infection is caused by virus or by bacteria. But doctors have found that younger children most often have an infection from bacteria called *Haemophilus influenza*, whereas older kids more often get one from bacteria called *pneumococcus*. So doctors generally give kids below six or seven *amphicillin*, an antibiotic that kills lots of different bacteria. And they give kids over six or seven penicillin because it works very well against pneumococcus bacteria.

Ear infections can be caused by several different viruses as well as by bacteria. About three out of ten ear infections are caused by viruses. Even though antibiotics don't work against viruses, doctors treat all ear infections with antibiotics for about 10 days. This is because a few children whose ear infections are not treated may develop other more serious problems, such as hearing loss or an infection of the mastoid bone behind the ear.

Sometimes an ear infection doesn't clear up with the antibiotic the doctor prescribes. The doctor can tell if this is happening by looking in the ears again. If the drums are still red and swollen, the doctor will prescribe a different antibiotic. Some doctors have you take *all* of the first antibiotic before they recheck your ears. Other doctors have you come back in three or four days if you aren't feeling much better. If your eardrums show no improvement, they may switch to a second antibiotic right away or add a drug called sulfa to the first antibiotic. Normally children feel much better within 12 hours after starting antibiotics, and they can return to regular activities, including school, within a day or two. But they should go to sleep early and exercise less than usual.

Doctors used to prescribe a *decongestant* along with the antibiotic. Decongestants are drugs that shrink the lining of the Eustachian tubes and the nose. Decongestants often have side effects and make kids either sleepy or nervous and excited. Recent studies have shown that they really don't speed the healing of ear infections that much, so many doctors are not prescribing them anymore.

If a child is in *severe* pain with an ear infection, the doctor may prescribe codeine syrup. Codeine is a powerful drug that will actually put most children to sleep. Also, if the eardrum has popped or ruptured, the doctor may prescribe antibiotic ear drops.

Prevention

Early treatment of a cold probably helps to prevent ear infections. Kids who have had several ear infections within a year should take special care if they appear to be catching a cold. They should learn to blow their noses in a steady, easy way so that they don't force mucus up into their Eustachian tubes. They should sleep with their heads up on pillows to help keep fluid draining from the middle ear. And some kids find it's important to keep their ears covered in cold, windy weather—especially if they feel as if they are catching cold.

Swimmer's ear (external otitis)

What's happening

Swimmer's ear is a disease in which the skin lining the ear canal becomes red and swollen. It can result from scratching your ears or cleaning them too firmly, but is most often caused by water being in the ear canal for a long time. The water lessens the skin's normal acidity and causes the top layer of skin cells to come off.

People ordinarily get swimmer's ear in the summer when they are in and out of pools many times a day. Chlorine that is added to pool water to kill unhealthy bacteria also kills helpful bacteria that live in the ear canal.

The combination of the lack of acid, lack of helpful bacteria, and loss of skin cells means the skin has lost its normal protection. It then becomes red and raw, which causes pain and itching in the outer ear. At this point the skin can become infected with pseudomonas bacteria.

Helping yourself

You can probably cure a mild case of swimmer's ear at home. Don't scratch or clean your ear, and if you are swimming a lot, stop. Wash out the ear with a warm solution of one tablespoon white vinegar and one tablespoon water, or with Vosol from the drugstore. This will clear out wax and dead skin cells, and will allow the ear to dry. It will also help the skin maintain its normal acid level.

The doctor

If the problem doesn't begin to clear up in several days or is very painful, see the doctor. The doctor may wash your ear out with acetic acid (vinegar) and water, then give you a prescription for ear drops. The drops are put in three to four times a day for five or six days. The drops contain steroids to reduce the swelling, which in turn relieves the pain and itching. The drops also contain an antibiotic in case there is a bacterial infection. It may be more comfortable to warm the ear drops before putting them in. Hold the bottle in your hand or put it in warm water for a few minutes.

Signs and symptoms

Pain in the ear

Itching in the ear

Pain when the ear is moved

Skin flakes and wax plugging the ear

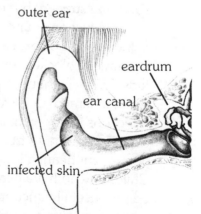

Swimmer's ear is an infection of the skin lining the outer ear canal. It is caused by water being in the canal too long and irritating the skin.

Prevention

Be very gentle when you clean your ears, and never use sharp objects to do it. In fact, doctors now recommend that you do not even use cotton swabs since ear wax comes out by itself. It's enough just to wash your outer ears with a washcloth. Cotton swabs can irritate the lining of your ears.

Whenever you swim, make sure you get all the water out of your ears when you come out of the water. If one of your ears is blocked with water, try tugging at your earlobe or tilt your head to that side and hop up and down on the foot on that side. You will feel when the water comes out.

Some doctors recommend that children who have gotten swimmer's ear several times put two or three drops of equal parts of vinegar and 70 percent alcohol in their ears before and after swimming. Doctors also warn against using cotton or poor-fitting earplugs.

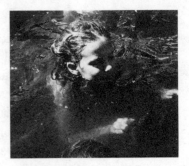

When kids develop swimmer's ear, it's a good idea for them to keep their ears out of water until they're better.

Glue ear (serous otitis media)

What's happening

"Glue ear" is a condition in which the middle ear (the area behind the eardrum) stays full of fluid because the Eustachian tubes leading from the middle ear to the back of the nose are plugged up. When the Eustachian tubes can't drain, the body removes air from the middle ear, which creates a suction effect. In order to balance this pressure, the goblet cells in the middle ear secrete fluid into the enclosed space (see diagram, page 200). This fluid makes it harder for the eardrum to move and transmit sound to the bones of the inner ear. So children feel as if they are hearing sounds underwater. Sometimes young kids don't even realize that things are sounding strange, but most older kids notice it fairly quickly. Glue ear can occur in just one ear or in both.

Generally doctors can't figure out what keeps the Eustachian tubes continually blocked, causing glue ear. It may be that the shape of some kids' Eustachian tubes is narrow or twisted. Sometimes allergies keep kids' tubes inflamed and swollen for long periods. Also, it seems that several ear infections in a row may lead to fluid-filled ears.

It is important to treat glue ear in order to prevent the possibility of any permanent hearing loss and to avoid problems that may arise at school. Children who have hearing loss from glue ear are sometimes thought to be purposefully uncooperative, daydreamy, or just plain stupid. Kids with a history of glue ear should always be seated near the teacher to make it easier for them to hear what's going on. Most kids with glue ear seem to outgrow it by the time they are 12. Very few kids have permanent loss of hearing ability.

Helping yourself

Kids with a history of glue ear should learn how to make their ears "pop," which tends to gently force open the Eustachian tubes. There are several

Signs and symptoms

Trouble hearing

A little pain in the ear

A feeling of fullness in the ear

ways to do this. One is to hold your nose and close your lips, puff your cheeks out hard with air, then let go of your nose and swallow. It sounds complicated, but it isn't once you get used to it. Another funny way to pop your ears if you feel pressure building up in them is to hold your nose and blow up a balloon. Sometimes swallowing several times in a row, chewing gum, or pressing on the outer flap of your ear will clear your Eustachian tubes.

The doctor

The doctor can tell if kids have glue ear by looking into their ears with an otoscope, a special machine that shines a bright light on the eardrum. The drum will appear pale, not shiny and healthy. Sometimes the doctor will even be able to see a shadow of the fluid that is blocked up behind the drum. Also, if the doctor blows a little blast of air against the drum, it won't move as it would normally. The doctor may even test to see if there is any loss of hearing, since this also indicates that there may be fluid instead of air in the middle ear.

If there is a lot of fluid in the middle ear, the doctor may send the child to a doctor who only treats ear, nose, and throat problems. That doctor may make a small opening in the eardrum. This process is called a *myringotomy*. It can be done in the doctor's office or in the hospital. After making the little hole, the doctor will then suction out the fluid, which may be uncomfortable. Finally, the doctor may put a tiny plastic tube into the hole in the eardrum. This tube keeps the hole from closing up and allows new fluid to drain out. It breaks the suction in the middle ear and allows air to get in. The tube is usually left in for about six weeks at a time, and may be put in more than once. While the tube is in, the eardrum cannot move as easily as usual, which means hearing is not as good as usual. After the tube is removed, the eardrum heals by itself within several weeks. Some doctors believe that the tubes are very helpful; some use them only if the ears stay plugged up for a long time.

Prevention

Early treatment of ear infections and allergies may prevent continuing fluid buildup in the middle ear. Kids who have a history of glue ear should learn to "pop" open their Eustachian tubes (see "Helping Yourself"). This is important when kids have colds and have to blow their noses, and when flying, driving up steep hills, and riding in elevators.

Allergies

Hay fever (and other allergies)

Signs and symptoms

> Itchy nose
>
> Sneezing
>
> Stuffy or running nose
>
> Red eyes
>
> Itchy eyes
>
> Teary eyes

What's happening

Some kids are allergic to certain tiny dust particles in the air. When these children breathe in the *allergen,* or particle that they are allergic to, a whole set of things happens in their bodies which do not happen to kids who are not allergic. Doctors don't know why, but allergic children's bodies overreact to the particle. In fact, their bodies react to the particles as if they were dangerous germs. Their white blood cells rapidly begin to make special proteins called antibodies. These antibodies "lock onto" the dust particles and hook them onto *mast cells* in the lining of the nose. Then, an amazing thing happens: The mast cells produce an explosion of chemicals. One of these chemicals is called *histamine.* It causes the lining of the nose to (1) swell, (2) increase blood flow, and (3) produce a lot of mucus. The result is a stuffed nose, a runny nose, and sneezing. Allergic kids' eyes and noses also itch and become red from rubbing.

The most common thing that kids are allergic to is *pollen.* Pollen is the male seed released by flowers. The seeds are so tiny they can blow in the wind. Millions of these seeds are in the air when a particular kind of plant is "going to seed." Different plants go to seed at different times of the year —trees in winter and spring, grasses in spring and summer, and weeds in summer and fall. Children's reactions to pollen can vary from one year to the next, even from day to day, depending upon how much pollen is around.

If people are allergic to pollen in certain seasons only, their allergy is called *hay fever.* If kids have stuffy, runny noses most of the time, they are usually allergic to household dust, which is around all year. Household dust contains lots of strange things including animal dander (skin scales), fungus, molds, and tiny pieces of insects, plants, and animals. People can be allergic to one or many of the things in household dust. This kind of allergy is worse in the winter when heating systems blow hot air around and kids spend more time indoors.

Grown-ups usually don't have as much trouble with their allergies as they did when they were young. And a quarter of all allergic children eventually outgrow their allergies.

Helping yourself

The basic treatmemt is to keep allergic kids away from whatever they are allergic to. If a child is allergic to something in household dust, the house must be kept very clean and free of animals, wool, or other allergens (see the Household allergy control chart, page 329). If a child is allergic to pollens, nearby plants should be removed if possible and air conditioning should be used in the pollen season (see Pollen control chart, page 327).

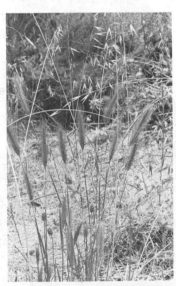

Children who have hay fever need to learn which pollens they're allergic to and try to avoid them.

Pollen control chart

East Coast

Trees—February–June
  Elm—March–April
  Maple, poplar, birch—March–May
  Oak, walnut, hickory—April–June
Grass—mid-May–mid-July
Weeds, ragweed—August–October

Southeast

Trees—February–May
  Pecan, gum, maples, oak—March–May
Grass, Bermuda grass—March–September
Ragweed—August–October

Central Plains

Trees—January–May
  Ash, oak—January–May
  Walnut, mulberry, pecan—March–May
Grass—Same as East and South
Weeds, ragweed—August–October

Rocky Mountains

Trees—January–June
  Elm—February–April
  Alder—March–April
  Poplar—April–May
Grass—May–July (Decrease with altitude)
Weeds—Few above 5,000 feet

Southwest

Trees—February–April (Ash, poplar, cypress, mesquite)
Grass—All warm months
Weeds, ragweed—July–October

California

Trees—January–April (Alder, acacia, poplar)
Grass—March–November
Weeds, ragweed—July–October

Northwest Coast

Trees—January–June
  Alder, willow, ash—February–April
  Birch, poplar, elm—March–June
Grass—May–August
Weeds, ragweed—August–September (Low amounts—almost ragweed-free)

Reducing exposure to pollens

After a rain, pollen is low.

After long periods of fair weather, pollen is higher.

Ragweed grows in fields, parking areas, vacant lots.

Avoid hiking in fields during peak season.

Avoid planting trees to which children are allergic. Plant insect-pollinated varieties such as locust, Norway maple, and so on.

Close windows during pollen season.

Use air conditioning and filters if necessary.

Electrostatic cleaners can help some children, but are expensive.

The doctor

If kids still have bad allergic symptoms after removing or avoiding the allergen, the doctor may prescribe a plain antihistamine or an antihistamine combined with a decongestant (see page 379). Antihistamines block the histamine reaction and decongestants help to relieve stuffiness. But antihistamines often make people feel sleepy and cranky and make their mouths feel dry. These side effects may be such a bother that many people would rather not take them. Doctors may also prescribe epinephrinelike medicines such as Sudafed or Ephedrine, which shrink the membranes lining the nose. Doctors do not advise using nose drops or aerosol sprays for a long time because they can cause damage to the delicate membrane lining the nose.

Sometimes doctors recommend a series of allergy shots for kids who are very allergic or who have ear problems (see Glue ear, page 324) caused by their allergy. The idea is to get the body "used to" the allergen by starting with tiny amounts and building up. Some doctors feel that allergy shots work so well that they suggest that anyone with hay fever get them.

Prevention

Hay fever and household-dust allergies often are inherited from parents. Doctors now think that some allergies may be avoided if mothers in allergic households avoid having babies in late autumn, breastfeed, avoid eating allergic foods while pregnant and nursing, and avoid giving allergic foods to their babies for the first year. Doctors also say that families who have histories of allergies or eczema (see page 295) should avoid having animals and control the house for dust until the baby is a year old. Smoking shouldn't be permitted in the house. Older children who are already allergic may prevent symptoms by avoiding whatever they are allergic to (see Household dust and pollen control charts).

Household allergy control

Concentrate on rooms where the child spends most of his or her time (bedroom, TV room, dining room).

Eliminate dust catchers in the bedroom, such as books and clothes.

Bedding should be washable and synthetic; avoid flannel and wool.

Curtains should be smooth and washable.

Avoid long pile carpet or shaggy rugs.

Frequent vacuuming and cleaning of surfaces are useful. (Dust daily with a damp cloth.)

Allergic children should not help to dust.

Pillows should be polyester or encased in plastic.

Heating units in the child's room should be closed at night if possible.

Heating ducts should be cleaned periodically.

Mattresses should be covered in plastic, then with a pad.

Moist areas should be washed with Lysol or Clorox to eliminate molds and fungi (every three months).

Sometimes crawl spaces or basements can be cleaned and washed if the child is especially allergic to molds and fungi.

Keep pets outdoors or out of the child's bedroom.

Do not brush animals in the house.

Avoid fur coats.

Avoid furniture stuffed with animal-hair, down pillows in the child's bedroom.

The child should bathe after playing in weeds.

Eliminate flowering plants next to the child's window, and close windows during pollen season.

Avoid pyrethrum and Kapok.

Vent clothes dryer outside.

Avoid all smoking in the house.

Food allergies

What's happening

A few children are allergic to certain foods that don't bother most other children. When they eat these foods they may get a rash, their eyes may swell, or they may even have trouble breathing. Some children vomit or have diarrhea from the food they're allergic to. These allergic reactions come on within an hour or two of eating the food. What the children are reacting to is one protein or substance in a food, not the whole food. When children are allergic to one kind of food—oranges, for example— they are often allergic to other foods in the same family, such as grape-fruits. This is especially true with fruit and vegetable allergies.

If children have very strong allergic reactions it is usually fairly easy to figure out the food to which they are allergic. But if their symptoms are mild, it is much harder to determine which food is causing the reaction.

Many so-called food allergies aren't really allergies at all. The symptoms are caused by other chemicals in the food rather than by allergic nutrients. These chemicals don't cause a true allergic reaction; they make the body sick like side effects from a drug. One example is chocolate. It contains caffeine, which can cause headaches, nervousness, and stomachaches. If kids don't feel well after eating a certain food or don't like its taste, it does *not* necessarily mean that they are allergic to that food.

Food allergies work in the same way as other allergies (see page 326). The allergic protein, or antigen, is recognized by the body and causes white blood cells to make antibodies. The antibodies attach themselves to the antigens and then lock on to mast cells in the skin, intestines, and lining of the nose and lungs. The mast cells send out large amounts of

Signs and symptoms

Mild

Skin rash

Itchy eyes

Swollen eyes

Diarrhea

Vomiting

Tiredness

Joint aches

Crankiness

Severe (This is an emergency—call the doctor)

Trouble breathing

Fainting

Itching all over

Foods that act like drugs

Bananas, tomatoes, avocados, pineapples, and cheese (cheddar, Camembert) have proteins that change blood flow.

Chocolate can cause headaches.

Coffee, cocoa, tea, cola, Dr Pepper, Mountain Dew, and chocolate have caffeine, which can cause headaches, nervousness, and stomachaches.

Artificial colors can cause hyperactivity in a few children who are allergic.

Foods with monosodium glutamate (MSG) can cause headaches and chest and face pains.

Very large amounts of licorice can cause high blood pressure and heart disease.

Allergic foods

Citrus—oranges, lemons, grapefruit

Cola—chocolate, cola

Gourds—melons, cucumber, squash

Grains—wheat, corn, rye, oats, rice

Legumes—peanuts, peas, alfalfa, clover, licorice

Poultry—turkey, chicken, duck and/or their eggs

Fish—flounder, halibut

Meat—cow, goat, sheep, and/or their milk

Food dyes, aspirin, preservatives (benzoic acid)

histamine, which causes swelling and increases blood flow and mucous production. This is how a food can cause a rash, swollen eyes, diarrhea, or breathing trouble.

Helping yourself

If children have a severe allergic reaction to a particular food, they should *not* be given that food again and the doctor should be called. The treat-

Isolating a food allergy

Eliminate a single suspicious food for seven to ten days (watch for this food in processed foods), then reintroduce it.

Eliminate other members of that food family at the same time; for example, *all* fish.

Eliminate several foods at once—for example, milk, chocolate, cola. Do this for two weeks. If symptoms disappear you can reintroduce the foods one at a time.

Keep track of symptoms during each food trial period.

You must read labels to really eliminate a food.

A parent can give a child an "allergic food" in the morning and watch the child for one day to see if the child is really allergic. This should *not* be done if the child has had a serious allergic reaction, like trouble breathing.

ment for food allergies is to have children avoid the food that gives them allergic reactions. At the same time, they need to eat other foods that can give them the same vitamins, minerals, and proteins. It's important to be sure children are really allergic to a food before they are told never to eat it.

The doctor

When children have very severe allergic reactions to a food it can be a true medical emergency (see Bee stings, page 344). The doctor will give epinephrine and antihistamines to stop the allergic reaction and make breathing easier.

Most doctors determine whether children are allergic to a food by having them stop eating it and watching to see if the allergic reaction stops. If the allergic reaction is very mild, the doctor may tell the children to try the food again and have their parents write down exactly what happens when they eat the food. If it is really hard to figure out what food is causing the allergic reaction, the doctor may tell the parents to withhold whole groups of foods, one after another, until the problem food is identified.

Prevention

Once children are allergic, the only way to prevent food allergies is to avoid the food.

Asthma

What's happening

Children who have asthma sometimes have trouble breathing. Most of the time these kids breathe normally, but once in a while they have an attack during which they find it hard to breathe because the air passages, or tubes, in their lungs temporarily become smaller.

Three things make the lung passages smaller: (1) The lining of the passages swells up; (2) the swollen passages put out a thick mucus, and (3) the muscles around the passages tighten and squeeze the tubes. Doctors think that these three events occur because the lining of asthmatic kids' air passages is very sensitive. These children react to things around them that don't bother other kids. They may be allergic to tiny particles they breathe in, like dust, or to certain foods they eat, like chocolate; or they may react to other conditions, like having a cold or becoming upset. Any of these situations may alert the lining of the sensitive passages. The lining reacts by releasing a chemical called histamine. It is the histamine that causes the lining to swell, tighten, and produce mucus.

When the passages start to close down, it becomes hard for the children

Signs and symptoms

Trouble breathing, especially breathing out

Wheezing

Coughing

to breathe out. The air going out makes a squeaky sound, like air going out of the narrow part of a whistle. This wheezing noise and difficulty breathing always happen during an asthma attack.

Most asthmatic kids begin to have attacks or periods of breathing difficulty before they are six. Kids vary a lot in how often they get attacks and how bad the attacks are, just as they vary in what sets off an attack.

With good care many asthmatic children can completely prevent asthma attacks. A third to a half of all asthmatic kids stop having attacks by the time they are teen-agers. Another group stops having asthma attacks but continues to be allergic to dust, pollens, or certain foods.

Helping yourself

Different things cause asthma attacks in different children. In order to treat asthma and avoid attacks, kids and their parents need to learn what situations usually set off an attack. Parents and kids should limit or remove only whatever causes the attacks. This gives asthmatic children the most freedom and involves the least work. For example, a child whose attacks are *only* set off by hard running probably won't have to live in a dust-free house. Moreover, that child may not have to avoid all sports, just ones that require lots of running.

It is good for asthmatic kids to drink lots of fluids all the time, and especially when they have a cough. Fluids help to thin out the mucus in their lungs and make it easier to cough it up.

All kids who have asthma tend to become upset and afraid during attacks. Doctors have found that being upset makes the air passages close down. So it's important for asthmatic kids to learn to relax and not be afraid when they are having trouble breathing. Relaxing actually makes breathing easier. Many asthmatic kids find it helpful to learn and practice relaxation exercises when they are *not* having an attack, so they'll be able to relax automatically if they start to have difficulty breathing.

Like all diseases, asthma is affected by what and how kids think. Doctors have found that some kids will have an attack if they *think* they are going to. A study was done in which children had plain water sprayed in their noses, but they were told that it was the pollen that they were allergic to. A number of children then had attacks. These kids quickly got better when more water was sprayed in their noses and they were told it was their asthma medicine. These kids were really allergic to pollen, and they did have sensitive air passages. But these experiments show how much control the *mind* can have over asthma.

When asthmatic children know that they can have some influence over their attacks, they are better able to relax and practice the kind of deep breathing that will make them better. It is very important that older children realize just how much control they have over their attacks, and take care to avoid whatever sets off their attacks, and practice relaxing and deep breathing when they occur. Doctors have also found that asthmatic

Causes of asthma attacks

Allergy—foods, dust, insects, insect bites, fungi, molds, drugs

Irritation—paint fumes, hair sprays, chemicals, air pollution, smoke, perfumes, cold air

Weather changes

Viral infections

Exercise—running, bike riding, cross-country skiing

Emotion

Chemicals—aspirin, yellow dye #5

Combinations of the above

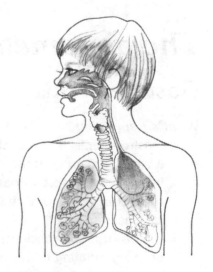

When people have asthma attacks, the air passages in their lungs swell and fill with mucus. This makes it harder for them to breathe.

kids tend to get better when family problems are solved, and the household becomes less hectic and tense.

The doctor

The doctor has many powerful medicines that can help children breathe during an asthma attack. Some medicines, called *broncodilators,* open up the air passages. They come in liquid or pill form, or in inhalers.

If an asthma attack doesn't get better with home treatment, it can be a real medical emergency and the children *must* be seen by a doctor. The doctor will give a shot of epinephrine, which will immediately make the children's breathing easier. Epinephrine relaxes the muscles around the air passages and reduces the swelling of the passage lining. In serious attacks, children may even have to be put in the hospital and given oxygen to breathe as well as intravenous fluids and medicine.

Prevention

Because doctors still don't know exactly what causes asthma, they can't stop kids from becoming asthmatic. But asthmatic kids and their parents can learn to control the disease and prevent attacks. Prevention involves learning and avoiding what sets off attacks. This includes household control and lowering stress. Learning to relax and picture calm scenes has helped many kids improve their asthma. It is also important to treat colds promptly because they can set off attacks in some children.

The abdomen

Gastroenteritis

What's happening

Gastroenteritis is an infection of the digestive system caused by bacteria or a virus. It often goes along with a head cold or cough, but it can occur by itself. Just as a sore throat, runny nose, and cough are symptoms of a head cold, so a stomachache, vomiting, and diarrhea are typical signs of a stomach flu.

The viruses or bacteria produce chemical substances called toxins that are very irritating to the lining of the digestive tract. Occasionally foods that are rotten or very spicy can have the same effect. Even worry or nervousness, which causes the stomach to secrete acid, can produce the same signs or symptoms.

When the lining of the digestive tract becomes irritated, tiny glands in the wall produce mucus to protect the lining. At the same time, the

Signs and symptoms

Stomachache

Nausea

Vomiting

Diarrhea

Fever

Loss of appetite

Muscle aches

Tiredness

Cold symptoms (maybe)

muscles in the wall contract strongly. The contractions lead to another set of movements that tend to push the food backward and up. Then partly digested food from the upper intestine may be pushed backward into the stomach. Meanwhile, nerves in the walls of the stomach and upper intestine send messages of nausea to the brain and trigger the vomiting reflex. The passage to the lungs is automatically closed off, the valve at the top of the stomach opens, and the stomach and diaphragm squeeze sharply, sending the food up and out.

If the irritation isn't strong enough to cause the food to be pushed back, it may cause the food to travel on through the intestines very quickly. Because there is no time for water to be absorbed in the intestines, the person has diarrhea. Stomach flu usually gets better within several days. The body has powerful antibodies that kill the bacteria or viruses. Then the lining of the digestive tract returns to normal.

Helping yourself

The basic treatment for stomach flu is to let the digestive tract rest and heal itself. After vomiting or diarrhea, children should not eat solid foods until their symptoms stop. For vomiting, children should drink *small* amounts of clear fluids, like water or apple juice. Children who have diarrhea should drink as much fluid as they can. If necessary the liquid diet can be continued for up to two days.

As the symptoms get better and the children become hungry, they can begin to eat small amounts of bland foods like dry toast. Until they are completely better, they should avoid large meals, fruits, milk, and spicy, irritating foods.

Diet for stomach flu

For vomiting
Give very small amounts of clear fluids until vomiting slows, then start bland foods.

For diarrhea
Stop solid foods and start clear fluids—water, soda (flat, without bubbles), apple juice, bouillon.

Continue clear fluids for up to two days.

Stop milk, which is hard to digest.

When diarrhea slows, start feeding bland foods such as rice, bananas, applesauce, crackers, toast, dry cereals without sugar.

Stop fruits (apricots, prunes) that can cause loose stools.

The doctor

The doctor is rarely needed to treat gastroenteritis. But the doctor should be called if the parents think the child is losing more fluid than he or she is taking in. A child who loses large amounts of fluids can become dehydrated, or low in water. This rarely happens to children over two. Doctors have powerful drugs that can stop vomiting and diarrhea in severe cases.

Prevention

There is no way to prevent stomach flu, but children who eat well and get enough rest and exercise are probably less likely to catch it. Stomach flu is generally very contagious, and kids who have it should stay home so they don't pass it to others. While children are sick they can easily spread the virus or bacteria if they don't wash their hands after they go to the bathroom. The germs from the digestive tract come out when they throw up or have diarrhea. When children wipe themselves or clean up, it's easy for the germs to pass to their hands and to other people. This is what makes cleanliness so important. In countries that don't have running water to wash with, diarrhea spreads easily and can be a serious disease among babies.

Childhood diseases

Chicken pox

What's happening

Chicken pox is a childhood disease caused by a virus. It is so easy to catch that nine out of ten kids get it when they are exposed to it for the first time, which means they almost always get it while they are young.

Generally kids get a runny nose, a slight fever, and tiredness, but sometimes they may not have, or may not notice, these early symptoms. One or two days later they get a rash; it starts as red dots, which then turn into tiny, clear, fluid-filled pimples, like water drops on a red base. Eventually the pimples burst, scab over, and finally disappear. The rash starts on the middle of the body and appears later on the face, arms, and legs. At one point all the different stages of the pimples can be seen—dots, drops, scabs. New pimples keep appearing for three or four days and can take two weeks to disappear completely. Even though the pimples look strange, they disappear without a scar unless they become infected. Pimples sometimes become infected when they are scratched.

Kids with chicken pox can spread the virus to others for 5 days before the rash and 6 days after. Kids get sick 2 to 3 weeks (11 to 21 days) after they've been exposed to someone who has chicken pox. Once people

Signs and symptoms

Rash with red dots, fluid-filled pimples, and scabs on the middle of the body first, then the arms, legs, face

Runny nose

Fever

Tiredness

have had chicken pox, their bodies make special antibodies and they can never catch it again.

Helping yourself

Chicken pox can range from a few dots to many. If it is a mild case with few dots, or if the child is not uncomfortable, no help is necessary. If children are very itchy they may find it makes them more comfortable if they take a cool bath with a cup of baking soda in the water or put on calamine lotion. Also, if kids cover up with lightweight clothes they may forget the pimples and feel less itchy. Kids should remember not to scratch because the pimples might become infected. And they should wash their hands often with soap and water, and keep their fingernails trimmed and clean.

The doctor

The doctor is usually not necessary to diagnose or treat chicken pox, but should be called if a child seems extremely sick or has pimples that become badly infected.

Prevention

There is no vaccine to prevent chicken pox. Little can be done aside from staying away from kids who are contagious. Although the disease is very easy to catch its symptoms are usually mild.

The chicken pox rash begins on the middle of the body and later appears on the face, arms, and legs.

Mumps

What's happening

Mumps is an infection of one or both of the big saliva glands, the *parotids*, which are located under the ears. It is caused by a virus. Kids with mumps have a lot of swelling where the back of the jaw meets the ear. The swelling is often painful and can make swallowing uncomfortable. The swelling increases for two or three days and goes away within a week. Kids sometimes develop a fever and cold symptoms, too.

Mumps is very contagious, but almost half the kids who get it never show any symptoms, so they don't know they have had it. Kids can spread mumps virus from 6 days before to 9 days after the swelling begins. Kids develop mumps 12 to 26 days after they come into contact with the virus.

Once kids have the mumps, whether on one or both sides, their bodies build up antibodies so they can't get it again. Because mumps can be more uncomfortable when kids are older, some doctors now suggest that

Signs and symptoms

Swelling where the jaw meets the ear (possibly painful)

Trouble swallowing

Fever

10- to 12-year-olds get a shot of mumps vaccine if they have not yet had the disease.

Helping yourself

Generally no treatment is necessary for mumps. Your body heals itself automatically. If a child is uncomfortable, aspirin may help to relieve the pain. Kids should eat soft foods that don't require much chewing. It may also be good to avoid acid foods like oranges and grapefruits because they may make the parotid glands produce more saliva.

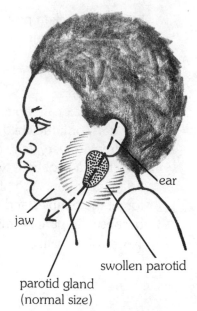

The doctor

The doctor isn't needed for mumps unless a child is very sick, especially with a headache, backache, or stomachache. These may be signs that the infection has spread to other parts of the body. This is very unusual and not likely to be dangerous.

Mumps is an infection of the parotid salivary gland, which is located where the back of the jaw meets the ear. The gland becomes swollen, making it uncomfortable to swallow.

Prevention

A vaccine is now available that is generally given to babies during the second year. Older kids who have not been vaccinated and have not had mumps should either stay away from kids who are contagious or be vaccinated.

Measles, German measles

We have not included discussions of measles and German measles because almost all children between the ages of 5 and 12 have been immunized against these diseases.

Chapter 9

Common accidents

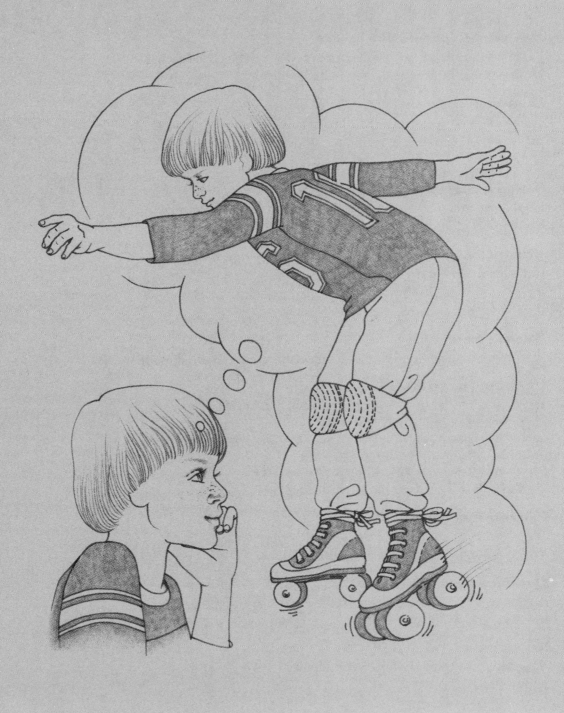

Quick emergency first-aid

For further emergency instructions turn to the pages listed below.

Animal bites (page 341)
Wash carefully, identify the animal.

Bee stings (page 344)
Remove the stinger, apply ice or cool water. If the child has trouble breathing or itches all over, call the doctor.

Bleeding and cuts (page 351)
Take out large sticks, glass, and so on, wash with a lot of water, press on cut with gauze or cloth to stop bleeding. Soak a puncture wound.

Blood under the nail (page 358)
Heat a paperclip to hot and lightly touch it to the nail over the black area.

Bumps, sprains, and broken bones (page 345)
Put a splint on a possible break, then raise the affected area above the body if possible. Put ice on a bump or sprain, raise above the body and rest.

Burns (page 349)
Put on ice or ice water (if a large area is affected, call the doctor).

Choking (page 365)
Put the child over your knees face down and whack the center of his or her back four times. If this does not work, turn child over and press on the center of the lower rib cage hard three times.

Drowning or electric shock (page 367)
If breathing or heartbeat stops, do resuscitation, call for help.

Eye injuries (page 355)
Wash out the eye, look for the object by opening the eyelid. Touch it lightly with a cotton swab to remove.

Head injuries (page 359)
Apply ice on bump, call doctor if the child is unconscious or behaves unusually after regaining consciousness.

Nosebleeds (page 362)
Squeeze nose firmly between thumb and forefinger for five minutes.

Emergency advice

Most accidents are not serious and they do not have to be dealt with in seconds. This means there is plenty of time for the parent and child to calm down. Relaxation should be the first step in treating all accidents except when a child has actually stopped breathing or is bleeding severely.

Many accidents can be prevented. Awareness is the key to prevention. Accidents frequently happen during periods of family stress. Fatigue and tension often play a role. Parents should resolve potential problems such as open fire pits, children's access to beehives, and boards with nails sticking out. And children need to learn safety rules for bike riding and using sharp tools like knives. The most common cause of severe illness and death in the 5- to 12-year-old age group is automobile accidents. So the single most important thing parents and children can do to prevent injury is to wear seat belts.

Emergency advice for the parent and child

Being calm will help you handle the emergency more effectively and will help the child's natural healing mechanisms set to work. It will also make both of you feel better.

Relax: Take several deep breaths. With each breath, let your body relax. With each breath, feel calmness and confidence flow into your body. Feel quiet and clarity surround you. Whenever you feel upset, picture the most peaceful scene you can think of for a brief moment.

Tell the child: You are all right. Your body knows what to do. You can help your body by being calm and breathing in slowly and evenly. Let your body feel as if it's floating. Imagine the hurt going out of your body every time you breathe out. Imagine the bleeding stopping the way a faucet stops dripping. Rest quietly and imagine a favorite scene.

Animal bites

What's happening

Most animal bites are not serious. In fact, many do not even break the skin. Bites are a bit more susceptible to infection than regular cuts, because an animal's saliva may have germs. But most animal diseases can't be caught by people. Surprisingly, human bites (from other children)

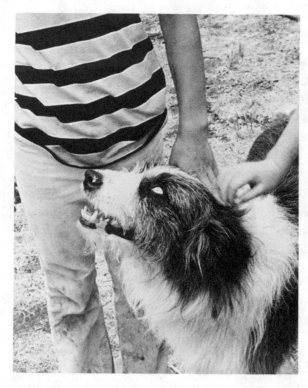

Unfamiliar animals should be treated with careful consideration to avoid being bitten.

are even more likely to get infected. This is because human saliva carries many germs, all of which other people can catch.

The most serious disease people can get from an animal bite is *rabies*. Rabies is very rare among pet animals in the United States, and animals who are vaccinated can't give you rabies. But wild animals can, especially skunks, bats, and foxes. Rabies is a virus that affects the nervous system. The virus is carried in the saliva of rabid animals. To transmit the virus, the bite must break the skin. An animal who is sick with rabies will behave strangely. It may walk in an unusual manner, act irritable, or chew on objects like dirt, stones, and sticks. The saliva around its mouth may be frothy.

Only one or two cases of people with rabies are reported in this country each year. But it is important to identify any animal that has bitten someone. If it is a household pet, the owner should be called to make sure the animal has been vaccinated. If it is a wild animal, it should be trapped or shot. The county health department will send someone out to catch the animal and test it for rabies.

Helping yourself

All bites should be carefully scrubbed with soap and warm water. First the wound should be held under running water for several minutes, then it should be submerged in a bucket or sinkful of warm soapy water for several more minutes.

Most animal bites that do not tear will not bleed badly. Bleeding can be stopped by pressing a bandage or tissues directly over the wound. Usually bite wounds tend to close by themselves. So the biggest problem is "locking in" germs that will cause infection. The bleeding actually helps to carry out the germs and clean the wound. To prevent infection, an animal bite should be soaked in warm water for 10 to 15 minutes at a time, several times a day. This is especially important if there are any signs of infection, such as redness or swelling.

The doctor

Any bite from a wild animal or from an unidentified pet should be reported to a doctor. Any bite that is torn or that is very deep should be seen by a doctor. The doctor will clean the wound very carefully, possibly even squirting an antiseptic solution into the teeth marks. If the bite leaves a big gaping wound, the doctor will probably put in sutures or stitches to close it.

The doctor will give the child a tetanus booster if it has been more than five years since the last shot. If there is some question of rabies, the doctor may give a single shot of human immune serum in the arm. In those rare cases in which rabies is proven in an animal or strongly suspected, a person may be given a shot of antirabies serum and a series of 14 to 21 shots of a rabies vaccine, which was first developed by Louis Pasteur. This treatment is not begun until the animal has been quarantined and observed.

Prevention

Many animal bites can be avoided if children learn the right way to treat animals and what to expect from them. It's only common sense that an animal will growl and possibly bite if you step on it, disturb it while it is eating, or tease it. And just because your dog or cat loves to be wrestled with doesn't mean you can expect the same thing of a strange animal. Never approach a dog with your hand over its head—the dog may react as though you are about to hit it. If you are trying to make friends with a strange dog, hold your hand out low so the animal can sniff your hand, *then* pat the dog on the back. And with a cat, stop playing when it begins to snap its tail back and forth. Don't wait until it hisses or pounces.

If you see an animal that is acting strangely but hasn't bitten anyone, don't hesitate to report it. If the animal is rabid, you will be helping to stop the spread of the disease. And just as important, make sure your own animals are properly vaccinated every year. Vaccination of cats and dogs is the most important part of rabies prevention in this country.

Bee stings

What's happening

Almost everyone gets stung by a bee, yellow jacket, or hornet at some time. Being stung can hurt a lot and be scary, but usually it's not serious. The insect's stinger, which is like a tiny needle, is connected to a venom sac. The little bit of venom squirted under the skin causes nearby blood cells to break, makes pain nerves hurt, and causes small blood vessels to leak out fluid. This is what causes the redness, pain, and swelling of a sting. The bee's stinger has a barb, or hook, on the end, which makes the stinger stay in. Losing its stinger kills the bee. Wasps, yellow jackets, and hornets don't have barbs and don't lose their stingers.

A few people gradually become very allergic to bee and wasp venom. These people react as if the sting were really dangerous. Their whole body releases a chemical called histamine which makes them red and itchy. Often allergic people will swell under their eyes, and sometimes they even have trouble breathing. *An allergic reaction to a sting can be a true medical emergency.* The doctor should be called immediately.

Helping yourself

A simple bite gets better by itself, but there are several measures that will make a person more comfortable. If it is a bee bite, the stinger can be removed with tweezers. To keep the swelling down and numb the area, an ice pack can be held against the bite. Calamine lotion or a paste of baking soda and water will help to stop the itching.

The doctor

A doctor should be called immediately if the child develops an allergic reaction to the bite. A lot of itching or swelling *far away from* the bite, feeling sick to the stomach, or any trouble breathing are signs of allergic reaction. The doctor will give the child a shot of epinephrine, which stops the swelling and makes breathing easier. Often the doctor will tie a tourniquet or a cuff above the bite to keep the venom from getting to the rest of the body. He may also give the child an antihistamine, another drug that helps to stop the allergic reaction.

If it is a serious allergic reaction, the doctor will give the child a special emergency kit that contains a premeasured shot of epinephrine, a tourniquet, and an antihistamine pill. The doctor will teach the child how to use the needle and when it is necessary to use it. Many doctors also recommend a series of allergy shots, which tend to make people less and less allergic to bee stings.

Prevention

Children should learn to identify insects that sting and should know not to tease them or play around them. When a number of bees or wasps are seen nearby, parents should find the nest. A ground nest can be destroyed by pouring in gas and setting it afire. This should be done after dark when all the insects are in the nest. A beehive can be removed by an exterminator or a beekeeper.

Bumps, sprains, and broken bones

What's happening

Kids between 6 and 12 tend to have lots of physical energy, which they pour out in running, climbing, bike riding, skating, and sports. And at some point these activities result in accidents. Kids fall, bump into something, or "land wrong."

Generally these accidents are minor and result in bumps, black-and-blue marks, or sore muscles. Doctors call this mild kind of injury a *contusion*. Skin and muscle are soft body tissues. When they are hit or squeezed hard, the tiny blood vessels inside break. Blood leaks out of the vessels and goes into the spaces between muscle and skin cells. The blood cells die and darken. This is what causes the common color of the black-and-blue mark. Most hard bumps also involve swelling. The injury starts the release of histamine, a natural chemical that causes large amounts of fluid to come out of the cells in the hurt area. The fluid clots and walls off the injury, protecting the rest of the body. Within a few minutes, white blood cells pour into the area and begin to carry off the dead and injured cells. Eventually this clears up the swelling and the black-and-blue mark completely. But a large bruise can take a week or more to go away totally.

Another kind of injury children get is a *sprain* or *strain*. A sprain is actually the stretching of a ligament—the strong band of tissue that holds joints together. A strain occurs when a muscle gets stretched too far. Most strains and sprains affect the knee or the ankle. Once in a while a joint can be stretched so far the bones pull apart. Doctors call this a *dislocation*. These injuries happen when kids bend in the wrong way or stretch too far. The most common dislocations happen to the elbow. Dislocations also cause broken blood vessels and swelling, which can make the joint tender and difficult to move. Strains and sprains can take days, weeks, or even months to heal, depending on whether a muscle or ligament is torn.

Occasionally when children fall with a great deal of force or at a strange angle, they fracture or break a bone. Sometimes a break is obvious because the bone is in an unusual position. If the bone is not broken all the way through, the break may not be so obvious, and may be hard to distinguish from a sprain, strain, or bruise. Generally a break is a more severe injury. *There are certain signs that make it more likely that a break has happened: if the bone is crooked, if it is very difficult to move, if it is very sore in one place, or if there is a lot of swelling.*

The body has amazing abilities to heal broken bones. Most of the healing is completed within a matter of weeks. And in less than a year there is no trace of the break. Like a bruise or a sprain, a break causes swelling and broken blood vessels. Dead blood and tissue cells are cleared up within several days by the body's white blood cells. Meanwhile special cells grow across the break. These cells form a mixture of bone and soft cartilage, a temporary "splint," which holds the ends of the bone in place. It is called a *callus*. In time, bone cells fill in where they were before, and the rest of the callus is dissolved. Finally, the bone regains the same strength and shape that it had before (see Bone healing, pages 235–36).

Helping yourself

Bumps: Mild black-and-blue marks need no treatment. The body heals itself within a matter of days. Bumps that are really painful and swollen should be treated with an ice pack. The cold slows blood flow to the area and that keeps down the swelling. The less swelling there is, the easier it is later to move the muscles and ligaments in the injured area. An ice pack can be made by putting ice cubes in a plastic bag and wrapping it in a towel. To really reduce swelling, an ice pack should be applied soon after the injury and kept on for at least 15 minutes.

Sprains: If there is a great deal of pain and swelling, see the doctor or go to an emergency room. To make the person as comfortable as possible and to prevent further injury on the way to the doctor, the joint should be immobilized with a splint.

This X-ray shows a break of both the radius and the ulna in the forearm of an eight-year-old.

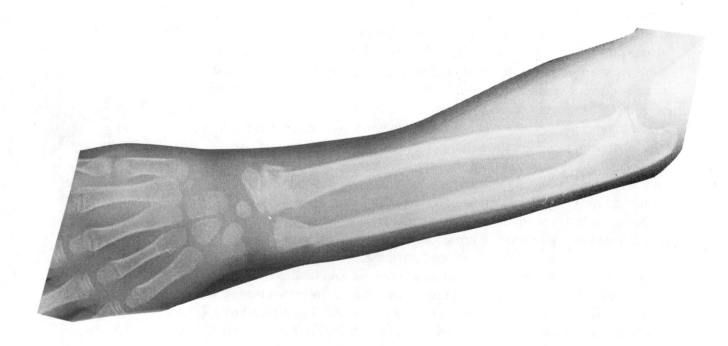

With a sprain, which usually has a great deal of swelling, the ice pack should be left on for at least a half hour. The joint that has been hurt should be raised in a comfortable position that is higher than the heart to reduce swelling. A twisted knee or ankle should be placed on pillows on a chair or in bed. A twisted wrist should be rested on a pillow on a table. The injured area should be allowed to rest until it can be moved without hurting. By about the second day, warm soaks or a heating pad can be applied for 15 minutes at a time. This will increase blood flow and promote healing once the swelling has stopped.

Fractures: If, in addition to pain and swelling, the bones look out of place, a *fracture,* or dislocation, is possible. The doctor should be called and the child should be splinted. Unless the child is in *shock* (very pale, confused, with cold moist skin) or not breathing, a break is not an emergency in which seconds or minutes count. In fact, the first thing is to make the child more comfortable, and help *everyone* to relax. The child should be reassured that broken bones heal readily, especially in children, that it will not take long to "set" the break, and that there will be less pain as soon as the bone is set.

The doctor

First the doctor will look at the injury and ask questions about how it happened. The doctor will gently feel all around and move the injured

This X-ray shows the same arm after it has been set and has been healing for about three weeks. In another three weeks the cast will be removed.

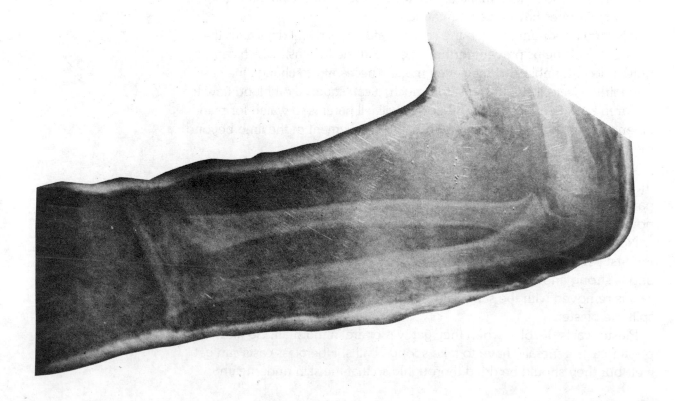

area. Based on this exam, the doctor will have X-rays taken if he suspects there is a break. Often, the X-ray technician will take a forward and a side view of an injured limb, and a top view of the other limb to compare them with. This is necessary because children's bones are still growing and their X-rays are harder to "read" or understand.

If a child simply has a mild sprain or strain, the doctor will put on an elastic bandage and possibly a splint to keep the limb from moving and to keep the swelling down. An injured wrist or elbow will be put in a sling. If a knee or ankle is injured, the child may be given crutches in order to help keep weight off the injured area.

A severe sprain or a fracture will be put in a cast which simply keeps the area from moving while the body heals the torn ligaments or broken bone. If a bone is broken, the doctor will straighten the ends if they are not in line. Doctors call this "reducing" the break. The child is given pain medicine and then the doctor aligns the break with a quick tug. It hurts for a moment, then feels much better. A tubelike sock is put over the broken bone, then rolls of soft padding are wound around. Rolls of moist plaster or fiberglass are wound over the padding. The limb is held in a position of relaxation for a short time while the cast material hardens. This is done so it will be easier to move the area when the cast comes off some weeks later. Then the bone is re-X-rayed to make sure it is aligned properly. Finally, the doctor splits the outer layer of the cast with a special vibrating saw. The blade simply shakes back and forth, so it can even be touched directly to a fingernail and it will not cut it. But the blade can get hot from the vibration and it does make a very loud noise. Older saws make a lot of dust; newer ones have a vacuum attached.

It is very important to keep the cast elevated for several days after the accident. This helps prevent further swelling inside the cast, which can be quite uncomfortable and may even make it necessary to change the cast. If the limb swells inside the cast too much, it can squeeze off blood flow to the area and be dangerous. The doctor will tell parents to watch for pain, paleness, tingling or numbness, and painful movement of the limb beyond the cast (usually the fingers or toes).

Often a child with a break will feel uncomfortable for a day or two after the accident and may even run a fever. The doctor may prescribe a mild pain medicine. Usually by the third day a child will begin to feel almost normal and soon be ready to return to school.

Nowadays a plaster cast is often changed to a smaller, lighter cast after the first several weeks. By this time the bone has already begun to heal and is strong enough to hold together while the cast is being changed. The cast is removed with the same vibrating saw that was originally used to split the plaster.

Plaster casts dissolve when they get wet or are in moist air. So kids with plaster casts generally have to take sponge baths. Fiberglass casts can get wet, but they should be dried thoroughly so that the skin underneath doesn't develop sores. It takes about 15 minutes with a hair dryer to completely dry a fiberglass cast and the sock underneath. The cast is dry when the inside no longer feels cool to the child.

While a cast is on, the child can run and play pretty much as usual. But, for about six weeks after the cast comes off, the child must be careful of rebreaking the bone. By the time the cast is removed, a bridge has formed between the broken ends, but it isn't made entirely of hard bone. That happens only as slight pressure is put on the break. Keeping the cast on longer doesn't help because it is the pressure from moving or carrying weight that causes the hard bone to grow. The bone callus, or bump, around the break actually gets bigger for several months after the cast comes off, but finally it dissolves and leaves the bone exactly as it was before the break.

Prevention

Many accidents are avoidable. Children should learn that they can cause or prevent their own accidents. Most accidents happen when children are tired, under stress, or careless. A parent can't always be around to warn kids; they have to learn for themselves to pay attention and not to do things for which they are physically unprepared. Strenuous activities are great when kids have developed the necessary balance and flexibility. But it's crazy to roller skate down a long hill the first time you skate, and it doesn't take a parent to understand that. Kids who are good at hard physical activities have generally built up to them over a long period of time.

Unfortunately many of the most severe bumps, sprains, and breaks take place in automobile accidents. Children and adults are much less likely to have serious injuries if they wear seat belts whenever they ride in a car. More kids are seriously hurt in car accidents than from all rare diseases.

Burns

What's happening

Because burns are much less common than cuts, even minor burns may be very frightening to both kids and parents. But minor burns tend to heal well and are easy to treat. Burns generally go through a series of strange-looking stages as they heal. This is normal and isn't a cause for concern unless the burn becomes infected. Increasing redness, swelling, heat, and pain after the first day are signs of infection.

Burns are divided into three categories based on how serious they are, not on what caused them. The seriousness of a burn depends upon how deep it is and, to some extent, on where it is.

First-degree burns are the least serious. They only involve damage to the outer, or superficial, layers of the skin. First-degree burns appear pink or red, and will turn white (blanch) when pressed on. First-degree burns can be quite painful because they affect the pain nerve endings just under the skin (see diagram, page 131). Such burns are generally the result of a sunburn, a minor scald, or briefly touching a very hot object.

Second-degree burns involve deeper layers of skin and are more serious. A second-degree burn looks blistered or moist and is painful to touch. Second-degree burns are generally caused by scalding liquids or a fire. Both first- and second-degree burns rarely become infected and they tend to heal with little or no scarring.

Third-degree burns are quite serious. They involve all the layers of skin and can even affect muscles or organs under the skin. Third-degree burns actually appear white, dry, or charred. They are painless at first because the nearby pain endings have been destroyed. Third-degree burns can be caused by contact with steam, an open flame, electric current, or strong chemicals.

Helping yourself

First- and second-degree burns that involve only small areas are minor and can be treated at home. The first step is to cool the area as rapidly as possible. Put the burned area under cold running water or apply clean cloths soaked in cold water or ice. Change the cloths frequently to keep them cold. This may be uncomfortable at first, but eventually it will help to relieve the pain and it definitely tends to reduce damage to the skin. Blisters that form should not be removed or popped. They make an ideal protective bandage for the healing area. Moist areas can be covered with clean dry bandages to keep the area clean. Provided the burns are small and do not involve the face, hands, or feet, they can be treated at home with clean bandages every 48 hours.

Large areas of second- or third-degree burns are a medical emergency. They should be briefly washed with cool water and the doctor or the rescue squad should be called immediately. Then the child should be wrapped in a clean sheet and taken to a hospital emergency room.

The doctor

The doctor should be seen for any third-degree burn, as well as for any second-degree burn that covers a big area or involves the face, hands, feet, or genitals. Important body structures lie just under the skin in these areas and the scars that result can affect movement.

If the burns are not too severe, the doctor will wash them and cover them with bandages that contain antibiotics. These gauze pads are changed every two days for about a week.

The doctor will hospitalize anyone with large, serious burns or burns in the special areas mentioned. The person will be given antibiotics to prevent infection and the burn will be cleaned daily to remove dead skin and scabs. This may hurt but it promotes the fastest healing with the least amount of scarring.

Prevention

The most common burns that kids get are from stoves, heaters, and open flames from fires, barbecues, candles, and matches. Electrical wires and caustic chemicals can also cause serious burns. People can even be scalded by hot water from the faucet if a water heater is set too high. Parents need to do everything they can to burn-proof their house, but kids have to learn how burns happen and what they can do to prevent them.

Cuts, scrapes, and puncture wounds

What's happening

The skin is the body's protective covering. Whenever you rub against anything scratchy or sharp, the skin is likely to be broken. Because the skin covers the whole body and because kids are generally very active, all kids get *scrapes*, *cuts* or *puncture wounds* once in a while. Fortunately, most of the skin accidents of childhood are not serious and don't need to be treated by a doctor. The body itself has fantastic powers to stop bleeding and heal cuts in the skin.

The most common and least serious skin accident is a scrape. Only the topmost layers of skin are broken. This is usually caused by rubbing or sliding against something scratchy. Kids fall when they are running or riding bikes and scratch their skin against the pavement or the ground. Although scrapes are the least serious, they can be bloody looking if many little blood vessels are broken. And it can be scary. But that kind of surface bleeding generally stops by itself and doesn't need to be treated by a doctor. Scrapes can be painful because they affect a lot of nerve endings if they cover a large area.

Puncture wounds are breaks in the skin made by sharp, pointed objects. Kids sometimes step on nails or poke themselves with needles or tools like screwdrivers. These wounds leave very little mark on the skin. They can be deep, but most puncture wounds are shallow enough so that they don't require a doctor's treatment. Puncture wounds generally don't bleed much because they don't involve very many blood vessels, and for this reason they don't clean themselves out well. Because the opening is so small, they are hard for you to clean out. So they often become slightly infected by the second day, which makes them sore.

Doctors call cuts *lacerations*. Most lacerations involve only the top layer of skin. Cuts bleed from the broken blood vessels along the edge. When cuts are shallow they don't bleed much and usually stop by themselves. A cut is considered deep if the sides of the cut do not stay together but gap

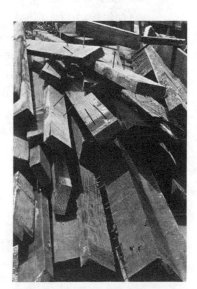

Most puncture wounds are caused by rusty nails.

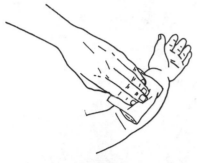

To stop heavy bleeding, put a gauze pad or a clean cloth over the wound and press on it firmly until the bleeding stops. Pressure helps squeeze shut the blood vessels and gives the body time to form a clot.

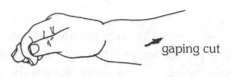

If the sides of a cut do not stay together but gape and look like an open smile, the doctor should be seen.

and look like an open smile. Very deep cuts or lacerations can injure blood vessels, nerves, or tendons underneath the skin. If a tendon is injured, movement will be affected. If a nerve is injured, there may not be feeling in that area. If an artery is injured, blood will come out of the cut in forceful spurts.

As soon as any tiny blood vessel is cut, the muscles in the vessel wall automatically squeeze down, which slows the bleeding. The vessel stays clamped down for about a half hour. This gives smaller cuts time to clot (see Blood clotting, page 232).

Your body can heal a clean cut fairly easily. But if a cut has dirt, pebbles, or glass chips left in it, your body has a harder time healing the cut. Such foreign particles make it more likely the cut will become infected. The body sends extra white blood cells to the area to clean up the foreign particles. This is what causes the swelling, redness, and pus from an infection.

A few hours after a clot is formed, new skin begins to grow from the top down into the cut. Within a week or so the new skin joins both sides of the cut together again.

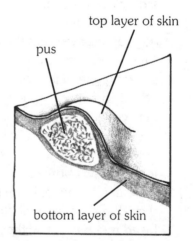

A skin infection is caused by germs getting under the skin and growing there. White blood cells come to eat the germs. Dead skin cells, germs, and white blood cells make up pus.

Helping yourself

The first step is to remove any large pieces of dirt, wood, or glass from the cut. The next step is to see that the bleeding is stopped. The body stops almost all bleeding by itself. But if there is a lot of bleeding, you can help the body by putting a gauze pad or clean cloth over the wound and pressing on it firmly. This pressure helps to squeeze the blood vessel shut,

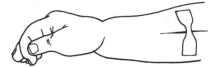

steristrip bandage   stitch (suture)

A steristrip is a kind of bandage that is put on with adhesive glue. It is sometimes strong enough to hold the sides of a cut together without using stitches.

A doctor treats a deep cut with little stitches called sutures. This holds the sides of the cut together while the body heals itself.

giving the clotting process time to work. The pressure should be kept up until the bleeding stops. It also helps to slow bleeding if the wounded area is held higher than the heart. With most cuts, raising and pressing on them will stop the bleeding within 15 minutes. This drops the blood flow in that area and makes it easier for the blood vessels to clamp down and a clot to form. In rare cases where bleeding can't be stopped with direct pressure on the wound, pressure should be put on the area "above" the wound, closer to the heart. This will slow blood from getting to the cut. If the bleeding is at all difficult to stop, the emergency squad or a doctor should be called.

Minor cuts, scrapes, and puncture wounds should be washed carefully with soap and water. The best, and least uncomfortable, way is to soak the cut in a bowl of warm, soapy water. The dirtier the cut, the longer you should soak it. If several minutes of soaking and swishing the cut doesn't remove all the dirt, hold the cut under a stream of running water or rub it gently with a clean washcloth. Careful cleaning lowers the chance of infection.

Redness, swelling, pus, and soreness are signs of infection. Most mild infections will clear up if the injured area is soaked in warm water 2 or 3 times a day for 15 minutes. Warmth increases blood flow to the area, which means more white blood cells are brought in to fight the infection. Soaking is especially important with puncture wounds because they are hard to clean and they often feel sore.

Most small scrapes, cuts, or puncture wounds need no bandage and, in fact, are better off without one. Being exposed to the air helps the cut to dry and scab over. A scab is a natural kind of Band-Aid that falls off when it is no longer needed because new skin has grown underneath it. A bandage may be useful if the cut is likely to be bumped or to get dirt in it. Sometimes kids like to put on a bandage just to cover up the cut. This is not necessary, but probably does no harm.

The doctor

A child should be taken to the doctor or emergency room for any deep puncture wound, especially of the hand, head, chest, or abdomen. The doctor should also be seen for any gaping cut that might need stitches. This is very important for cuts that involve the face or hands. Careful repair of cuts in these areas will minimize scarring and loss of movement. The doctor should definitely be called if a flap of skin such as a fingertip is cut off. Pressure should be applied to the cut to stop the bleeding. Meanwhile the skin flap should immediately be put in ice cold water or salt water (one-half teaspoon of salt to one quart of water). If the skin flap is transported to the doctor in this way, it is likely that a plastic surgeon can stitch it back into place.

The doctor will first evaluate the injury and control the bleeding if necessary. Then the doctor will remove any foreign particles like dirt or glass, and clean the wound thoroughly with a greenish antiseptic solution. If the cut gapes a little but is in an area that doesn't move—like the forehead—the doctor may apply a special bandage called a *steristrip*. This is a kind of adhesive tape that is put on with liquid glue. A steristrip won't stretch or break, so it can keep the two sides of a cut together without using stitches. If the two sides are not brought together, new skin must grow across a larger area, and the scar that is left will be bigger. Because the scar is narrower with a steristrip, the wound will also tend to heal more quickly. A steristrip is left on for 3 to 14 days, until the body has had a chance to close the wound naturally. Then the steristrip is simply peeled off.

If a cut is in an area of movement or is too long or too deep, the doctor will close the wound with stitches, or sutures. Before beginning to put in the sutures, the doctor will numb the pain nerves in the area by injecting an anesthetic into the sides of the wound. This may be a bit uncomfortable for a minute, but it means the stitches won't hurt and the doctor can take the time to put them in carefully. If the wound is very deep, the doctor may put in a layer of stitches under the skin. Each stitch is put in separately, knotted, and then cut off. The stitches are put in at equal distances. In certain areas, like the face, many stitches of fine thread are put in close together because that leaves less of a scar.

The actual number of stitches is not really important because the wound does not heal from end to end, but from one side of the cut to the other. So a three-inch cut will heal no faster than a six-inch cut. Wounds, especially deep ones, should be sutured within a few hours if possible. If sutures are not put in for many hours, the chances of infection increase, and healing tends to be slower. A sutured wound is usually bandaged to protect it and keep out dirt.

Depending on where the cut is, the stitches will be taken out between the fourth and tenth days. Only outside stitches are removed. The doctor simply lifts the stitch a little with tweezers, cuts it with scissors, then gives a little tug with the tweezers to pull out the thread. This whole process doesn't hurt. In fact, some people say it feels itchy.

Usually a child who is brought to the doctor for a cut will be given a tetanus shot to protect against infection from tetanus bacteria, which live in the soil. If the child had a basic tetanus series as a baby, he or she will simply be given a booster or helper shot. If a tetanus shot has never been given, the child will receive a special immunization.

If the wound shows any signs of infection like redness, swelling, heat, or pus, the doctor will prescribe an antibiotic. Occasionally, if a wound develops a large white *abscess,* which is a bump filled with pus, the doctor will prick it to drain out the pus and help speed healing.

Prevention

Getting cuts, scrapes, and even puncture wounds seems to be an unavoidable part of growing up. Most of the wounds are not serious and are not easily prevented. Certainly a child shouldn't refuse to ride a bike for fear of falling and getting scraped. But kids and parents should take some care to avoid serious or needless accidents. Children should not play in areas where there are dangerous nails or pointed objects that could cause puncture wounds. And kids should learn the proper way to handle tools like knives, scissors, screwdrivers, and saws.

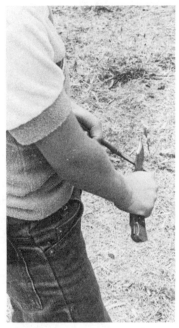

Children need to learn how to work with sharp tools safely.

Eye injuries

What's happening

The eyes are naturally protected by the eyelids and eyelashes, and by a reflex action that automatically causes the eyes to blink whenever something comes very close to them. But children occasionally get something in the eye like dirt, sand, or sawdust. The eye naturally reacts to such a foreign body by trying to get rid of it. A reflex immediately starts tears to flow from the tear gland at the upper, outer corner of the eye (see page 196). The tears wash across the eye and down into a duct in the inner corner of the eye. This duct drains into the back of the nose.

Usually such tearing is very effective and washes out the object, but sometimes the object remains. When something is stuck in the eye, little nerve endings send pain signals to your brain. These nerve endings make it so uncomfortable to have something caught in your eye that you have to do something about it. This protects you from leaving something in your eye that could really hurt it.

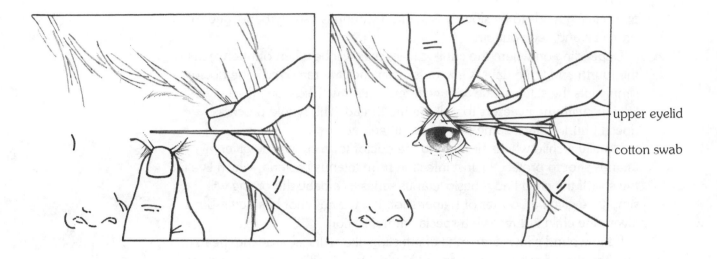

upper eyelid

cotton swab

Occasionally serious injuries to the eye can endanger a person's sight. A cut of the eye or eyelid, a splinter stuck in the eye, chemicals in the eye, or burns near the eye are cause for concern. Blood in the eye caused by a hit or a fall can also be serious. If any of these things happen, you should immediately tell your parents, and a doctor should be called. Most eye injuries are not serious, but there is no sense in taking chances with your sight.

To find something stuck under the upper eyelid, roll the lid up over a cotton swab.

Helping yourself

If your eye can't naturally remove a foreign body with its tears, you may be able to do it yourself. First try to wash it out with cool water. Use an eyecup or cup your clean hand under your open eye and let the water flow into it. Blink several times, then gently rub your finger across your eyelid from the outer corner toward the nose. Often this frees an object that is stuck under the top lid.

If a foreign body can't be washed out in this way, the next step is to try to find it. Tell your parents exactly where it *feels* like the object is. If it's in the middle of your eye, one of your parents may be able to see it by spreading your eyelids apart and having you slowly look in all directions. If it's under the lower lid, he or she can probably lift it out quite easily by pulling out your lower lid and touching the object with a handkerchief or a cotton swab.

Most foreign bodies that are really stuck are caught under the upper lid. To see them and get them out, the upper lid has to be flipped over (see illustration above). Once the object has been located, it usually can be lifted out quite easily with a cotton swab. The swab is moistened slightly and touched very lightly to the particle, then rolled out and away. The swab itself should never be rubbed or pushed across the eye.

If you ever get any kind of chemical or household cleaner sprayed in your eyes, immediately wash your eyes with large amounts of cool water. Cup your hands under your eyes and let the water run into your open eyes for at least five minutes. Meanwhile, someone else should call the doctor.

The doctor

The doctor should be called if you get any kind of strong chemicals in your eyes or if a foreign body remains stuck in your eye. If there is pain and continuous tearing for more than half an hour, also check with your doctor.

The doctor can evaluate whether a chemical has done any harm to your eye, and will have experience in removing foreign bodies. To help locate something stuck in your eye the doctor may put in a colored dye called *fluorescein,* which makes an object glow a greenish color under a light that emits only ultraviolet rays. An ophthalmologist, a doctor who specializes in eyes, may also look at your eye with a slit lamp, which is a very powerful magnifier with a very bright light.

Prevention

Most serious eye accidents and many minor ones can be prevented by good safety habits. Children should wear safety goggles for all kinds of shop work, such as sanding and cutting, especially when it involves metal. And all long sharp objects (like fishing poles) and sharp tools should be used carefully. Tools are not toys; nor are eyes.

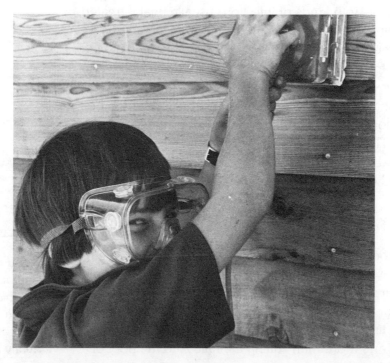

Many eye injuries can be prevented. Safety goggles are recommended for any kind of work that makes dust or chips.

Injuries and infections of the fingers and toes

What's happening

Kids often hurt their fingers and toes by hitting or cutting them or catching them in doors. Very few of these accidents involve broken bones or big cuts. More common is blood under the nail, which happens when a blood vessel breaks inside because of a hard blow or pinch. This is called a *subungual hematoma*, which means bleeding under the nail. Since the nail is hard, the area underneath it can't swell in the usual way. The blood forms a little pool under the nail and that presses on all the pain nerve endings. This pressure can be intensely painful.

Occasionally kids get infections of the finger or toe. An infection near the edge of a nail is called a *paronychia,* or *runaround*. An infection on the bottom of the finger or toe is called a *felon*. Both kinds of infections are caused by staphylococcus bacteria. The first sign is a red, warm, swollen area. Pus may also appear. Since a nail is in the way, these infections can't swell or drain easily and are very painful. Because they are close to the bone, they can be serious if they are not treated.

Helping yourself

If the blue-black blood under the nail does not hurt, nothing has to be done about a subungual hematoma. In a few weeks the body will absorb all of the blood. If the finger or toe really hurts, a hole should be made in the nail to drain out the blood. A parent who is confident can do this at home (see below).

Infections of the fingers and toes should be treated early, before they become painful or serious. Both kinds of infections usually heal if treated with three or four 15-minute soaks a day. This can be done in a bowl or in the bathtub. Warm water will cause the blood vessels in the area to widen. This helps the infection to drain and brings in white blood cells to fight it. When a toenail or fingernail is infected, the nail becomes loose at the edge and starts to rub against the skin. When this happens the nail should be trimmed back slightly along the side and a tiny piece of cotton should be pushed under the nail. This will immediately relieve some of the pain and help the infection to heal. Some people find it also relieves the pressure if they cut a tiny V-shaped wedge out of the center of the nail.

The doctor

The doctor will drain blood from under the nail by a simple technique that instantly relieves most of the pain. It sounds and looks scary, but actually doesn't hurt. The doctor heats a straightened paper clip until it's red hot. Then he *touches* the hot end to the dark area of the nail; he does not push. The heat melts a tiny hole in the nail. The nail has no nerves, so this procedure doesn't hurt any more than cutting the nail. And the pool of

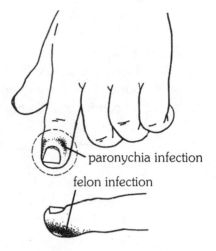

paronychia infection

felon infection

An infection near the edge of a nail is called a "runaround" or paronychia. An infection on the bottom of a finger or toe is called a felon. Both can be painful and should be seen by a doctor.

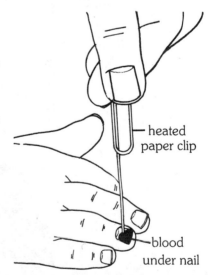

heated paper clip

blood under nail

A blood blister under a fingernail is drained by melting a hole in the nail with the end of a very hot paper clip. This doesn't hurt and instantly relieves the pain.

blood under the nail protects the skin underneath. Once the hole has been made in the nail, blood and clear fluid will slowly drain out for a day or so. To help keep the hole open to drain, the finger or toe should be soaked in warm water several times a day.

If an infected finger or toe becomes very painful or quite swollen, it should be seen by the doctor. The doctor will numb the area with an injection that temporarily stops the pain nerves from sending messages to the brain. Then the doctor will make a cut on the tip to let the infection drain.

Prevention

Subungual hematomas can be prevented by teaching kids to be careful when they are working with tools or lifting heavy objects.

Infections of the fingers and toes are best prevented by promptly treating small cuts and by keeping hangnails and nails trimmed. It's also important for kids to learn not to bite their nails.

Head injuries

What's happening

Once in a while kids hit their heads hard enough to cause concern. The most common ways in which this happens are falling from a bike, horse, or high place; hitting the windshield of a car; or being hit by a bat or a ball. Luckily, most of these accidents are not serious, and the kids recover by themselves. But such accidents are scary for both the kids and people watching.

In a minor head injury, the child hits his or her head and may be stunned, but does not become unconscious. Crying immediately after an accident doesn't necessarily mean the injury is serious. Actually it shows the child hasn't been unconscious, but is frightened or in pain. If the bump has been hard enough, an area may immediately swell up into an egg shape. This is caused by bleeding under the skin and clear fluid coming into the area from the nearby cells. The reason a bump on the head looks so big is because it can only swell out, not in, since the skull is made of bone.

In a medium-serious head injury, the child actually becomes unconscious for a few seconds or minutes. When people are unconscious, they don't move or talk. Their eyes are closed and they look as if they're asleep. Unconsciousness is caused by the soft brain bumping against the hard skull. Doctors call a head injury with unconsciousness a *concussion*. After a concussion a child may have a headache and feel dizzy, tired, and cranky. It's not unusual for the child to be confused and not really remember much about how the accident happened. Sometimes the child may

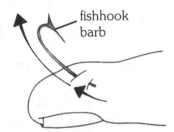

A fishhook caught in the skin can be removed by gently pushing it on through or by cutting off the end of the hook and pulling out the rest.

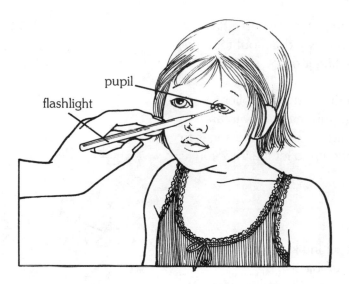

pupil

flashlight

After a head injury, parents are often told to shine a light in the child's eyes to make sure the pupils close down normally.

even throw up or run a fever. Generally a concussion gets better in a day or two, but the doctor should always be called.

In a serious head injury a child is unconscious for more than a few minutes. Later the child may be very cranky or very sleepy for periods of time on and off. The child's headache will get worse and he or she may have difficulty moving arms, legs, or eyes. All of these signs are caused by the brain swelling and pressing on nerves. The child may become unconscious *again,* as much as two days later. Of course, any child with a serious head injury should be seen by a doctor in a hospital.

Helping yourself

A mild head injury gets better by itself. An ice pack can be put on a goose egg to keep down the swelling. One or two ice cubes should be put in a plastic bag, wrapped in a towel, and gently held on the bump for at least 15 minutes.

The doctor

The doctor should be called about any head injury in which a child becomes unconscious or acts strangely after the accident. The doctor will ask questions about the accident and do a special examination of the child's nervous system. The doctor will have the child move his or her arms, legs, and eyes, testing the nerves' automatic reactions, or reflexes (see The physical exam, page 372). One of these is the pupil reflex of the eyes. The child's pupils should shut down normally when a flashlight is shined at them.

If doctors don't see any immediate signs of brain injury, they will generally send the child home with special instructions for the parents. If the injury is more serious, the doctor will put the child in the hospital and have the child watched closely. In the most serious cases doctors may take skull X-rays or CAT brain scans to figure out what is happening. Swelling of the brain can be brought down with drugs. Pressure from bleeding in the brain can be removed with surgery. The actual number of cases this serious is very small. And most of these kids recover very well.

Prevention

Many head injuries can be prevented. Seat belts should always be worn when riding in cars. (Car accidents are the single greatest cause of serious injury in children between 6 and 12.) Kids who play sports, ride horses, or skateboard should wear safety helmets. Such safety measures may take getting used to, but they will certainly be worthwhile if an accident occurs.

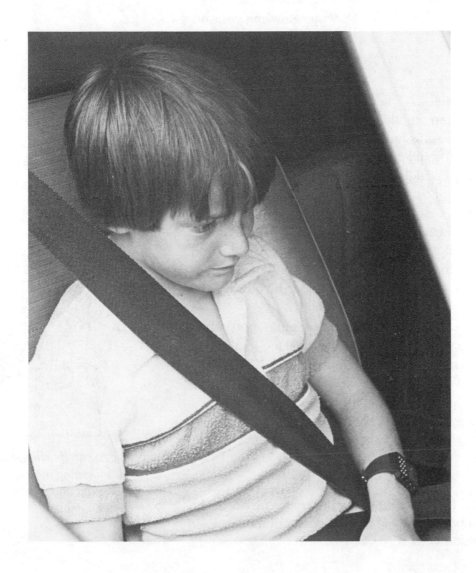

Wearing seat belts is the single most important thing kids can do to prevent being seriously injured.

Nosebleeds

What's happening

Lots of kids get nosebleeds. They are almost never dangerous, but they are often scary because it seems as if a lot of blood is being lost. Really, though, it is a very small amount. Nosebleeds are caused by tiny blood vessels breaking in the lining of the nose. Almost always they are from the *septum,* the center wall that separates the two nostrils. These blood vessels are very close to the surface and are fairly easily hurt. Nosebleeds can be caused by hitting or falling on your nose, by scratching your nose, or even by blowing your nose strongly. When the lining of the nose is thinner than usual because it is dry or you have a cold, then nosebleeds sometimes happen by themselves. Some kids never seem to get nosebleeds; others may get them fairly often during a period of time.

Nosebleeds don't hurt your body and they are usually not hard to stop with firm pressure. The muscles of the little blood vessels squeeze themselves closed and a clot forms (see Blood clotting, page 232). The whole process can take place in three to six minutes. But the clot can only finish forming when bleeding slows. Otherwise the bleeding washes away the chemicals in the blood that make the clot. This is why squeezing your nose speeds up clotting.

Helping yourself

Many nosebleeds stop by themselves. The rest will stop quickly if you do the following: First, sit up and lean slightly forward so you don't swallow the blood. Then squeeze your nostrils firmly between your thumb and forefinger. Keep squeezing—without letting go—for at least three full minutes. Often this will be long enough. If not, it means you are not pressing hard enough or in the right place. Change your position slightly and squeeze again for five, and, if necessary, ten full minutes.

By pressing on your nose, you keep the blood from coming out and give your body time to form a clot, which plugs the tiny hole in the blood vessel. It is important not to bump or scratch your nose for a little while after the bleeding stops, because the clot is delicate and can be broken easily.

If pressure doesn't stop the bleeding after 10 to 15 minutes, you can apply a medicine that tends to shrink the membrane, or lining, of the nose. A good medicine happens to be the main ingredient in Neo-Synephrine nose drops. First blow your nose to clear out the old clots that aren't working. Then put a little ball of cotton moistened with Neo-Synephrine into your nostril and again press firmly on your nose for ten minutes.

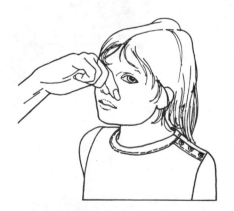

A nosebleed can be stopped by firmly squeezing the nose between thumb and forefinger for three minutes. This gives the body time to form a clot.

The doctor

The doctor should be called if the bleeding just won't stop. The doctor has more experience in applying pressure and has very powerful medicines to shrink the membrane and blood vessels.

Prevention

Don't blow your nose hard or scratch the lining—especially if you have a cold or have a runny nose from allergies. If you get nosebleeds frequently and the lining of your nose tends to be very dry, try moistening your nose with a little Vaseline and using a vaporizer at night.

Resuscitation—basic life support

What's happening

There are several kinds of accidents that can cause people to stop breathing and possibly stop their heartbeat. In children the accidents that might cause this are near-drowning, auto accidents, smoke inhalation, choking, and severe electric shock. Among older people, a heart attack can cause breathing and heartbeat to stop. Fortunately, such situations among children are so rare that most people will never have to deal with one. But, it's important to know what to do because in these rare situations this knowledge could save a life.

To stay alive, people have to take in oxygen through the lungs and send it to the brain by way of the bloodstream. They take oxygen in by breathing in and out. To send oxygen to the brain, the heart must pump and circulate the blood. Normally people's bodies do these things automatically. But if there is a serious accident, another person can do the work of an injured person's heart and lungs. Doctors call this whole technique *cardiopulmonary resuscitation* (CPR). It consists of *rescue breathing* and *artificial circulation*. Ideally it should be done by a trained person. Children who are interested can learn the technique by taking a course in CPR through their local fire department or Red Cross. If the technique is done properly, a person can be kept alive until help arrives.

Helping yourself

Briefly, here are the steps recommended by the American Heart Association: (1) Check to see if the person is unconscious. An unconscious person is limp and doesn't cry or awaken when tapped or shaken. If the person can be awakened, he or she doesn't need CPR. If the person is conscious but having trouble breathing, the airway needs to be cleared (see page 364). (2) If the person is unconscious or having trouble breathing, call for help. Someone should *immediately* call the Rescue Squad, Fire Department, or Police. They will send out a trained person. (3) The injured person should be placed back down on a hard surface, not a bed. If there is any possibility of a head or neck injury, the person's head should be held so it can't roll or move.

CPR (Cardiopulmonary Resuscitation)

Opening the airway

Place one hand under the person's neck and the other hand on his or her forehead. Lift the neck slightly and push the forehead down slightly. This moves away the tongue so the windpipe is open.

Or push the forehead down with one hand and carefully lift the bony part of the jaw near the chin, keeping the mouth open slightly.

Place your ear over the person's mouth and nose and look at the chest and stomach. The person is breathing if you see the chest rise and fall and hear air from the nose and mouth.

If the person is not breathing or the lips are blue, start rescue breathing.

Rescue breathing

Put your mouth over the mouth of the injured person and pinch his or her nose closed with thumb and index finger.

Take a deep breath and blow four gentle breaths, one after another, into the person's mouth. If the airway is not obstructed, the chest will rise and fall. (If the chest doesn't rise, reposition the person's head and try this step again. If the second attempt doesn't work, see *Choking.*)

Feel gently for the pulse in the groove between the windpipe and the muscles on either side of the neck. (If a pulse is not present, begin *artificial circulation* as well as rescue breathing.)

Breathe into the person's mouth once every 4 seconds, or 15 times a minute. You should see the chest rise with each breath, and feel air exhaling from the person's mouth and nose.

After each breath turn your head and get a breath of fresh air.

Artificial circulation

Feel gently for a pulse in the groove between the windpipe and muscles in the side of the neck.

If a pulse cannot be felt, start artificial circulation.

Make sure person is lying on a firm surface (ground or floor).

Locate notch in the center of the chest above the bottom of the ribs with the middle finger.

Push down the heel of one hand (fingers off the chest) to compress the chest 1 to 1½ inches, then release. Do this 80 times per minute smoothly without sudden, jerky movements.

Rescue breathing must be done with artificial circulation. This is the pattern: Push chest, count one, two, three, four, five, then breathe. Another person should check the pulse in the neck to see if artificial circulation is working.

Choking

If the person can cough, encourage him to do so.

If he cannot cough and has blue lips, his or her airway is blocked.

Kneel on the floor and put the person across your thighs, head down.

Hit the person four times with the heel of your hand, between the shoulder blades.

Now roll the person onto the floor and find the notch in the center of the chest above the bottom of the ribs.

With the heel of one hand push down on the chest one inch and release. Do this four times.

If you can't see the object, do *not* stick your finger down the throat because it can push the object further down.

If the person is an infant or a child, do *not* squeeze the tummy below the ribs because the liver or other organs can be injured.

Drowning

Get to the drowning person as quickly as possible.

Start mouth-to-mouth breathing in the water if it is shallow.

Support the neck if a diving injury may have occurred.

Drowning children have been resuscitated in spite of being under water for a half hour or more, so always do CPR unless you *know* the child has been under water for over an hour.

Then someone should do the ABC's of CPR: *airway, breathing,* and *circulation* (see chart). All these steps should be performed as quickly as possible.

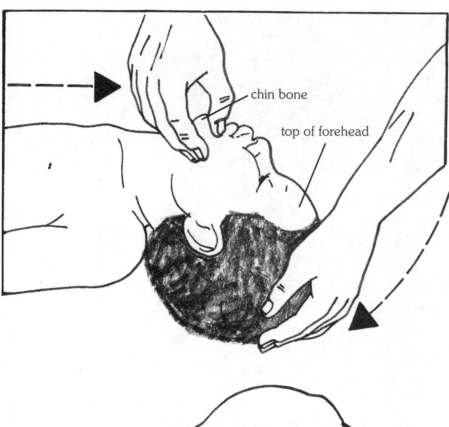

Open the person's airway by lifting the chin with one hand and pushing down on the forehead with the other.

chin bone

top of forehead

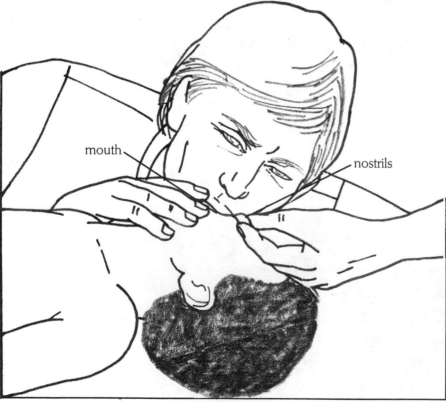

Take a deep breath, pinch the child's nose closed with one hand, and blow into his or her mouth until the chest actually rises. Repeat this 15 times per minute.

mouth

nostrils

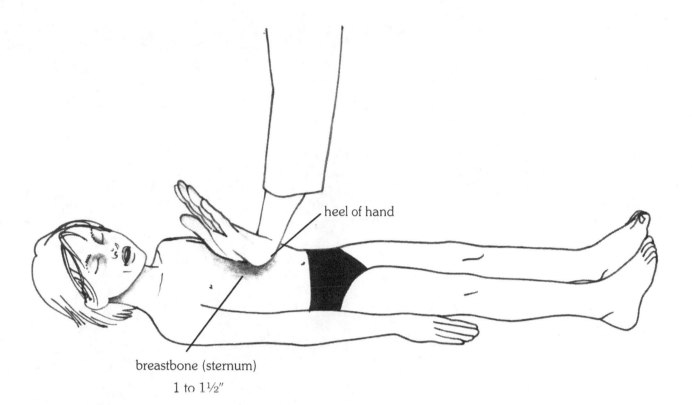

heel of hand

breastbone (sternum)
1 to 1½″

The doctor

The rescue squad or doctor has special tools and skills to deal with such emergencies. They have a machine that can deliver oxygen. If necessary a doctor can insert a tube to make breathing easier and can give drugs to help breathing and circulation.

Prevention

Most of the situations that might cause a child's heart and breathing to stop are preventable. Children who can't swim should be carefully supervised around pools, lakes, or the ocean. They should learn to wear water wings or life jackets until they can swim, and they should learn to swim as soon as possible. Children in cars should wear seat belts routinely as soon as they become too old for safety seats. Kids should learn basic fire safety and the proper use of matches. And parents should install smoke alarms and regularly clean and check furnaces, water heaters, and wood stoves. Any wiring problems should be checked immediately and fixed by a person who knows about electricity. Kids should know that a regular electrical outlet or cord carries enough electricity to be dangerous. And kids should learn never to work on or take apart any electrical appliance that is plugged in.

Locate the notch below the child's breastbone. Put the heel of one hand on the breastbone just above the notch, and push down on the chest 1 to 1½ inches, then release. Repeat this 80 times per minute.

To dislodge an object stuck in a child's throat, first hit the child between the shoulder blades four times with the heel of your hand. Then roll the child onto his or her back and press down the chest several times with the movement just described.

Chapter 10

Using the doctor

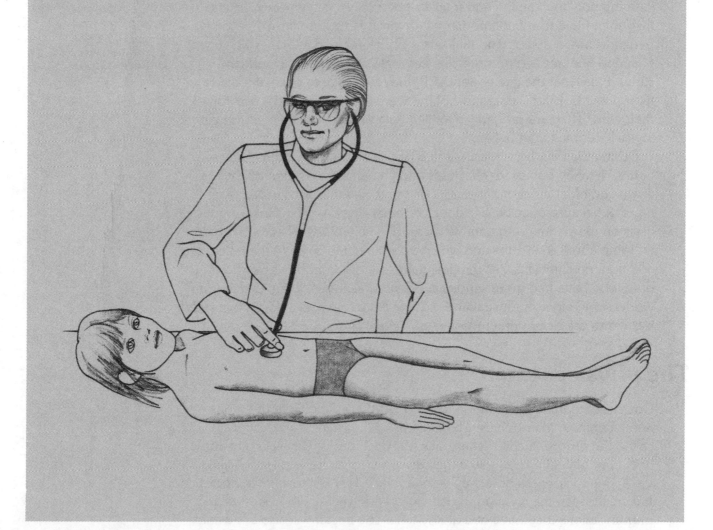

Going to the doctor

Most children from 6 to 12 don't go to the doctor very often. And they don't remember much about going to the doctor when they were babies. So a doctor visit is unusual. Many children don't know their doctor very well and feel a little uneasy with him or her. Often kids will have to wait quite a while before they are even seen. The more children understand about why they go to the doctor and what the doctor does, the more comfortable they will be with their visit.

Who the doctor is

Doctors are men and women who have studied medicine. In high school they were probably interested in science and may have first considered the idea of becoming a doctor. Then they went on to college where they took courses in biology, chemistry, physics, and math to prepare themselves for medical school. After four years of college, they spent four more years in medical school. Half of this time is spent learning how the body works and what diseases people get. The other half of the time is spent in a hospital learning how to examine and treat sick people. To get a medical license they then have to spend another year working in a hospital. To become a pediatrician—a doctor who takes care of children and infants—they have to spend another two or three years in a special program of work and study. Finally, at the age of about 30, they are ready to open an office and treat patients. By this time most of them are married and have children of their own. They are probably a lot like your parents, but their job is helping sick people to get better.

During the day, pediatricians see a large number of children. They see young, healthy babies for checkups and immunizations; they do physical exams on older children for school or camp; and they see children who are sick because of colds, accidents, or other illnesses. They answer questions on the phone from parents (or kids!) who wonder what they can do at home about a sickness and whether they need to come to the office. In addition, pediatricians visit the hospital to see newborn babies and children who have had more serious accidents or illnesses. Every pediatrician works some nights and weekends so that there is always a doctor available if children are sick during those times.

The physical exam

Doctors determine if children are sick or well by asking them questions and examining their bodies. The first part of the exam, the questions, is called the *history*. If children are sick, the doctor asks what is wrong and how long have they been ill. If they are there for a checkup (a well-child visit), the doctor asks how they've been since their last visit; if the doctor has never seen the children, he or she will ask what (if any) illnesses and immunizations they have had at any time. The doctor will also ask what

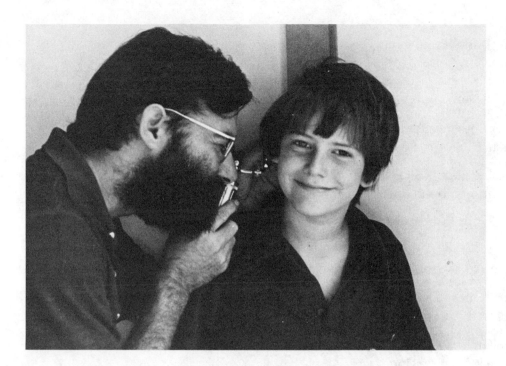

Doctors can see the eardrum with a special tool called an otoscope.

the children eat, how much they sleep, how they do in school, and what their families are like.

The doctor listens carefully to the answers to the questions, taking note of anything that might indicate a problem. In medical school doctors learn the stories of all the illnesses children get. Because they have learned what pains or problems go along with each illness, how it starts and what happens next, they can generally tell from a child's story what is wrong. The simple questions doctors ask are really quite useful in figuring out what the problem is. So it's important that parents and children answer the questions carefully.

If the visit is for a well-child checkup, children are weighed and their height is measured to see how they're growing. This is frequently done by the nurse before the doctor comes in. Children vary a lot in size and in the speed at which they're growing. But every child grows steadily and follows a predictable pattern.

If children come to the doctor because they don't feel well, the nurse will also take their temperature. Then the doctor will simply *look* at them. Sick kids generally look tired, droopy, or in pain. The doctor can tell a lot by just how sick children look.

Next the doctor looks at their skin to see if there are any rashes, cuts, or swollen areas. By looking at the skin the doctor can see if children have poison ivy, cuts, mumps, chicken pox, flea bites, or a skin infection.

The eyes are checked to see if they're red or have pus and to see if they move together. Looking at the eye tells the doctor if children have an eye infection or a sty. The doctor may also flash a light at each eye to see whether the pupils close down properly (see page 360). This is especially important after people have hit their heads. In a well-child checkup the

How to use the doctor

The more you understand about what's going on, the more comfortable you'll feel.

Tell the doctor *yourself* what the problem is, as clearly as you can.

Try to ask the doctor any questions you have. Don't be afraid to say, "I don't understand," or to keep repeating your questions.

If you're uncomfortable about, or afraid of, something say, "That bothers me. Tell me more about what you're going to do."

If you can't get the doctor to explain more, ask your parents to talk to him or her.

Don't be embarrassed to ask to talk to the doctor alone.

Answer questions as honestly and completely as you can; it will help the doctor give you better treatment.

Always report any allergic reactions to medicines, or problems you've had before taking a medicine.

Make sure you understand the doctor's instructions and tell him or her any problems you might have following them.

Call the doctor if you have any further problems once you are home.

If you are going to the doctor for a specific illness, read about it beforehand if you can.

doctor may have children read briefly from an eye chart. If they have difficulty reading the lines, the doctor will refer them to an eye doctor. Sometimes the doctor will look into the eyes with a special light with magnifying lenses in it. This machine, called an *ophthalmoscope*, actually lets the doctor see the blood vessels on the retina, the lining at the back of the eye.

Next the doctor checks the nose with a flashlight to see if the inside lining is swollen and red. This might show the doctor if the child has a cold, allergy, or nosebleed. The doctor will also look in the throat, using a tongue blade to push the tongue out of the way for a clear look. If the throat is red, swollen, or has pus on it, the child may have a cold or a strep throat. While the doctor is looking in the mouth, he or she will also check to see if there are brown spots on the teeth. This may mean the child has cavities. Such brown spots should be seen by a dentist.

The doctor checks the ears with a special flashlight called an otoscope. This machine has a magnifying glass and a funnel that points the light into the ear. With the otoscope, the doctor can see the skin lining the ear canal and the eardrum. If the drum is red or swollen, the child has an infection of the middle ear; if the skin in the canal is red or swollen, the child has an outer ear infection (see page 323).

The doctor feels the sides of the neck to see if the child has swollen or tender lymph nodes. Very swollen nodes mean the child may have an infection like a sore throat or an ear infection.

Next the doctor listens to the heart and lungs with a *stethoscope,* which is simply a long tube that brings body sounds to the doctor's ears. The end of it has a funnel that picks up low, rumbly noises and a flat disk that picks up high, scratchy noises. When the doctor listens to the heart, he or she can hear the sounds of the valves closing as blood moves from one chamber of the heart to another. The doctor moves the stethoscope to hear different areas of the heart. This tells the doctor how strongly and steadily the heart is pumping.

The doctor moves the stethoscope to the child's back in order to hear breathing sounds from the lungs and the bronchi, the tubes leading to the lungs. Regular breathing sounds like air going into a balloon. If a child has a chest cold, the doctor will hear noises like bubbles popping. These noises are caused by mucus rattling around in the air tubes. If a child is having an asthma attack, the doctor will hear squeaky wheezing sounds. This is caused by air going through passages that have swelled and become narrow. Sometimes doctors will tap with their fingers on children's backs. Because the lungs are full of air, the tapping makes a hollow sound like a drum. If mucus is in the lungs, the sounds are duller like hitting something hard.

The doctor checks the child's belly or abdomen by pressing lightly all over to see if there are any areas that are tender or sore. By doing this the doctor can tell if a stomachache is serious. The doctor may even listen to the sounds of the digestive tract with a stethoscope. If a child has a stomach flu, the sounds will be noisier than usual.

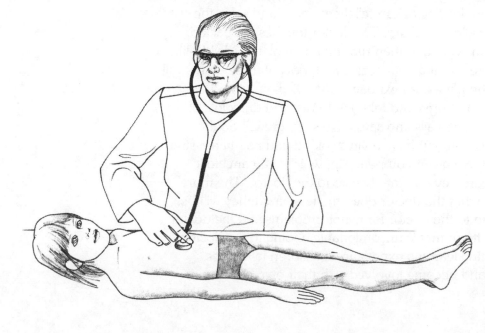

The doctor uses a stethoscope to listen to your heart and lungs.

The doctor may also look at a child's penis or vagina to see if they are growing normally. The doctor looks to see if children are beginning to develop body hair and determines whether the children are where they should be in terms of their growth spurt and adult development.

Finally the doctor looks at the child's arms and legs to see if they are moving and developing normally. The doctor may also tap some of the child's tendons, or muscle endings, with a hammer. When tapped, the tendons automatically cause muscles to tighten and move. Such movements are called reflexes. They show if the child's nerves and muscles are working properly (see page 188).

If the doctor is still not sure what's wrong after the physical exam, he or she may do laboratory tests or take an X-ray. An X-ray will show whether a bone is broken. Other laboratory tests can tell if there is an infection and what it is due to.

Really the doctor is like a detective. The doctor asks questions and looks all over the body for *clues* about how the body is working. For example, say you go to the doctor complaining that you don't feel well. This tells the doctor you're sick, but it doesn't tell what's wrong. Then the doctor discovers that your temperature is 102°F. That's a clue that you're really sick and that the doctor should look carefully to see what's making you sick. When the doctor asks if anything hurts, you say your throat is sore and it's hard to swallow. During the physical exam, the doctor looks very carefully at your throat, sees that the back of it is red and swollen, and finds the lymph nodes in the sides of your neck are swollen and sore. Those are two more clues. But the doctor finds nothing wrong with your ears, and your lungs sound good. Those are clues too, but they're "no" clues, whereas the others are "yes" clues. Out of all these yes and no clues, doctors get an idea of what's wrong. They were taught in medical school that a fever, a sore, red throat, and swollen lymph nodes with everything else normal is a sign of a sore throat caused by a virus cold or a strep cold. The only way the doctor can tell them apart, and solve the mystery, is to do a test called a *culture*. The doctor touches the back of your throat with a cotton swab and then rubs that on a plate of Jell-O-like food. If strep bacteria are causing your sore throat, dots of these germs will be visible growing on the plate the next day.

So the doctor sends you home and tells you to rest and drink lots of fluid. The next day he or she calls and says, "No strep grew." So the answer to the mystery is that you have a virus cold. If you had had a strep cold the doctor would have given you penicillin, which is an antibiotic.

Many children are scared every time they go to the doctor. The more they understand about what the doctor does, the less afraid they will be. Generally kids are going to the doctor for minor problems and the doctor doesn't do anything to them that is uncomfortable. Going to the doctor can become an interesting learning experience if children talk to the doctor, ask questions, and become involved with their own health care.

Chapter 11

Common drugs

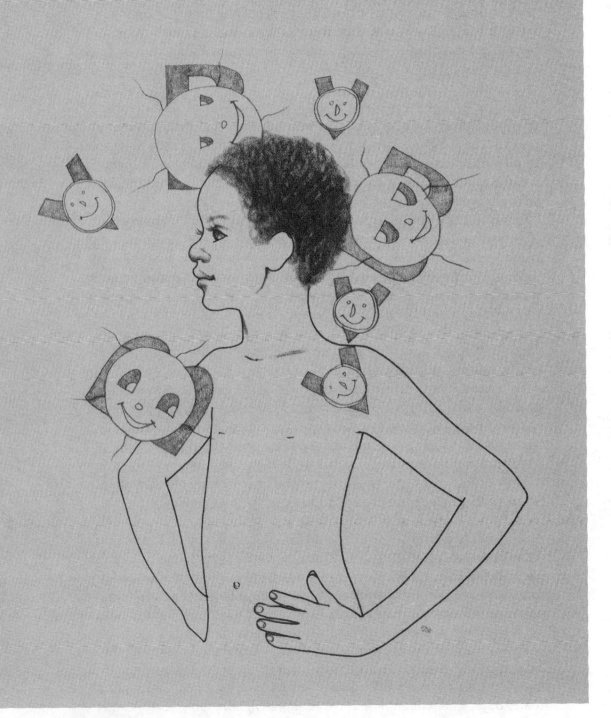

Drugs are powerful medicines

Children don't get sick very often. Five to twelve is one of the healthiest of all age groups. Even when children do get sick, their bodies usually heal by themselves. But sometimes when children are sick, drugs can *help* them heal and make them feel more comfortable. There are very few drugs, however, that are absolutely needed. Most of the drugs children take are given out of habit.

New drugs are very powerful medicines. So doctors are very careful when they give them to children. Parents and children should be very careful about the amount, or *dose,* they take of any drug. Children's bodies are so much smaller than those of adults that it's much easier for them to get too much of a drug. Because too much of some drugs can be very dangerous, doctors decide how much of a drug to give based on how much a child weighs.

Every drug is given to do a particular job. Some drugs lower temperature, some drugs kill bacteria, and so on. But almost all drugs do more than just the job they are supposed to do. For example, a drug that stops a runny nose may also make a child sleepy. This is called a *side effect.* Some side effects aren't even noticed, some are just annoying, and some can be more serious or more of a problem than the illness itself.

Often children and their parents have been taught by TV commercials that they *need* drugs to get better and that the drugs will *always* cure them instantly. Neither of these ideas is really true. In fact, most drugs taken by children don't even affect what's causing the illness, so they can't cure the illness. The drugs just make children feel better for a little while. For example, aspirin doesn't kill virus, so it can't cure a virus cold. It does help bring a child's fever down, but this isn't absolutely necessary. Often the child doesn't even feel bad. It's important that children realize that their *bodies* are the healers, not the medicine.

To a large extent, medicines work because people *believe* they will work. In fact, doctors have found that people can take sugar pills *(placebos)* and have pain go away or a runny nose stop. What actually happened was their *minds* made the pain or runny nose stop. If you concentrate, you can make your mind do the same thing.

Most drugs were first made from natural things like plants or molds. Some of them were discovered thousands of years ago. Now scientists have figured out just what part of the plant was helping people get well. And they make just that part in chemical laboratories. In the last twenty years scientists have been able to make many new drugs that don't exist naturally. Unfortunately, more and more of these drugs are now being found to have serious side effects. Several drugs have even been found to cause cancer (*see* A personal cancer plan chart, page 96). For this reason no one should take drugs unless they really *need* to.

People can get drugs in two ways. Powerful or dangerous drugs have to be prescribed by a doctor. The doctor writes down the name of a particular drug, how much should be taken each time, how often, and for how many days. The written note is called a *prescription.* Only doctors and dentists can write prescriptions.

Alternatives to drugs

Drug	Alternatives
Aspirin or Tylenol for fever	Put on less clothing. Sponge with lukewarm water. If comfortable, do nothing.
Aspirin or Tylenol for muscle aches	Relax. Rub muscles. Take a warm bath (if you don't have a fever).
Aspirin for a headache	Massage next to eyes, and muscles in back of neck. Relax. Rest in a dark room.
Cough syrup (suppressant)	Drink lots of liquids. Drink warm herb tea (no caffeine) with honey.
Nasal decongestants	Drink lots of liquids. Hold your face next to hot running water to relieve stuffiness.
Antacids for a stomachache	Relax. Drink milk or soda water. Eat a few plain crackers.
Antidiarrhea drugs	Stop solid foods and milk but drink plenty of clear liquids. Later eat dry toast or crackers.
Medicated skin creams	If irritated skin is *moist,* expose it to sunlight and air. Apply water, then oil, if area is dry —reapply frequently and cover if dryness continues.
Nonprescription eye drops	Bathe eyes with clear water.

When a prescription is given to a specially trained person in a drugstore, he or she can then give you the drug the doctor has ordered. There is no other way to get these drugs. This is done because many drugs are so powerful that they can seriously hurt people if they are not used properly.

There are some drugs that can be bought "over the counter"; that is, without a prescription. These drugs are usually mild enough that if they are taken according to instructions, they are not very dangerous. But they are still powerful enough to cause side effects and make people sick. All drugs can be dangerous if too much is taken at one time. For example, too much aspirin can poison a person. Some drugs can be dangerous if taken for too long a period of time. For example, antihistamines can injure cells in the lining of the nose if taken for too many days in a row. And some drugs have bad side effects even if they are taken according to instructions. Aspirin, for example, causes the stomach lining to bleed, and antihistamines make people sleepy.

Aspirin

The active part of aspirin, called *salicylic acid,* was first found in the bark of willow trees. People used to chew a little bit of the bark to bring down a fever. Aspirin lowers the body temperature by resetting the body thermo-stat, the hypothalamus in the center of the brain (see page 190). When people are sick, toxins, or poisons, made by the viruses or bacteria set the brain's thermostat higher. The brain tells the body not to sweat or send blood up to the skin, so the body doesn't cool off as it normally does. It gets hotter and hotter. A fever probably helps to kill the bacteria or viruses. But the aspirin sets the thermostat back down as if the body weren't sick. Then the body sweats and sends blood to the skin in order to cool off.

Aspirin also relieves certain kinds of pain. It works for headaches and muscle aches, but not for stomachaches. Aspirin works against pain for over half the people who take it. But when sugar pills were secretly given to people who thought they were taking aspirin, the sugar pills worked almost as well. This shows that pain will often go away if people expect it to. In fact, the brain itself produces a chemical called *endorphin,* which relieves pain better than aspirin.

Aspirin is such a powerful drug that it would probably require a prescription if it were just introduced. It affects practically all parts of the body and it also has side effects that bother people sometimes. Aspirin makes people's muscle cells use more oxygen, which makes them breathe more. It makes the whole body more acid. And, most importantly, it eats tiny holes in the lining of the stomach, and they bleed. This is why people sometimes get a stomachache when they take aspirin.

Aspirin does *not* make colds better. It does *not* kill bacteria or viruses. It simply makes people feel less uncomfortable. Aspirin should not be taken for a cold unless people are very uncomfortable and can't make themselves feel better without it.

Recommended dose: 5 to 7 years: ½ of an adult tablet (5 grain), or 2 or 3 baby aspirin tablets (1¼ grain), *every* 3 to 4 hours. 8 to 12 years: 1 adult tablet or 4 baby tablets, *every* 3 to 4 hours.

Acetaminophen (Tempera Drops or Tylenol)

This drug also relieves fever and mild aches. It works on the brain's thermostat in the same way that aspirin does. Like aspirin, it also affects the whole body, but it has fewer side effects than aspirin. It does not make the body acid and it doesn't make the lining of the stomach bleed. Also like aspirin, it cannot cure a cold because it does not kill bacteria or viruses.

Recommended dosage: 6 to 12: ½ to 1 tablet (325 milligrams), 3 times per day.

Antihistamines

Antihistamines relieve swelling and itching in allergies and they slow a runny nose somewhat. The body itself makes histamine, a chemical that makes the tiny blood vessels open wider all over the body. This causes redness of the skin and nasal lining. It also causes clear fluid to leak out between the cells, which causes swelling. Histamine causes itching because it excites nerve endings in the skin. The body sends out histamine when it is injured or when it's allergic to something.

Drug companies make chemicals called *anti*histamines, which stop all the things that histamine does by blocking the places where histamine attaches to cells. That means that antihistamines can stop swelling, redness, and itching when someone has an allergic reaction. It helps stop the runny nose, itchy eyes, and sneezing of hay fever.

In spite of what many people think, antihistamines are not really useful for treating a cold. They don't kill viruses or bacteria; they just slow a runny nose a little.

Antihistamines have strong side effects. They dull the brain and make people sleepy. They also can make people sick to their stomachs and make their mouths dry.

Recommended dosage: There are over 50 different kinds of antihistamines. They are taken in different amounts, so instructions should be followed carefully. The most common ones given to children are Actifed, Sudafed, Chlor-Trimeton, and Phenergan.

Antibiotics

Antibiotics are chemicals produced by microscopic plants or animals such as fungi or bacteria. These chemicals kill other microscopic plants or animals. Antibiotics have been used a long time. Two thousand years ago the Chinese put moldy soybeans on skin infections. But antibiotics didn't come into wide use until after 1928 when Dr. Alexander Fleming discovered that a particular kind of mold killed the bacteria he was growing. This mold was penicillin. Since that time many other antibiotics have been discovered. Antibiotics have saved many lives by killing the bacteria causing severe infections in people. In fact, these drugs are probably the most important tools of modern medicine.

Penicillin works by stopping growing bacteria from making an outside wall. This allows water to leak in and makes the bacteria explode. Penicillin doesn't actually kill adult bacteria, it just stops young ones from growing up. This is why you have to take penicillin for several days. Bacteria have very short lives—they live only a few hours. Adult bacteria die by themselves, but they are quickly replaced by a new crop of babies.

Antibiotics don't cure infections all by themselves. They lower the number of bacteria so that the body's own white blood cells can eat the remaining ones. In fact, antibiotics don't always cure people with infections who have no white blood cells of their own. Antibiotics don't kill viruses at all, so they don't work against the common cold. Different antibiotics kill different kinds of bacteria. So doctors prescribe different antibiotics according to what type of bacteria is causing an infection.

Like other drugs, antibiotics do have side effects, so they should be taken only for serious infections. People can become allergic to some antibiotics. In severe allergic reactions, people can even go into shock (see page 344). Also, antibiotics kill the helpful bacteria in the body. These include intestinal bacteria that make vitamins, and bacteria that protect you from other bacteria. Some antibiotics have other side effects as well. Tetracycline can cause tooth enamel to darken while teeth are still developing under the gum, and should not be given to young children. Ampicillin often causes diarrhea.

Recommended dosage: The dosage varies with the particular antibiotic and according to the severity of the infection, so the doctor's instructions should be followed carefully. Yogurt may be eaten to help replace intestinal bacteria. The most common antibiotics given to children are penicillins, erythromycins, and sulfas.

Steroids

The outer part of the body's adrenal glands produces hormones called steroids. They are powerful chemicals that affect the whole body (see page 206). Cortisone, one of these steroids, actually stops the body from defending itself when it is hurt. It stops swelling, redness, and tenderness

Problems with common drugs

Drug	Possible problems
Aspirin	Stomachache
Cough syrups	Drowsiness due to alcohol content Allergic reactions to the artificial color
Decongestants	Drowsiness (side effect)
Amphicillin (an antibiotic usually given for ear infections)	Repeated episodes of diarrhea
Steroid creams	Absorbed through the skin—can affect amount of adrenal hormones if used for long periods
Food coloring	Children can react to the red or orange food colorings put in many drugs by being nervous, irritable, and unable to sleep, by getting a rash, and so on.
Many drugs—including aspirin, antibiotics, and anti-histamines. Penicillin and sulfa drugs are most common.	Allergic reaction—itching and red dots or raised red areas like hives anywhere on the body. Fever. *Discontinue medicine immediately and call doctor.* In future, always report this reaction to any doctor.

from asthma, allergies, or wounds. It stops white blood cells from coming in and keeps new cells from growing. In other words, it stops healing. This is very useful in an emergency when the body needs to keep working. For children, cortisone is most commonly used in creams that are put on the skin for diseases like eczema or poison ivy. Cortisone does not affect what caused these illnesses, it just stops the symptoms. This often gives the body a chance to heal itself.

When people take steroids, their own adrenal glands make fewer natural steroids to keep the body in balance. So if people suddenly stop taking the steroids, their body won't have enough of them to work properly. This is why doctors instruct people to take fewer and fewer steroid pills for the last six or seven days. Because steroids affect every cell in the body, they are very dangerous if they are not taken in the right amounts and for the right reasons. Even creams can affect the whole body because they are absorbed through the skin into the blood in small amounts. For this reason the creams are given only for a short time for serious skin problems.

Notes

Chapter 1. Stress

1. Thomas, L. *The Lives of a Cell* (New York: Viking Press, 1974), p. 82.

2. Hinkle, L. E. "Illness, Life Experience, and Social Environment," *Annals of Internal Medicine* 49:1873 (1958).

3. Ibid.

4. Meyer, R. "Streptococcal Infections in Families," *Pediatrics* 29:539.

5. Roghmann, K. J. "Daily Stress, Illness, and Use of Health Services in Young Families," *Pediatric Research* 7:520 (1973).

6. Holmes, T. H. and Rahe, R. H. "The Social Readjustment Rating Scale," *Journal of Psychosomatic Research* 11:213–18 (1967).

7. Coddington, R. D. "The Significance of Life Events as Etiological Factors in the Diseases of Children," *Journal of Psychosomatic Research* 16:7, 205.

8. Heisel, J. S. "The Significance of Life Events as Contributing Factors in the Diseases of Children," *Journal of Pediatrics* 83:119 (1973).

9. Padilla, B. R. "Predicting Accident Frequency in Children," *Pediatrics* 58:223 (1976).

10. Jackson, G. G. "Susceptibility and Immunity to Common Upper Respiratory Viral Infection—The Common Cold," *Annals of Internal Medicine* 53:2, 719 (1960).

11. Kroger, W. S. *Hypnosis and Behavior Modification: Imagery Conditioning* (Philadelphia: J. B. Lippincott, 1976).

12. Barber, T. "Hypnosis, Suggestion, and Psychosomatic Phenomenon: A New Look from the Standpoint of Recent Experimental Studies," *American Journal of Clinical Hypnosis* 21:1 (1978).

13. Jung, C. Introduction to *The Inner World of Childhood* (New York: New American Library, 1968), pp. xvii, xix.

14. Wickes, F. G. *The Inner World of Childhood* (New York: New American Library, 1968), p. 40.

15. Skipper, J. K. "Children, Stress, and Hospitalization," *Journal of Health and Social Behavior* 9:278 (1968).

16. Nuckolls, Katherine et al. "Psychosocial Assets, Life Crises and the Prognosis of Pregnancy," *American Journal of Epidemiology* 95:431–41 (1972).

17. Brown, G. W. et al. "Social Class and Psychiatric Disturbance Among Women in an Urban Population," *Sociology* 9:225–54 (1975).

18. Cobb, S. "Social Support as a Moderator of Life Stress," *Psychosomatic Medicine* 38:300–14 (1976).

19. Bourne, P. G. "Altered Adrenal Function in Two Combat Situations in Vietnam," in B. E. Eleftheriou, *The Physiology of Aggression and Defeat* (New York: Plenum Press, 1971).

20. Spitz, R. *Hospitalism in Psychoanalytic Study of the Child* (New York: International Universities Press, 1947).

21. Bruhn, J. et al. "Social Aspects of Coronary Heart Disease in Two Adjacent Ethnically-Different Communities," *American Journal of Public Health* 56:1493–1506 (1966).

22. Moos, R. H. *The Human Context—Environmental Determinants of Behavior* (New York: John Wiley & Sons, 1976), pp. 320–50. Note p. 330 ff.

23. Kaplan, B. H. et al. *Family and Health: An Epidemiological Approach* (Chapel Hill: University of North Carolina Press, 1975), p. 18.

24. Ibid., pp. 63–87.

25. Friedman, M. and Rosenman, R. H. *Type A Behavior and Your Heart* (Greenwich, Conn.: Fawcett, 1975).

26. Henry, J. P. and Stephens, P. M. *Stress, Health, and the Social Environment* (New York: Springer-Verlag, 1977), p. 196.

27. Ibid., p. 202.

28. Benson, H. *The Relaxation Response* (New York: William Morrow, 1975).

29. De Rosis, H. *Women and Anxiety* (New York: Delacorte, 1979).

30. Luthe, W. *Autogenic Therapy*, vol. 4. (New York: Grune Stratton, 1970), p. 12.

31. Beary, J. F. and Benson, H. "A Simple Psychophysiologic Technique Which Elicits the Hypometabolic Changes of the Relaxation Response," *Psychosomatic Medicine*, vol. 36, no. 2 (March–April 1974).

32. Jones, G. E. "Physiological Responses During Self-Generated Imagery of Contextually Complete Stimuli," *Psychophysiology* 15:438 (1978).

33. Chamberlain, R. W. "Approaches to Child Rearing: Early Recognition and Modification of Vicious-Circle Parent-Child Relationships," *Clinical Pediatrics* 6:2, 469 (1967).

34. Gordon, T. *Parent Effective Training* (New York: Peter H. Wyden, 1970).

35. Moos, op cit., p. 234.

36. Wahler, R. G. et al. "Mothers as Behavior Therapists for Their Own Children," *Behavior Research and Therapy*, vol. 3, pp. 113–24 (1965).

37. Pelletier, K. *Toward a Science of Consciousness* (New York: Delta, 1978), p. 136.

38. Bentov, I. *Stalking the Wild Pendulum* (New York: Bantam Books, 1979), p. 92.

Chapter 2. Nutrition

1. Yperman, A. "Factors Associated with Children's Food Habits," *Journal of Nutrition Education* 11:2 (1979).

2. Lowenberg, M. A. "The Development of Food Patterns in Young Children," in Pipes, P., *Nutrition in Infancy and Childhood* (St. Louis: C. V. Mosby, 1977).

3. Eppright, E. S. "Nutrition Knowledge and Attitudes of Mothers," *Journal of Home Economics* 62:327 (1970).

4. Gussow, J. "Counternutritional Messages of TV Ads Aimed at Children," *Journal of Nutrition Education* 4:48 (1972).

5. Nizel, A. E. "Preventing Dental Caries: The Nutritional Factors," *Pediatric Clinics of North America* 24:141 (1977).

6. McLaren, D. S. *Textbook of Paediatric Nutrition* (New York: Churchill Livingstone, 1976).

7. Neumann, C. G. "Obesity in Pediatric Practice: Obesity in the Preschool and School-Age Child," *Pediatric Clinics of North America* 24:118 (1977).

8. Editorial, *American Journal of Clinical Nutrition* 31:9, p. 1712 (1978).

9. American Academy of Pediatrics Committee on Nutrition. "Megavitamin Therapy for Childhood Psychoses and Learning Disorders," *Pediatrics* 58:6, p. 910 (1978).

10. Peterkin, B. "Diets That Meet the Dietary Goals," *Journal of Nutrition Education* 10:1 (1979).

11. McLaren, D. S., op. cit.

12. Pipes, P. "Between Infancy and Adolescence," in *Nutrition in Infancy and Childhood* (St. Louis: C. V. Mosby, 1977), p. 122.

Chapter 3. Chemicals

1. Griffin, A., and Shaw, C. *Carcinogens: Identification and Mechanisms of Action* (New York: Raven Press, 1979), p. 458.

2. Higginson, J. "A Hazardous Society? Individual Versus Community Responsibility in Cancer Prevention," *American Journal of Public Health* 66, 4:361 (April 1976).

3. Ibid.

4. Miller, E. "Some Current Perspectives on Chemical Carcinogenesis in Humans and Experimental Animals," *Cancer Research* 38:1479, p. 1482 (June 1978).

5. Higginson, op. cit., pp. 364–65.

6. Griffin, A. and Shaw, C., op. cit., p. 54.

7. Epstein, S. S. *The Politics of Cancer* (Garden City, N.Y.: Anchor Press/Doubleday, 1979), p. 473.

8. Ibid., p. 484.

9. U.S. Academy of Science. *Journal of Nutrition Education* 11:2.

10. Epstein, op. cit., p. 488.

11. The Environmental Defense Fund and Boyle, R. H. *Malignant Neglect* (New York: Knopf, 1979), p. 133.

Chapter 4. Exercise

1. Astrand, P. O. *Textbook of Work Physiology* (New York: McGraw-Hill, 1970).

2. Cooper, K. *The New Aerobics* (New York: Bantam, 1975).

3. Bailey, D. A. "Exercise, Fitness and Physical Education for the Growing Child—A Concern," *Canadian Journal of Public Health* 64:423 (1973).

4. Falkner, F. *Human Growth* (New York: Plenum Press, 1978).

5. Bailey, D. A., op. cit., p. 425.

6. Ibid., p. 427.

7. Ibid., p. 421.

8. Ibid., p. 429.

9. Kannel, W. B. "Habitual Level of Physical Activity and Risk of Coronary Heart Disease: The Framingham Study," *Canadian Medical Association Journal* 96:811 (1967).

10. Cooper, K., op. cit., p. 29.

11. American Academy of Pediatrics, 1968 Guidelines in Athletics for Elementary Age Children.

12. Cooper, K., op. cit., p. 144.

13. Hendricks, G. and Wills, R. *The Centering Book* (Englewood Cliffs, N.J.: Prentice-Hall, 1957).

14. Feldenkrais, Moshe. *Awareness Through Movement* (New York: Harper & Row, 1972).

15. Barlow, W. *The Alexander Technique* (New York: Warner Books, 1973).

16. Bailey, D. A., op. cit., p. 430.

17. Ibid., p. 425.

Bibliography and recommended reading

Allison, L. *Blood and Guts: A Working Guide to Your Own Insides.* Boston: Little, Brown, 1976.

American Academy of Pediatrics, 1968 Guidelines in Athletics for Elementary Age Children.

American Academy of Pediatrics Committee on Nutrition. "Megavitamin Therapy for Childhood Psychoses and Learning Disorders," *Pediatrics* 58:6, 1978.

Astrand, P. O. *Textbook of Work Physiology.* New York: McGraw-Hill, 1970.

Bailey, D. A. "Exercise, Fitness and Physical Education for the Growing Child—A Concern," *Canadian Journal of Public Health* 64:423, 1973.

Barber, T. "Hypnosis, Suggestion, and Psychosomatic Phenomenon: A New Look from the Standpoint of Recent Experimental Studies," *American Journal of Clinical Hypnosis* 21:1, 1978.

Barlow, W. *The Alexander Technique.* New York: Warner Books, 1973.

Beary, J. F., and Benson, H. "A Simple Psychophysiologic Technique Which Elicits the Hypometabolic Changes of the Relaxation Response," *Psychosomatic Medicine,* vol. 36, no. 2 (March–April 1974).

Beck, W. S. *Human Design.* New York: Harcourt Brace Jovanovich, 1971.

Benson, H. *The Relaxation Response.* New York: William Morrow, 1975.

Bentov, I. *Stalking the Wild Pendulum.* New York: Bantam Books, 1979.

Bierman, C. *Allergic Diseases of Infancy and Childhood and Adolescence.* Philadelphia: W. B. Saunders, 1980.

Blough, G. *Elementary School Science.* New York: Holt, Rinehart & Winston, 1964.

Bourne, P. G. "Altered Adrenal Function in Two Combat Situations in Vietnam." In B. E. Eleftheriou, *The Physiology of Aggression and Defeat.* New York: Plenum Press, 1971.

Brown, G. W. et al. "Social Class and Psychiatric Disturbance Among Women in an Urban Population," *Sociology* 9:225–54, 1975.

Bruhn, J. et al. "Social Aspects of Coronary Heart Disease in Two Adjacent Ethnically-Different Communities," *American Journal of Public Health* 56:1493–1506, 1966.

Chamberlain, R. W. "Approaches to Child Rearing: Early Recognition and Modification of Vicious-Circle Parent-Child Relationships," *Clinical Pediatrics* 6:2, 1967.

Cheki Haney, E., and Richards, R. *Yoga for Children.* Indianapolis: Bobbs-Merrill, 1973.

Cobb, S. "Social Support As a Moderator of Life Stress," *Psychosomatic Medicine* 38:300–14, 1976.

Coddington, R. D. "The Significance of Life Events as Etiological Factors in the Diseases of Children," *Journal of Psychosomatic Research* 16:7.

Cooper, K. *The New Aerobics.* New York: Bantam, 1975.

De Rosis, H. *Women and Anxiety.* New York: Delacorte, 1979.

Editorial, *American Journal of Clinical Nutrition* 31:9, 1978.

The Environmental Defense Fund and Boyle, R. H. *Malignant Neglect.* New York: Knopf, 1979.

Eppright, E. S. "Nutrition Knowledge and Attitudes of Mothers," *Journal of Home Economics* 62:327, 1970.

Epstein, S. S. *The Politics of Cancer.* Garden City, N.Y.: Anchor Press/Doubleday, 1979.

Falkner, F. *Human Growth.* New York: Plenum Press, 1978.

Feldenkrais, Moshe. *Awareness Through Movement.* New York: Harper & Row, 1972.

Friedman, M., and Rosenman, R. H. *Type A Behavior and Your Heart.* Greenwich, Conn.: Fawcett, 1975.

Goodman, L., and Gillman, F. *The Pharmacological Basis of Therapeutics.* New York: Macmillan, 1980.

Gordon, T. *Parent Effective Training.* New York: Peter H. Wyden, 1970.

Griffin, A. *Carcinogens: Identification and Mechanisms of Action.* New York: Raven Press, 1979.

Gussow, J. "Counternutritional Messages of TV Ads Aimed at Children," *Journal of Nutrition Education* 4:48, 1972.

Guyton, A. *Physiology of the Human Body.* Philadelphia: W. B. Saunders, 1979.

Guyton, A. *Textbook of Medical Physiology.* Philadelphia: W. B. Saunders, 1980.

Healthy People: Report of the U.S. Surgeon General, 1980.

Heisel, J. S. "The Significance of Life Events as Contributing Factors in the Diseases of Children," *Journal of Pediatrics* 83:119, 1973.

Hendricks, G., and Wills, R. *The Centering Book.* Englewood Cliffs, N. J.: Prentice-Hall, 1957.

Henry, J. P., and Stephens, P. M. *Stress, Health, and the Social Environment.* New York: Springer-Verlag, 1977.

Higginson, J. "A Hazardous Society? Individual Versus Community Responsibility in Cancer Prevention," *American Journal of Public Health* 66,4:361, April 1976.

Hinkle, L. E. "Illness, Life Experience, and Social Environment," *Annals of Internal Medicine* 49:1873, 1958.

Holmes, T. H., and Rahe, R. H. "The Social Readjustment Rating Scale," *Journal of Psychosomatic Research* 11:213–18, 1967.

Jackson, G. G. "Susceptibility and Immunity to Common Upper Respiratory Viral Infection—The Common Cold," *Annals of Internal Medicine* 53:2, 1960.

Jacobson, E. *Progressive Relaxation.* Chicago: University of Chicago Press, 1942.

Jones, G. E. "Physiological Responses During Self-Generated Imagery of Contextually Complete Stimuli," *Psychophysiology* 15:438, 1978.

Jung, C. Introduction, *The Inner World of Childhood.* New York: New American Library, 1968.

Kannel, W. B. "Habitual Level of Physical Activity and Risk of Coronary Heart Disease: The Framingham Study," *Canadian Medical Association Journal* 96:811, 1967.

Kapit, Wynn. *The Anatomy Coloring Book.* New York: Canfield Press/ Barnes & Noble, 1977.

Kaplan, B. H. et al. *Family and Health: An Epidemiological Approach.* Chapel Hill, N.C.: University of North Carolina Press, 1975.

Kempe, C. H. *Current Pediatric Diagnosis and Treatment.* Los Altos, Calif: Lange Medical Publications, 1980.

Kessel, R. *Tissues and Organs: A Text-Atlas of Scanning Electron Microscopy.* San Francisco: W. H. Freeman, 1979.

Kroger, W. S. *Hypnosis and Behavior Modification: Imagery Conditioning.* Philadelphia: J. B. Lippincott, 1976.

Krugman, S. *Infectious Diseases of Children.* St. Louis: C. V. Mosby, 1977.

Langley, L. *Dynamic Anatomy and Physiology.* New York: McGraw-Hill, 1980.

Lauer, R. M. *Childhood Prevention of Atherosclerosis and Hypertension.* New York: Raven Press, 1980.

Lowenberg, M. A. "The Development of Food Patterns in Young Children." In P. Pipes, *Nutrition in Infancy and Childhood.* St. Louis: C. V. Mosby, 1977.

Luthe, W. *Autogenic Therapy,* vol. 4. New York: Grune Stratton, 1970.

McIntyre, K. "1979 National Conference on Cardio-Pulmonary Resuscitation and Emergency Cardiac Care," *Emergency Medicine,* 12, 14:24–202.

McLaren, D. S. *Textbook of Paediatric Nutrition.* New York: Churchill Livingstone, 1976.

Medalie, J. H. *Family Medicine.* Baltimore: Williams & Wilkins, 1978.

Meyer, R. "Streptococcal Infections in Families," *Pediatrics* 29:539.

Miller, E. "Some Current Perspectives on Chemical Carcinogenesis in Humans and Experimental Animals," *Cancer Research* 38:1479, June 1978.

Moos, R. H. *The Human Context—Environmental Determinants of Behavior*. New York: Wiley & Sons, 1976.

Nelson, W. *Textbook of Pediatrics*. Philadelphia: W. B. Saunders, 1964.

Neumann, C. G. "Obesity in Pediatric Practice: Obesity in the Preschool and School-Age Child,"*Pediatric Clinics of North America* 24:118, 1977.

Nizel, A. E. "Preventing Dental Caries: The Nutritional Factors," *Pediatric Clinics of North America* 24:141, 1977.

Nossal, G. *Antibodies and Immunity*. New York: Basic Books, 1978.

Nuckolls, Katherine et al. "Phychosocial Assets, Life Crisis and the Prognosis of Pregnancy," *American Journal of Epidemiology* 95:431–41, 1972.

Padilla, B. R. "Predicting Accident Frequency in Children," *Pediatrics* 58:223, 1976.

Pelletier, K. *Toward a Science of Consciousness*. New York: Delta, 1978.

Peterkin, B. "Diets That Meet the Dietary Goals," *Journal of Nutrition Education* 10:1, 1979.

Physicians Desk Reference. Oradell, N.J.: Litton Publications.

Pipes, P. "Between Infancy and Adolescence." In *Nutrition in Infancy and Childhood*. St. Louis: C. V. Mosby, 1977.

Roghmann, K. "Daily Stress, Illness, and Use of Health Services in Young Families," *Pediatric Research* 7:520, 1973.

Samuels, M., and Bennett, H. *The Well Body Book*. New York: Bookworks/Random House, 1972.

Samuels, M., and Samuels, N. *Seeing With the Mind's Eye*. New York: Bookworks/Random House, 1975.

Samuels, M., and Samuels, N. *The Well Baby Book*. New York: Summit Books, 1979.

Satchidananda, Swami. *Integral Yoga Hatha*. New York: Holt, Rinehart & Winston, 1970.

Schaefer, C. E. *Therapies for Psychosomatic Disorders in Children*. San Francisco: Jossey Bass, 1979.

Sinclair, D. *Human Growth After Birth*. London: Oxford University Press, 1969.

Skipper, J. K. "Children, Stress, and Hospitalization," *Journal of Health and Social Behavior* 9:278, 1968.

Spitz, R. *Hospitalism in Psychoanalytic Study of the Child*. New York: International Universities Press, 1947.

Thomas, L. *The Lives of a Cell.* New York: Viking Press, 1974.

Valadian, I. *Physical Growth and Development.* Boston: Little, Brown, 1977.

Varga, C. *Pediatric Medical Emergencies.* St. Louis: C. V. Mosby, 1968.

Wahler, R. G. et al. "Mothers as Behavior Therapists for Their Own Children," *Behavior Research and Therapy,* 3:113–24, 1965.

Weisz, P. *The Science of Biology.* New York: McGraw-Hill, 1959.

Whipple, A. *Wound Healing.* Springfield, Ill.: Thomas, 1963.

Wickes, F. G. *The Inner World of Childhood.* New York: New American Library, 1968.

Yperman, A. "Factors Associated with Children's Food Habits," *Journal of Nutrition Education* 11:2, 1979.

Index

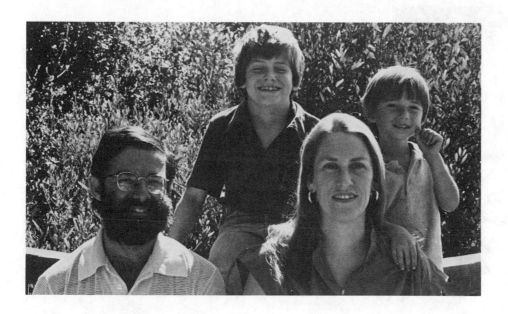

About the authors

Mike Samuels is a physician and author. He attended Brown University and New York University College of Medicine. After internship he chose to remain in family practice, first working on the Hopi Indian Reservation, then working for county public health. During this time he helped to set up one of the first holistic clinics in northern California and wrote the pioneering self-help book *The Well Body Book,* with Hal Z. Bennett. Since that time he has devoted himself to writing, research, and lecturing.

Nancy Harrison Samuels is a former nursery school teacher who now writes full-time with her husband. She attended Brown University and Bank Street College of Education. After several years of teaching she did editing on *The Well Body Book.* Subsequently she and Mike wrote *Seeing With the Mind's Eye* and *The Well Baby Book.*

Mike and Nancy are the parents of two boys, Rudy and Lewis. As their sons grew older, the Samuelses found that, much like other parents, they wanted to explain to their children how the body works, how it heals, and why people sometimes get sick. This book is a natural sequel to *The Well Baby Book* and part of a series of books on what people can do to learn about their bodies and improve their health.

Mike and Nancy live in a small seacoast town in northern California in a house they built themselves. They have a close family life and spend much of their free time doing things with their children, gardening, and working on their house. During the winter they write and actively partici-pate in the boys' schools. During the summer the Samuelses mix traveling and camping with working on the editing, illustration, and design of their books. At present they are cheerfully occupied with a coloring book to accompany *The Well Child Book.*

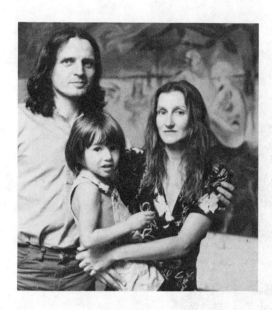

About the illustrator

Australian-born artist Wendy Frost has lived in London for four years and New York City for eleven years. She has worked for magazines, newspapers, and publishers in England, Europe, and the United States, and has also exhibited her paintings in London, Sydney, and New York. With her in the photograph are her son, Darcy Darwin, and his father, Terry O'Connor. They now live in Australia.